MANUAL EXAMINATION AND TREATMENT OF THE SPINE AND EXTREMITIES

D1377586

MANUAL EXAMINATION AND TREATMENT OF THE SPINE AND EXTREMITIES

Carolyn T. Wadsworth, L.P.T., M.S.

Lecturer
Physical Therapy Education
The University of Iowa
Iowa City, Iowa

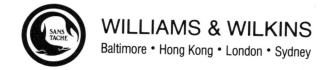

WILLIAMS & WILKINS
Baltimore • Hong Kong • London • Sydney

Editor: John P. Butler
Associate Editor: Victoria M. Vaughn
Copy Editor: Judy Minkove
Design: Saturn Graphics
Illustration Planning: Lorraine Wrzosek
Production: Raymond E. Reter
Cover Design: Bolton Graphics

Printed in the United States of America

Library of Congress Cataloging-in-Publication Data

Wadsworth, Carolyn T.
 Manual examination and treatment of the spine and extremities.

 Includes bibliographies and index.
 1. Physical therapy.   2. Musculoskeletal system—
Examination.   I. Title.   [DNLM: 1. Bone Diseases—
diagnosis.   2. Extremities.   3. Muscular Diseases—diagnosis.
4. Physical Examination.   5. Spine.
WE 141 W124m]
RM700.W32 1988   617′.3   87-14777
ISBN 0-683-08600-6

To John, of course.

PREFACE

Musculoskeletal impairment afflicts as many as 20,000,000 people in the United States (1). It affects the quality of life more frequently than any other disease and, because of lost earnings and services, is the most economically costly nonfatal illness (1). Twenty-five percent of all persons seeking medical attention have some type of musculoskeletal pathology. Eighty to 90% of these persons are not surgical candidates, and thus require other methods of management (2).

A major form of nonsurgical management of musculoskeletal pathology includes physical and manual therapy. This type of therapeutic intervention particularly benefits those with pain and impaired movement. Manual examination utilizes a thorough system based upon biomechanical principles of structural assessment, coupled with evaluation of a patient's clinical response to movement. The sensitivity and specificity with which a skilled manual therapist can execute such techniques as palpation and movement assessment are unmatched by other examination processes. Manual treatment involves application of mobilizing forces via the fingertips and palms, providing excellent control of procedures and offering immediate feedback so that a therapist can respond appropriately to a patient's status.

This text presents principles of the structure, function, and disorders of the musculoskeletal system. It addresses the needs of those dealing with patients who have orthopaedically based movement dysfunction. Initial chapters review the skeletal and articular systems and manual therapy theory. Following chapters devoted to the spine and extremity joints emphasize normal and pathologic movement, and restoration of function by manual means.

The "clinical anatomy and biomechanics" components of the spine and extremity chapters prepare the reader for recognizing normal anatomy and function, and for identifying and analyzing pathologic findings. These sections emphasize structures that have potential for limiting movement; they offer extensive references for those interested in more comprehensive coverage of anatomy and kinesiology.

The "examination" components of each chapter provide a detailed clinical examination form, accompanied by narrative describing the examination procedure, norms for various tests and measurements, and examples of abnormal findings. Since appropriate examination is vital to successful management, these sections include much detail—from taking a history to assessing passive movement. Photographs illustrate the specific positioning and hand placement necessary to execute many of the tests properly. A table summarizing the differential diagnosis of disorders common to each area with an outline of treatment (which is too lengthy to cover in detail) completes this part.

The "manual therapy techniques" components present the indications and procedures for performing selected joint mobilizations. A photograph depicts each technique, and each is also described in terms of patient position, therapist position, execution, and comments related to relieving pain or restoring movement.

It is my intention that this material will provide clinicians with fundamental concepts from which they can initiate manual examination and treatment of their patients. I hope that these concepts will serve as a stimulus for further investigation and clinical application, devoted to the continuing enhancement of patient care.

C. T. Wadsworth

References

1. Kelsey JL, Pastides H, Bisbee GE: *Musculoskeletal Disorders: Their Frequency of Occurrence and Their Impact on the Population of the U.S.* New York, Product Publishing Co, 1978.
2. Lipscomb PR: Orthopedics, orthopaedic surgery, musculoskeletology, orthopaedics. *J Bone Joint Surg* 57A:872–876, 1975.

ACKNOWLEDGMENTS

I happily express my gratitude to Judy Biderman for her painstaking efforts in preparing the original manuscript. I also wish to recognize Chanatip Suksang (Tai) for his artistic talent and expertise and Gina Harvey for her patience as a model during arduous photographic sessions. Finally, I want to thank John Wadsworth, L.P.T., M.A., Duane Williams, L.P.T., M.A., Stan Schlachter, L.P.T., and Mary Martin, L.P.T. for their professional collaboration in the initial development of this material that we used in teaching continuing education workshops.

CONTRIBUTORS

David Johnson, L.P.T.
Private Practice
Minneapolis, Minnesota
Co-authored Chapter 2 (*Basic Concepts of Orthopaedic Manual Therapy*); contributed to *Clinical Anatomy and Mechanics* section and wrote *Cervical Spine Examination* and *Mobilization* sections in Chapter 3 (*The Spine*).

Richard P. DiFabio, L.P.T., Ph.D.
Director of Physical Therapy
University of Wisconsin Hospital and Clinics
Madison, Wisconsin
Contributed *Joint Kinematics* and *Joint Neurology* in Chapter 1 (*The Skeletal and Articular Systems*); contributed to *Clinical Anatomy and Mechanics* section and wrote *Thoracolumbar* and *Sacroiliac Examination* sections in Chapter 3 (*The Spine*).

CONTENTS

THE SKELETAL AND ARTICULAR SYSTEMS

Carolyn T. Wadsworth, L.P.T., M.S.
Richard P. DiFabio, L.P.T., Ph.D.

HISTOGENESIS AND MORPHOLOGY

Connective Tissue

Four basic types of tissue comprise the human body. They are connective, nervous, epithelial, and muscle tissue. Each tissue contains cells, intercellular substance, and fluid (1). Cells are living elements; their nuclei and cytoplasm support metabolism, matrix formation, and reproduction. Intercellular substance (matrix) is nonliving, but organic. It provides a scaffold for cells, and a medium for diffusion of fluid and nutrients. The formed portion of the intercellular substance contains collagen, elastic, and reticular fibers which, depending upon their proportions and alignment, lend shape and other qualities that characterize the various tissues. The amorphous portion of the intercellular substance contains mucopolysaccharides, long chain polymers of protein-sugar complexes, which readily permit diffusion between cells and capillaries. The fluid component of tissues includes blood, intercellular fluid, and lymph.

The mesoderm germ layer of an embryo produces the connective tissue (CT). Connective tissues embrace a wide variety of specimens, including bone, cartilage, tendon, bursa, ligament, aponeurosis, and blood. These tissues provide structural and defensive properties that are essential to life. An abundance of matrix relative to the other components (cells and fluid) typifies most CT (2). Fibroblasts represent the basic cell of less differentiated forms of CT, elaborating the fibers and much of the amorphous content (3). Although fibroblasts become inactive in mature tissue, they retain the capacity for growth and regeneration when stimulated, e.g., wound healing (1). Macrophages are also abundant in some types of CT. They are agents of defense, characterized by mobility and phagocytic activity. Depending on the concentration and arrangement of fibers, CT may be categorized as loose, e.g., areolar, adipose, reticular; dense irregular, e.g., fascia, dermis, periosteum; dense regular, e.g., tendon, ligament; and specialized, e.g., cartilage, bone.

Cartilage. Cartilage represents a specialized type of CT. It is a relatively firm tissue which adapts in unique ways to mechanical demands upon the body. Cartilage emerges from the mesoderm around the 5th week of embryonic life (4). A sheet of mesenchymal cells differentiates into chondroblasts, which deposit intercellular material. As the intercellular material surrounds the cells, they enlarge into chondrocytes, and continue to extend the matrix. In this manner, relatively young cartilage grows interstitially, from the multiplication of existing cells and deposition of new matrix. Continued growth occurs appositionally, from an enveloping perichondrial membrane, which provides a source of mitotically active cells.

Chondrocytes represent the primary type of cartilage cell. They possess a rounded nucleus with one or more nucleoli. The younger cells are flattened, but become rounder and hypertrophied as they differentiate. They occupy lacunae within the cartilage matrix, in which they may proliferate. Cartilage amorphous substance consists principally of proteoglycans. The quality of the fibers in cartilage determines which of three forms it will assume.

Hyaline cartilage, the most abundant form, covers the articular surfaces of synovial joints, and forms the costal cartilages and cartilage of the larynx, nose, bronchi, and trachea (2,5). Collagen fibers predominate in hyaline cartilage. They are oriented randomly throughout the chondromucoprotein matrix. Hyaline cartilage matrix appears clear and almost homogeneous because the fibers are difficult to recognize. Elastic cartilage, the second form, has more flexibility, and occurs in the external ear and epiglottis. Elastic fibers are most numerous in this form of cartilage, imparting a yellow color to the tissue. Fibrocartilage, the third form, contains thick, white, compact bundles of collagenous fibers alligned in a parallel fashion (5). Fibrocartilage occurs in the interface between articular cartilage and ligamentous structures, and within labra, intervertebral discs, and joint menisci (4). Fibrocartilage has high tensile strength and toughness, but also possesses sufficient elasticity to withstand the long-term effects of pressure and friction (2).

Cartilage is an avascular tissue, depending on diffusion of metabolites from its surfaces for nutrition. Synovial fluid and subchondral bone are the two sources of nutrition for cartilage. Nutrients must permeate the cartilage matrix in order to reach the cells. As older cartilage becomes less cellular, nutrition diminishes. Adult chondrocytes display some metabolic activity in a process of continual matrix turnover to replace that lost by normal attrition. Chondrocytes are also capable of mitotic activity in response to certain stimuli, such as damage associated with osteoarthritis.

The healing of articular cartilage in response to trauma involves an initial stage of necrosis, during which there is death of cells and destruction of matrix at the site of injury. An inflammation stage, which normally follows the necrotic stage in the healing of other body tissues, is absent in articular cartilage because of its avascularity. As a consequence, there is no exudation nor fibrin clot, no additional cells nor a scaffold for growth of repair tissue. The existing chondrocytes alone must replace the injured tissue if repair is to occur. Given their limited metabolic activity, repair is tenuous.

The location and depth of injury play a major role in determining the healing capability of articular cartilage. Following experimental *superficial* lacerations, investigators noted cellular necrosis, a burst of mitotic activity within 24 hours lasting 1–2 weeks, then no further healing over time (6,7). This type of lesion does not necessarily progress to degenerative joint disease (6). In contrast, a *deep* laceration that penetrates subchondral bone produces a defect that is filled in with a blood clot; later ingrowth of fibroblasts and capillaries leads to production of granulation tissue. Bone eventually replaces the subchondral defect; a mixture of fibro- and hyaline cartilage replaces the cartilaginous defect, which may nevertheless degenerate with wear over time. Defects of less than 3 mm wide tend to repair completely, whereas those greater than 9 mm do not (6).

Researchers propose that continuous passive motion enhances healing of chondral defects by stimulating the rate of metaplasia and differentiation of mesenchymal tissue to hyaline cartilage. Full thickness cartilage defects in rabbits were healed by hyaline cartilage in approximately 50% of the subjects receiving CPM, as compared with 8% in subjects whose knees were immobilized or permitted intermittent active motion (8).

Aside from traumatic lesions of articular cartilage, a more subtle, but equally debilitating, destructive process can result from altered mechanics. Since the only source of nourishment for the superficial layers of articular cartilage is the synovial fluid, the joint surfaces depend on intermittent compression and a changing area of contact for proper lubrication and nutrition. Mechanical changes and immobilization may interfere with this process and lead to cartilage degeneration.

Investigators have found that prolonged immobilization may produce:

1. progressive contracture of capsular and pericapsular structures;
2. encroachment by fibrofatty connective tissue, which blends with articular cartilage and obliterates the joint;
3. cystic defects in areas of direct contact, which repair by ossification and ankylosis;
4. fibrillation of cartilage in areas without surface contact;
5. decreased production of mucopolysaccharides or proteoglycans, which function to lubricate the collagen fiber interface and minimize cross-linking;
6. adhesion of synovial membrane to underlying articular cartilage (9–12).

Alteration of joint mechanics similarly interferes with joint nutrition and can result in destruction of cartilage, and eventually, degenerative joint disease. The logical approach to management of such patients with loss or alteration of motion is restoration of normal mechanics. Patients must regain accessory as well as physiologic movement in order to establish proper joint function.

Bone. Bone is also a specialized type of CT. It is the only tissue (except tooth) in which a portion of the matrix is inorganic. The inorganic constituents (lime salts) produce the hardness and rigidity of bone, and account for approximately two-thirds of its weight (1). Mucopolysaccharides comprise the organic portion of bone matrix. Collagenous fibers imbedded in the matrix contribute to bone's strength and resilience (13). Osteoblasts constitute the primary type of cells of developing bone and in areas of remodelling. These cells contain a single, large nucleolus, in addition to enzymes and basophilic proteins, which contribute to bone matrix synthesis and calcification. Once osteoblasts become entrapped in bone matrix, they become osteocytes. Osteocytes have an oval nucleus with one or more nucleoli. They inhabit lacunae in the matrix that are joined by an intricate system of canals (canaliculi). The canals provide access for the exchange of metabolites between the blood vessels and osteocytes (13). In areas of bone resorption, another cell type, the osteoclast, abounds. It is a multinucleated giant cell with a bone-erosive function (2).

Bone appears after the 7th week of embryonic life (4,14). Dense concentrations of mesenchymal cells assume the shape (model) of bones, which will derive through either intramembranous or intracartilaginous processes. Intramembranous bone formation produces the cranial vault, face, clavicles, mandible, carpals, and tarsals. Intramembranous formation is initiated as the condensed mesenchyme models become highly vascularized, stimulating cellular differentiation and proliferation. Osteoblasts and matrix form within the model constituting the organic component of the bone, i.e., osteoid. Mineral deposition within the osteoid produces calcified bone, which is initially of the immature or woven variety. Eventual remodelling with concentric deposition of matrix produces a mature or lamellar type of bone. Craniocleidodysostosis represents a developmental disorder in which intramembranous development is defective, resulting in clavicular or cranial anomalies.

Appositional bone growth (growth in width from osteoblasts derived from the periosteum) resembles intramembranous bone development, and is the only type of bone growth possible after skeletal maturity. Excessive growth of this type in adulthood is abnormal, but occurs in a pituitary gland-related disorder known as acromegaly.

Intracartilaginous (endochondral) bone formation creates most of the long bones and ribs. It requires the conversion of condensed mesenchyme to a hyaline cartilage model, then subsequent transformation to bone (Fig. 1.1). Hypertrophy of cartilage cells at the center of the model initiates this process. Then the cartilage cells degenerate and die, and the walls of the empty lacunae calcify. Perichondrial cells, surrounding the surface near the center of the model, hypertrophy, then differentiate into osteoblasts. These osteoblasts produce bone, forming a periosteal collar to strengthen the model. Vascular channels penetrate the collar, creating primary marrow spaces. Osteoblasts and osteoclasts invade the calcified cartilage matrix, and replace the matrix with osteoid, which later calcifies. (Cartilage does not change into bone, but is replaced by it.) This central area of bone formation is the primary ossification center. The periosteal bone collar acts as a buttress to support the central zone of resorbing cartilage, prior to its replacement by bone.

As the area of intracartilaginous ossification enlarges, the adjoining cartilaginous regions on both ends of

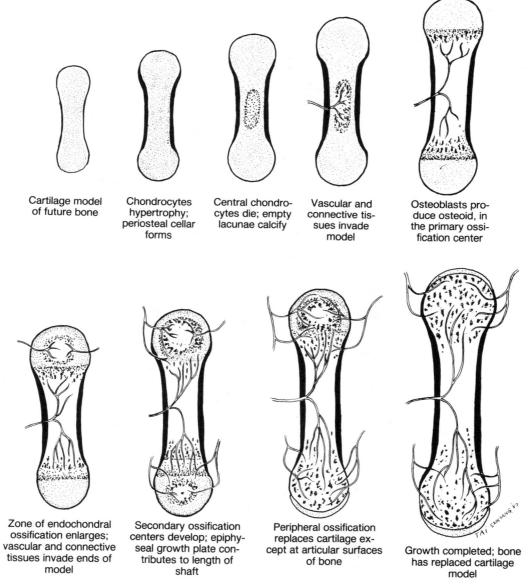

Cartilage model of future bone

Chondrocytes hypertrophy; periosteal cellar forms

Central chondrocytes die; empty lacunae calcify

Vascular and connective tissues invade model

Osteoblasts produce osteoid, in the primary ossification center

Zone of endochondral ossification enlarges; vascular and connective tissues invade ends of model

Secondary ossification centers develop; epiphyseal growth plate contributes to length of shaft

Peripheral ossification replaces cartilage except at articular surfaces of bone

Growth completed; bone has replaced cartilage model

Figure 1.1. Intracartilaginous bone formation.

the model undergo a progression of changes (Fig. 1.2). The transition area between the new bone and the cartilage model is the epiphyseal plate, or growth cartilage. It demonstrates a series of zones oriented longitudinally. The zones are responsible for growth in length of the bone. The germinal or resting zone, nearest to the epiphyseal plate, contains scattered, active, immature chondrocytes, and expands in all directions. The proliferation zone contains cells aligned in rows, parallel to the bone's long axis; active interstitial growth in this area lengthens the bone. The maturation zone is an area of cellular hypertrophy, degeneration, and death. The calcification zone includes the empty lacunae, the walls of which calcify. The ossification zone is an area where vascular mesenchyme enters and differentiates into osteoblasts which

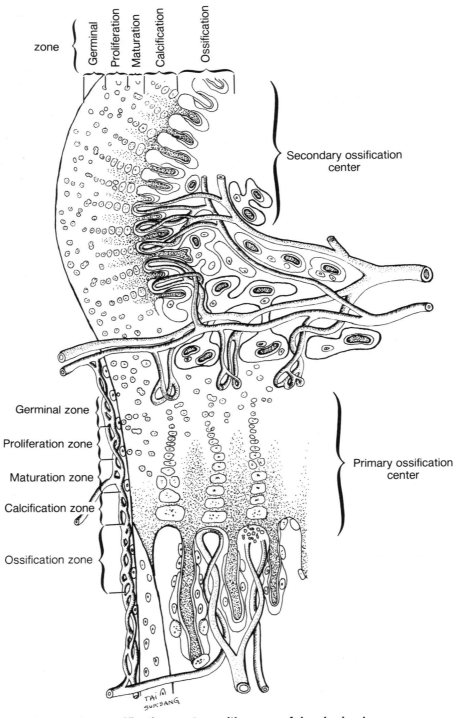

Figure 1.2.   Primary and secondary ossification centers with zones of developing bone.

form osteoid; calcified cartilage is resorbed and replaced by woven bone. While some bones contain only a single, primary center, one or more secondary ossification centers usually appear at the ends of the cartilage model and at other specific areas during the time period between birth and puberty. The appearance of each secondary center at a specified time for each particular bone is so predictable that clinicians are able to estimate a child's age from the presence of existing ossification sites. Zones, similar to those found at the primary ossification center, surround the secondary centers in a spherical fashion (Fig. 1.2). The articular cartilage supplies the cells which contribute to the growth of this epiphyseal region of the bone. Normal growth requires simultaneous enlargement of the epiphysis and the shaft (diaphysis). Periosteal growth

also contributes to a bone's circumferential shape. As a bone thickens, osteoclastic activity enlarges the marrow space within. When bone attains its final dimensions, the areas of ossification encroach upon the growth plate(s), which bony fusion finally eliminates. Achondroplastic dwarfism represents a defect in intracartilaginous bone development, which affects primarily the limbs rather than the axial skeleton.

Developing bone, and bone undergoing longitudinal growth or repair, is very cellular, demonstrating an irregular and less dense matrix. This immature or woven type of bone gradually transforms into mature or lamellar bone. In lamellar bone, cells deposit matrix in layers around Haversian canals (longitudinal channels containing neurovascular bundles—Fig. 1.3). The Haversian canal with its surrounding lamellae consti-

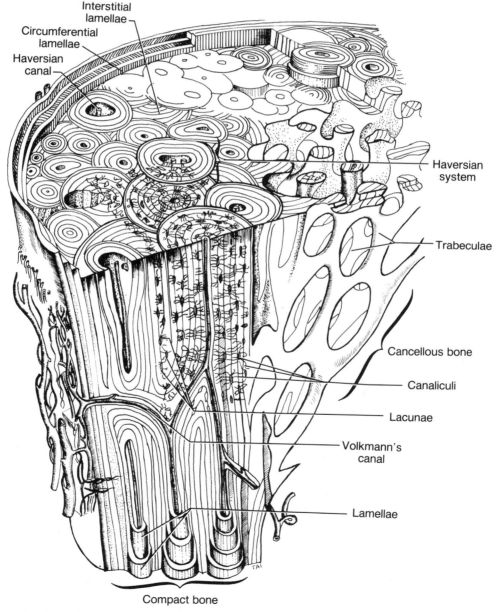

Interstitial lamellae
Circumferential lamellae
Haversian canal
Haversian system
Trabeculae
Cancellous bone
Canaliculi
Lacunae
Volkmann's canal
Lamellae
Compact bone

Figure 1.3. Macrostructure of bone.

tuteo Haversian system, the basic structure of compact bone. Lacunae, containing bone cells, occupy small spaces between the lamellae, and communicate with one another and the Haversian canal through fine, radiating channels called canaliculi. In addition to surrounding Haversian canals, lamellae also occupy crevices between canals (interstitial lamellae), and encircle the periosteal and endosteal bone surfaces (circumferential lamellae). Volkman's canals, which also contain neurovascular structures, are transverse channels which connect the Haversian canals with the endosteal and periosteal surfaces.

Compact bone, containing sheets of concentrically arranged lamellae, parallel to the longitudinal surface, comprises the cortex and most of the shaft or diaphysis of long bones. In contrast, cancellous bone predominates near the ends of the shaft (metaphysis) and in the epiphyseal areas where force is distributed over a large area (Fig. 1.3). In cancellous bone, a trabecular pattern emerges that corresponds to lines of mechanical stress. Trabeculae contain a fragmented lamellar system separated by intercommunicating spaces filled with marrow and blood vessels, which supply nutrition. Both compact and cancellous bone contain identical elements, but differ in spatial arrangement. Cancellous bone is lightweight and provides efficient support, but is 30 times weaker than an equal amount (by weight) of compact bone.

Bone functions as an organ in several capacities. Bone marrow is a chief source of blood cells. At birth red marrow exists throughout the skeleton in the cylindrical cavities of long bones and between the trabeculae of all bones (2). After the 5th year, yellow marrow begins replacing red marrow, and by the 25th year, hemopoietic (blood cell-forming) marrow remains only in flat bones such as the ribs, sternum, vertebrae, skull, and limb girdles.

The skeleton provides a major storehouse for calcium and phosphorous salts, undergoing constant exchange with blood and tissue fluids. Secretion of parathormone stimulates bone resorption, increases the serum calcium level, and decreases the serum phosphorous level. Vitamin D is necessary for calcium resorption from the gut, increasing the serum calcium level and promoting bone mineralization.

Another function of the skeleton is to provide structure and support for the body. Bone architecture, however, is never static: remodelling occurs throughout life. According to Wolff's law, bone responds to stress and functional demands by alterations in its internal architecture and its external configuration. Osetoclasts and osteoblasts continually remove and replace bone relative to mechanical stimuli.

Because bone is vascular and its cells remain alive and constantly nourished by tissue fluid, it retains unique powers of regeneration. The skeleton, unlike most other tissue, is able to repair itself with its own tissue, rather than by scar tissue. Bone repair is a nonspecific process, i.e., the same response occurs whether the stimulus is a fracture or a tumor. Reparative bone formation follows the same cellular progression as embryonic bone formation and growth. The periosteum greatly facilitates healing by serving as an osteogenic sleeve, if it is not damaged by the trauma to the bone.

Following a bone trauma (fracture, tumor, disease process, etc.), there may be hemorrhage, followed by clot formation, which provides a framework for repair. The trauma usually disrupts nutritive channels, producing cell death and necrosis. Necrotic material incites an inflammatory response, leading to the ingrowth of new vessels and cells. Fibroblasts produce granulation tissue, which becomes dense fibrous tissue known as callus. Callus contains elements of collagen, cartilage, and bone, and serves to unite the bone fragments. The periosteum, endosteum, and differentiating fibroblasts supply osteoblasts to the repair site. Osteoblasts form osteoid, which is mineralized, replacing the callus. At this stage there is clinical union of the bone, but a defect is still visible radiographically. Remodelling later creates lamellar bone and solid bony union.

Blood supply is a major determinant of cellular differentiation in bone repair. The vascularity of the bone and surrounding tissue directly affects the rate and certainty of repair. Osteogenic cells appear capable of producing either bone or cartilage in response to the degree of vascularization and subsequent oxygenation (15). With a low oxygen concentration, the cells behave as chrondroblasts which repair the defect with cartilage. High oxygen concentration stimulates differentiation of osteoblasts, which produce osseous tissue. Weightbearing and other forces on bone also stimulate osteogenesis, as long as motion across the defect is minimal. Impediments to healing include inadequate immobilization (allowing excessive motion), unsatisfactory reduction, infection, inactivity, and a poor nutritional state.

JOINT CLASSIFICATION

Joints occur at the junction of bones, and permit varying amounts of motion. Synarthroses are joints which allow relatively little motion, whereas diarthroses allow a greater range (Table 1.1). Comprising the synarthrodial classification are fibrous and cartilaginous categories of joints. In fibrous joints, dense connective tissue unites bones in a tightly knit arrangement. Examples include the sutures of the skull, gomphoses of the teeth, and syndesmoses, such as the distal tibiofibular joint. In cartilaginous joints, cartilage joins the bony articulations. Examples are the synchondroses, or temporary joints at epiphyseal plates, and the symphyses, such as the fibrocartilage-linked symphysis pubis and intervertebral discs. Embryologically, synarthroses form from differentiation of mesenchyme into uniting layers of connective tissue, cartilage, and bone (14,16).

Diarthrodial, or synovial, joints include uniaxial, biaxial, multiaxial, and plane categories (Table 1.1). This classification is useful for distinguishing general features of each category; however, joint surfaces are

Table 1.1.
Joint Classification

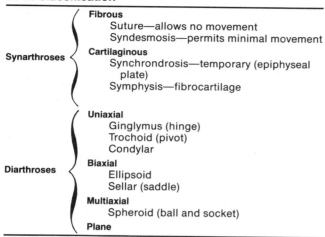

Synarthroses	**Fibrous**	
		Suture—allows no movement
		Syndesmosis—permits minimal movement
	Cartilaginous	
		Synchrondrosis—temporary (epiphyseal plate)
		Symphysis—fibrocartilage
Diarthroses	**Uniaxial**	
		Ginglymus (hinge)
		Trochoid (pivot)
		Condylar
	Biaxial	
		Ellipsoid
		Sellar (saddle)
	Multiaxial	
		Spheroid (ball and socket)
	Plane	

not perfectly congruent, flat, or exact replicas of spheres, ellipsoids, etc., as represented in this simplified classification. (A later section of this chapter describes the ovoid nature of joint surfaces.) Examples of uniaxial joints include ginglymus (hinge), trochoid (pivot), and condylar joints. Biaxial joints are depicted by ellipsoid and sellar joints. Multiaxial joints are spheroid (ball and socket) types. Plane joints have relatively flat surfaces and permit gliding in many directions.

Embryologically, diarthroses arise from clefts in the mesenchyme. Dense fibrous tissue, continuous with the bones' periosteum, forms joint capsules. Cells on the inner surface of the capsule differentiate and flatten similar to epithelial cells, producing synovial lining (4,14).

Diarthrodial joints contain a joint cavity and various other components. Articular cartilage, which is usually hyaline, covers a layer of compact bone, the subchondral bone plate, at the adjoining bone ends. Fibers in the matrix of articular cartilage align in three zones. The deepest zone is perpendicular to the bone plate; the middle zone is directed radially or obliquely; and the superficial zone is tangential to the surface. The deep layer is often calcified and may be penetrated by blood vessels.

Articular cartilage furnishes a bearing surface for joints. It provides a wear-resistant, low-friction, lubricated surface, both slightly compressible and elastic, which facilitates movement and accommodates enormous forces of shear and compression. Joint lubrication occurs through a combination of mechanisms. Hydrodynamic, or fluid film, lubrication occurs under conditions of low load, in which a layer of synovial fluid separates the articular surfaces. Special properties of synovial fluid and articular cartilage allow them to combine to a certain extent, enhancing lubricating properties in a boundary type of process. Elastodynamic or hydrostatic lubrication involves the weeping of synovial fluid under high loads, which squeeze it out of the porous articular surfaces, and then trap it between their deformable surfaces (3). Synovial fluid circulation is directly related to joint mobility; absolute

immobilization, excessive pressure, or lack of pressure, prevent fluid flow and cause death of the chondrocytes (17).

A joint capsule is present in all diarthrodial joints. Its outer layer, the stratum fibrosum, is formed of dense, fibrous CT, which is often reinforced by thickenings and ligaments. Sharpey's fibers unite the capsule to bone, and are of sufficient strength that stress often produces avulsion fractures rather than capsular tears. The stratum fibrosum is relatively inelastic, as its primary function is to maintain the mechanical integrity of a joint. It guides and restricts joint movement mechanically, as well as neurologically. A rich nerve supply renders the capsule sensitive to pain, position, and movement. Blood enters the capsule through sparse vessels from subchondral bone, but in general, vascularity is poor; thus a torn capsule heals slowly and poorly.

The inner capsular layer, the stratum synoviale, is also referred to as the synovial membrane. It lines nonarticular areas of the joint, as well as communicating bursae and tendon sheaths. The synovial membrane is richly vascularized and repairs well, being capable of complete regeneration within a few months. It produces synovial fluid, and thus regulates the entry of nutrients into the joint. The intimal portion of the membrane consists of a layer of specialized fibroblasts—synoviocytes—of which there are three types: Type A, which are phagocytic; Type B, which synthesize hyaluronic acid; and Type C, which represent a combination of Types A and B (3).

The nerve supply to synovial membrane is scanty; many are vasomotor and produce changes associated with inflammation, such as an increase in vascularity, followed by a proliferation of surface cells and a gradual fibrosis of subsynovial tissue. Posttraumatic synovitis is a response to minor trauma, in which an effusion occurs; if it remains, the membrane eventually becomes hypertrophied and sclerotic.

Synovial fluid resembles an ultrafiltrate of plasma with the addition of hyaluronate. It is clear, pale yellow, and does not clot (resembles egg white). It is quite sparse in normal joints, with intraarticular structures and fat pads taking up dead space and economizing on the amount of fluid necessary. One of the functions of synovial fluid is joint lubrication. A fluid film constantly separates joint surfaces, thus reducing cartilage wear. The hyaluronic acid is responsible for viscosity (thickness) of the fluid, which exhibits non-Newtonian properties: viscosity decreases as fluid shear rate increases. The viscosity is high at low rates of shear so that the joint is able to support heavy loads. At higher rates of movement, the viscosity falls so that the drag is reduced, but it can still bear heavy loads because the rate of movement offsets the fall of viscosity. Another function of the fluid is to provide nourishment for the avascular articular cartilage.

Examination of synovial fluid plays an important role in the diagnosis of joint disease. In synovitis, the fluid reflects the inflammatory reactions occurring in the membrane. There are increased levels of white blood cells, protein, and increased volume, with a fall in concentration of hyaluronate and decreased viscosity. If the fluid is cloudy, it is usually due to leukocytes, suggesting an infectious disorder. A ligamentous or capsular tear may produce bloody fluid. If bone marrow spicules or immature red cells are observed in the fluid, they can indicate a fracture. If fat globules are present, then possibly an intracapsular fracture or synovial tear exists (intracapsular extrasynovial adipose tissue).

Many joints contain intraarticular structures, such as ligaments, tendons, labra, discs, menisci, and fat pads. In addition to providing mechanical stability for the joint, they serve to fill in "dead" space between poorly congruent surfaces.

A variety of factors contributes to a joint's stability. For every plane of motion there are both primary and secondary static joint stabilizers. The primary restraints are the major ligamentous and capsular structures resisting movement in a particular direction; the secondary restraints resist movement if excessive laxity should occur in the primary system. Often the secondary structures are not designed to withstand such forces and may be stretched or torn by moderate stress. Joint geometry and compressive forces assist in maintaining alignment.

In addition to passive (static) stability afforded the joints by ligaments, dynamic factors also play a role. Musculotendinous units offer much control over a joint, and are intimately associated with joint movement through highly sensitive neurologic feedback mechanisms.

JOINT KINEMATICS

Osteokinematics and Degrees of Freedom

Motion of bony segments is referred to as osteokinematic (physiologic) movement (18). Flexion/extension, abduction/adduction, and rotation describe osteokinematic limb segment motion. In using these terms, the reference point for motion is the bone itself. Thus, the humerus abducts on the scapula, or the tibia rotates on the femur.

The movement of a bone about each primary axis of any given joint is called a degree of freedom. The hip and shoulder move in three planes, and both have three degrees of freedom, whereas the ulnohumeral joint, which moves in one plane, has only one. Two or more degrees of freedom can combine to produce other movements, such as circumduction.

Arthrokinematics

Incompatibility in the size, curvature, and precise shape of joint surfaces creates the need for movement at the joint surface to be different from movement of the limb segment (18–23). For example, in order for the upper limb to abduct, the humeral head must glide caudally in the glenoid fossa. Joint surface movement (arthrokinematic) is often referred to as component or accessory motion because it accompanies limb move-

ment (24). Types of accessory motion include glide, spin, distraction, compression, roll, and slide. Since it is difficult to clinically distinguish roll and slide from other accessory motions during joint mobilization, descriptions of roll and slide per se will not be incorporated into the assessment and treatment sections.

Glide is a motion at the joint surface which occurs as one joint member moves across another without any appreciable angular or rotary movement (2). During knee extension, the femoral condyles glide posteriorly on the tibial plateau. Glide allows the relatively large condyles to maintain articular contact with limited tibial surface area.

Spin is rotation of a joint member about its long axis. During the process of standing, medial rotation of the femur on the tibia occurs as accessory motion to lock the knee in extension. Therefore, spin is occurring at the junction of the femoral condyles and the tibial plateau.

Distraction is a separation or "gapping" of joint surfaces. Osteokinematic trunk rotation produces a distraction of the facet joint surfaces toward the side of rotation (Fig. 1.4). Manual or mechanical traction are examples of therapy to restore the gapping potential of a joint.

Compression is an approximation of joint surfaces seen normally in the lower extremities during weight-bearing activities. It also occurs in nonweightbearing joints in certain parts of their range of motion. Compression and distraction are necessary for the circulation of synovial fluid, and may be performed manually when indicated.

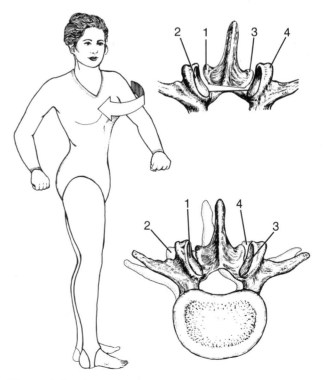

Figure 1.4.   Accessory motions: Distraction (between 1 and 2) and compression (between 3 and 4) of selected spinal facets during rotation of the trunk.

In addition to articular structure, muscle action plays a role in facilitating accessory motions. This can be seen in the shoulder where the rotator cuff muscles act to depress the humeral head during limb elevation for optimal utilization of available glenoid space (25–28). This mechanism produces a greater freedom of movement within a limited articular surface area.

Close- and Loose-Packed Positions

When joint members are fully congruent (approximating each other with a maximum surface area) and the periarticular structures are taut, then the joint is considered close-packed, and further accessory or physiologic motion is not possible (2). Examples of close-packed positions are:

1. The talocrural joint fully dorsiflexed;
2. The knee fully extended;
3. The shoulder abducted 90° and externally rotated; and
4. The metacarpophalangeal joint flexed 90°.

In cases of joint pathology, the close-packed position of a joint may be reached short of its normal range of motion due to adhesion, muscle spasm, or capsular scarring. As a joint is moved from close-packed to loose-packed, the potential for accessory motion between articular surfaces increases. Therefore, to produce accessory motion through manual application of force, the starting position is usually a loose-packed position.

Concave and Convex Joint Members

Manual therapists find it useful to view the majority of synovial joints as having a convex and a concave member. The concept of convex and concave components is derived from a geometrical model that describes joint surfaces as ovoid, i.e., a surface with a changing radius of curvature (2). Table 1.2 lists the convex members of some major synovial joints and their corresponding concave mates.

When a joint member contains a concave surface in one plane and a convex surface in another, perpendicular plane, the geometrical configuration assumes the form of a sellar (saddle) surface. For example, the first carpometacarpal joint is a "saddle" joint. Flexion and extension occur when the concave metacarpal base glides on the convex surface of the trapezium. In contrast, abduction and adduction occur when the convex portion of the metacarpal base glides on the concave portion of the trapezium.

Table 1.2.
Convex and Concave Joint Surfaces

Convex	Concave
humeral head	glenoid fossa
head of the proximal radius	ulnar notch
metacarpal head	phalangeal base
femoral head	acetabulum
femoral condyle	tibial plateau
dome of the talus	ankle mortise

Some joints do not fit the convex-concave classification scheme. Examples are the spinal facets, proximal tibiofibular, and individual intercarpal joints, which essentially have "flat" joint surfaces and glide as their primary movement. Manual therapists may also deal with nonsynovial joints which contribute a critical component of movement. Examples include the interbody vertebral joints, the scapulothracic articulations, and the ulnomeniscotriquetral junction.

Application of some manual therapeutic procedures is based on joint kinematics which determine relative directions of accessory and physiologic motions. The direction of accessory motion that accompanies a physiologic motion depends on which joint member is fixed and which is moving. In general, when a concave member is moving on a fixed convex mate, the accessory motion occurs in the same direction as the physiologic motion. When a convex member is moving on a fixed concave mate, the accessory motion is opposite to the physiologic motion. In Figure 1.5A, during flexion of an interphalangeal joint, the concave base of the middle phalanx would glide in the same direction as the physiologic motion. In Figure 1.5B, during abduction of the glenohumeral joint, the con-

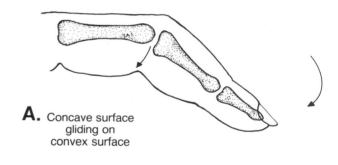

A. Concave surface gliding on convex surface

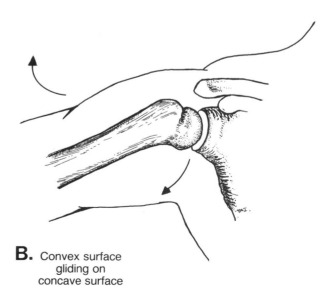

B. Convex surface gliding on concave surface

Figure 1.5. The directions of joint surface and limb segment movement. *A*, Concave joint member moving in flexion, *B*, Convex joint member moving in abduction.

vex humeral head would move in a direction opposite the physiologic motion.

When concave and convex members are readily identifiable, the kinematic rules governing the direction of physiologic and accessory motions can be applied as stated above. In special cases, such as spinal motion, the facet joints and intervertebral discs do not directly conform to a concave-convex model. However, some important similarities exist between spinal and peripheral limb kinematics (Fig. 1.6). Forward bending, backward bending, side-bending, and rotation of the trunk are physiologic osteokinematic motions and are defined in the same manner as peripheral limb movements (i.e., they focus on movements of bones and body segments rather than movements at the joint surface). Each physiologic spinal motion has underlying component arthrokinematic motions which must occur during voluntary movement. For example, forward bending of the trunk is accompanied by anterior glide of the vertebral bodies and rotation of the vertebral bodies about a left-right horizontal axis (Fig. 1.6B). This phenomenon is analogous to the posterior glide of the tibial plateau on the femoral condyles during knee flexion (Fig. 1.6B).

JOINT NEUROLOGY

Hilton's law states that the same nerve trunk furnishes a distribution to:

1. A group of muscles moving a given joint;
2. The skin over the insertion of those muscles; and
3. The interior of the joint being moved by the muscle group.

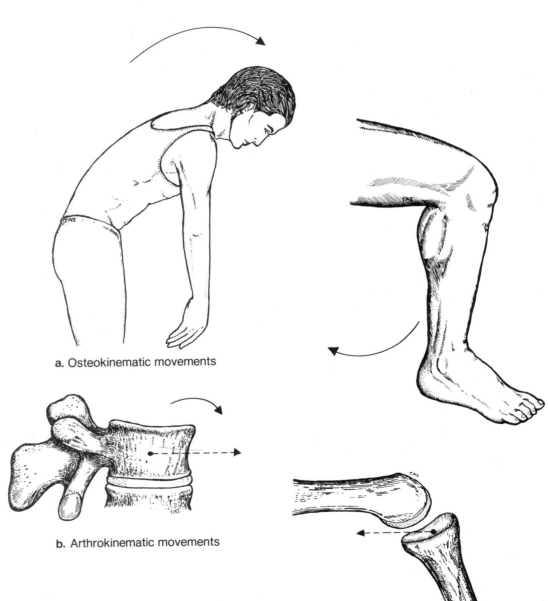

Figure 1.6. Similarities between spinal and peripheral limb kinematics. Osteokinematics describe gross movements of the trunk or limbs. Arthrokinematics describe movements at the joint surfaces.

a. Osteokinematic movements

b. Arthrokinematic movements

This arrangement creates an interdependence between skin sensation, muscle action, and joint movement. For example, mechanoreceptors located in the joint can influence muscle tone. All joints contain four varieties of receptor nerve endings (Table 1.3) (29).

Type I and Type II receptors occur in the joint capsule. In general, Type I receptors tonically (continuously) contribute to the regulation of the tone of muscle groups moving a particular joint. They respond to very small increments or decrements of tension when the part of the capsule in which they lie is stretched or relaxed. Their frequency of resting discharge is proportional to the degree of tension change (29). They are active at every position of the joint, even at rest. In contrast, Type II receptors rapidly adapt to changes in joint position by providing a brief burst of activity at the moment when tension increases. Therefore, the Type II receptors exercise a phasic influence on muscle tone.

Type III receptors are present in the peripheral joint ligaments. They are completely inactive when the joint is at rest and discharge only at the extreme end of motion, a position which stresses the ligaments. Muscle inhibition is the end result of Type III receptor discharge. Fisk has suggested that manual therapy leads to increased passive motion because joint mobilization triggers Type III mechanoreceptors and facilitates a reduction in muscle spasm (30). In the presence of spasm, however, mobilizing forces sufficient to activate the Type III receptors may produce too much pain. Therefore, one must use a less forceful technique that works through different mechanisms. (31)

Joint receptors also provide position and pain sensation. Type IV corpuscles represent free nerve endings in the fibrous joint capsule, and mediate a pain response. Type IV endings are not present in the synovial lining, menisci, or intervertebral discs (29). They are sensitive to noxious mechanical or chemical stimuli, but remain inactive under normal conditions. If a noxious stimulus is present, the Type IV receptors provoke nonadapting alphamortorneuron discharge (spasm). Mobilization in the painful range of motion could also provide the adequate stimulus for the Type IV receptors if applied too vigorously.

References

1. Leeson CR, Leeson TS: *Histology*. ed 4. Philadelphia, WB Saunders, 1985.
2. Warwick R, Williams PL: *Gray's Anatomy*. ed 35 (Brit). WB Saunders London, Longman, 1973.
3. Rodman CB (ed): Primer on the rheumatic diseases, ed 7. *JAMA* 224:7–24, 1973.
4. Turek SL: *Orthopaedics: Principles and Their Application*. ed 4. Philadelphia, JB Lippincott, 1984, vol 1.
5. Halkovich LR: Histology of cartilage. *Bulletin of the Orthopaedic Section, APTA* 3:15–17, 1978.
6. Mankin HJ: Current concepts review: The response of articular cartilage to mechanical injury. *J Bone Joint Surg* 64A:460–466, 1982.
7. Westers BM: Review of the repair of defects in articular cartilage, part II. *J Orthop Sports Phys Ther* 4:6–15, 1982.
8. Salter RB, Hamilton HW, Wedge JH, Tile M, Torode IP, O'Driscoll SW, Murnaghan JJ, Saringer JH: Clinical application of basic research on continuous passive motion for disorders and injuries of synovial joints: A preliminary report of a feasibility study. *J Orthop Res* 1:325–342, 1984.
9. Akeson WH, Savio L-YW, Amiel D, Matthews JV: Biomechanical and biochemical changes in the periarticular connective tissue during contracture development in the immobilized rabbit knee. *Connect Tissue Res* 2:315–323, 1974.
10. Enneking WF, Horowitz M: Intraarticular effects of immobilization on the human knee. *J Bone Joint Surg* 54A:973–985, 1972.
11. Meachim G, Emergy IA: Cartilage fibrillation in shoulder and hip joints in Liverpool necropsies. *J Anat* 116:161–197, 1973.
12. McDonough AL: Effects of immobilization and exercise on articular cartilage—A review of literature. *J Orthop Sports Phys Ther* 3:2–5, 1981.
13. Halkovich LR: Histology of bone. *Bulletin of the Sports and Orthopaedic Section, APTA* 3:6–8, 1977.
14. Halkovich LR: Embryological development of skeleton. *Bulletin of the Orthopaedic Section, APTA* 2:13–14, 1977.
15. Weeks P, Wray C: *Management of Acute Hand Injuries*, ed 2. St. Louis, CV Mosby, 1978.
16. Moore KL: *Clinically Oriented Anatomy*. Baltimore, Williams & Wilkins, 1980.
17. Westers BM: Review of the repair of defects in articular cartilage, part I. *J Orthop Sports Phys Ther* 3:186–192, 1982.
18. MacConnaill MA, Basmajian JV: *Muscles and Movements, a Basis for Human Kinesiology*. New York, Krieger, 1977.
19. Kapandji IA: *Physiology of the Joints*. London, Churchill Livingstone, 1970, vol 1.
20. Kapandji IA: *Physiology of the Joints*. London, Churchill Livingstone, 1970, vol 2.
21. Kessler RM, Hertling D: *Management of Common Musculoskeletal Disorders*. Philadelphia, Harper & Row, 1983, pp 30–34.
22. Saha AK: Mechanics of elevation of the glenohumeral joint. *Acta Orthop Scand* 44:668–678, 1973.
23. Steindler A: *Kinesiology of the Human Body Under Normal and Pathological Conditions*. Springfield, IL, Charles C Thomas, 1955.
24. Maitland GD: *Peripheral Manipulation*. Stoneham, MA, Butterworth, 1977.
25. Codman EA: *The Shoulder*. New York, G Miller Co., 1934.
26. Dvir Z, Berme N: The shoulder complex in elevation of the arm: A mechanism approach. *J Biomech* 11:219–225, 1978.
27. Lehmkuhl LD, Smith LK: Brunnstrom's Clinical Kinesiology. Philadelphia, FA Davis, 1983.
28. Saha AK: *Theory of Shoulder Mechanisms: Descriptive and Applied*. Springfield, IL, Charles C Thomas, 1961.
29. Wyke B: The neurology of joints. *Ann R Coll Surg Engl* 41:25–50, 1967.
30. Fisk JW: A controlled trial of manipulation in a selected group of patients with low back pain favouring one side. *NZ Med J* 10:288–291, 1979.
31. Zusman M: Reappraisal of a proposed neurophysiological mechanism for the relief of joint pain with passive joint movements. *Physiotherapy Practice*:64–70, 1985.

Table 1.3.
Classification of Articular Receptor Systems[a]

Type	Location	Characteristics
I	Fibrous joint capsule—superficial layer	static and dynamic, low threshold, slowly adapting mechanoreceptors
II	Fibrous joint capsule—deep layers	dynamic, low threshold, rapidly adapting mechanoreceptors
III	Intrinsic and extrinsic joint ligaments	dynamic, high threshold, slowly adapting mechanoreceptors
IV	Fibrous capsule, articular fat pads, ligaments, walls of blood vessels	nociceptive, high threshold, nonadapting mechanoreceptors

[a]Modified from Wyke B: The neurology of joints. *Ann R Coll Surg Engl* 41:25–50, 1967.

BASIC CONCEPTS OF ORTHOPAEDIC MANUAL THERAPY

Carolyn T. Wadsworth, L.P.T., M.S.
David Johnson, L.P.T.

INTRODUCTION

The scope of orthopaedics includes the art and science of prevention, investigation, and treatment of disorders and injuries of the musculoskeletal system by medical, surgical, and physical means (1). Orthopaedic manual therapy (OMT) extends this traditional specialty with emphasis on examination and treatment through the application of specific manual techniques. OMT deals with traumatic, developmental, and systemic musculoskeletal disorders of acute and chronic nature, and attempts to restore optimal function by relieving pain, increasing or decreasing mobility, and preventing dysfunction. Orthopaedic manual therapists utilize palpatory skills, dextrous application of passive joint movement, active or resisted muscle contractions, and other techniques to determine the quantity and quality of a patient's movement, and its effect on his symptoms.

Competence in OMT requires fine psychomotor skill, selective attention to the mechanical, nonverbal, and verbal (as in "Ouch!") responses of the patient, judgment regarding the degree of vigor or gentleness appropriate to a given problem, and awareness of potential hazards of such treatment. The therapist must demonstrate considerable manual skill in gently handling painful joints and ascertaining the directions of movement dysfunction. He must also develop sensitized digits in order to selectively palpate and recognize tissue changes (2). Advanced knowledge in biological, behavioral, biomechanical, and clinical sciences permits judicious application of manual therapeutic maneuvers to assess and relieve joint and soft tissue lesions.

Continuous analytical assessment of the patient's status is essential to the use of manual therapy procedures. No technique should be administered without accurately examining the patient prior to treatment, then reevaluating the patient's responses both during and following the treatment (3). The therapist must become adept in applying basic examination and treatment techniques, but more importantly must recognize the need for constantly monitoring the patient's status and modifying therapeutic techniques until an appropriate result occurs. He must also interpret the patient's signs and symptoms relative to his history, because characteristics of the onset and nature of the disorder affect its response to treatment.

A major aspect of OMT assessment is determining what movements or positions provoke or relieve the patient's symptoms. This information assists in both biomechanical and physiological analyses of the involved structures. To reproduce pain by passive stretch at the limit of motion, for example, alerts the examiner to the possibility of a specific joint lesion through biomechanical assessment. To elicit pain upon initial movement, prior to reaching an end feel of passive resistance depicts the physiological response of an acute, highly irritable structure.

Knowing the effects of movements or positions also assists a therapist in treatment planning. It informs him of which activities and postures to recommend and which to avoid. In the absence of a precise diagnosis, one may cautiously proceed with treatment by monitoring these clinical findings. Determining that a lesion has a mechanical etiology reinforces the need for manual restoration of function. Few, if any, treatment regimens other than OMT have the specificity and sensitivity for dealing with such mechanical disorders.

Pain and Movement

Pain and pathological joint movement are leading reasons why patients seek health care, and constitute the bulk of disorders which orthopaedic manual therapists treat. The manual therapist attempts to minimize, correct, or prevent pain and/or pathologic movement. Pain presents and behaves in seemingly infinite patterns (3). Lack of objective parameters for measuring pain, variability in terminology describing pain, and differences in pain responses to various procedures produce challenging obstacles to a therapist's accurate assessment of pain. A subsequent section of this chapter provides information about describing the site, nature, and behavior of a patient's pain.

Cyriax states that all pain arises from a lesion, and that treatment must reach the lesion to be beneficial (4). A challenge to evaluating and treating the exact site of the lesion is the existence of referred pain. Referred pain represents an error in perception, as the patient feels pain at a site apart from the lesion causing it. Referred pain occurs because the segmental derivation of dermatomes, myotomes, and sclerotomes in the embryo produces a singular representation of these diverse structures in the cerebral cortex. Consequently, a noxious stimulus of a muscle (myotome-derived) can be interpreted by the cortex as a stimulus arising from the skin (dermatome-derived), which develops in the same segment with that particular muscle, and receives the same nerve supply. Common clinical examples of referred pain include myocardial pain felt in the absent upper extremity of an amputee or felt after a brachial plexus block. Because of this phenomenon, practitioners frequently but erroneously treat the *area* where the patient experiences pain rather than the lesioned tissue(s) producing the pain. The therapist can avoid misidentifying the site of a lesion by examining the patient accurately.

In manual examination and treatment, joint movement may be physiological, i.e., that which a patient can perform voluntarily; or accessory, i.e., that which a patient cannot perform in isolation but that normally accompanies physiologic movement and may be produced by a force external to the joint. An example of physiological movement at the wrist joint is extension; accessory movement accompanying wrist extension is volar carpal glide. Physiological movement of an active or passive nature has been a mainstay of traditional therapy, and clinicians continue to use it in various evaluation and treatment procedures. Accessory movement at a joint is necessary, if that joint is to attain normal, painless physiologic range of motion (ROM); it is this intrinsic joint play which promotes efficiency of functional movements (5). Orthopaedic manual therapy incorporates evaluating and restoring accessory movement to obtain painless joint function.

Physiological and accessory movement may be normal, hypermobile, or hypomobile. The anatomical limit of joint ROM is the point where a joint's articular surfaces or other restraining components normally stop movement. A hypermobile joint, due to excessive laxity, moves beyond its anatomical limit. A hypomobile joint, due to tissue resistance, pain, or spasm ceases movement short of its anatomical limit, a point

called the pathological limit. Physiological and accessory treatment movements may be performed up to, and beyond the joint's pathological limit, but they cannot exceed its anatomical limit (6). Manual therapists grade the distance a joint moves through its total range. They generally measure physiological movement in degrees with a goniometer. They grade accessory movement on a scale of 0–6, as listed in Table 2.1.

The techniques therapists use to restore accessory movement are termed joint mobilization or manipulation. Generically, manipulation means passive movement of any kind. Some prefer, however, to use the term mobilization to denote passive movement performed slowly enough that preventing its occurrence remains within a patient's reaction time. Manipulation, in this context, would then denote only passive movement involving a high velocity, small amplitude thrust which proceeds quickly enough that a relaxed patient cannot prevent its occurrence. Thus, the speed of the technique—not necessarily the degree of force—differentiates the two categories of passive movement. Following this scheme, a therapist may grade passive treatment movement according to the amount of available range, or slack, that he takes up in the joint, and the velocity of techniques (Table 2.2) (3). Grade I is a small amplitude movement in the beginning of the ROM. Grade II is a large amplitude movement within the mid-ROM. Grade III is a large amplitude movement up to the pathological limit of motion. Grade IV is a small amplitude movement at the pathological limit of motion. Grade V is a small amplitude movement at the pathological limit of motion, delivered in a single quick thrust. The therapist may perform Grade I–Grade IV techniques in an oscillatory manner, with low to moderate velocity, maintaining a consistent position within the accessory range. He may progress deeper as muscles relax, pain subsides, or the barrier to motion recedes. Alternatively, he may sustain a more prolonged stretch on the tissues.

Orthopaedic manual therapy deals with lesions of both joints and soft tissues (6). Such pathological or traumatic lesions typically result in pain and movement disorders which may be involved in a vicious cycle. Joint disease causes secondary muscle changes, particularly atrophy and spasm (5). Spasm is an involuntary protective mechanism which attempts to prevent painful joint movements; lack of joint movement causes further joint disease. It is difficult to restore normal muscle function when joints are not free to

Table 2.1.
Grading Accessory Joint Movement

Grade	Joint Status
0	ankylosed
1	considerable hypomobility
2	slight hypomobility
3	normal
4	slight hypermobility
5	considerable hypermobility
6	unstable

Table 2.2.
Grading Passive Treatment Movement

Grade I:	small amplitude oscillation at the beginning of range; used to reduce pain
Grade II:	large amplitude oscillation within the range; used to reduce pain (doesn't move into resistance) or limit of range
Grade III:	large amplitude oscillation from mid- to end of range; used to increase mobility (reaches limit of range)
Grade IV:	small amplitude oscillation at the limit (end) of range; used to increase mobility
Grade V:	sharp thrust beyond the pathological limitation of range

move. Additionally, normal joint function depends upon movement; joint deterioration results from impaired mechanics and muscle action. Therefore, manual examination and treatment must consider both the joints and the soft tissues, and their relation to one another.

EXAMINATION

General Information

The goal of an examination is to define and clarify the source and nature of the patient's lesion. This information allows a clinician to implement appropriate treatment procedures, with a baseline for judging their effectiveness. The examiner also assesses the overall disability stemming from the patient's primary complaint, relates the disability to his underlying pathology, and plans for optimal restoration of function.

Much of an examination deals with attempting to reproduce the patient's signs and symptoms which relate to his primary complaint. The manifestation and behavior of these signs and symptoms may implicate or rule out any of a number of conditions, as well as suggest further testing. Manual examination is ideally suited to probing structural lesions, selectivity stressing tissues, coaxing passive movements, and similar procedures in an attempt to identify the basis of the patient's problem.

Examination formats vary, but regardless of the particular version one chooses, the examination should be thorough and accurate. The examiner should record all information as objectively as possible. The use of a recording form often contributes to the efficiency and completeness of an examination. The rest of this chapter describes a general examination format; chapters 3–9 present examples of formats that can be used for specific body areas. Two sections generally comprise an examination: a patient history and a physical examination. A history offers the patient an opportunity to subjectively describe the problem and his perception of the limitations it poses. A physical examination provides objective data necessary to confirm, refute, or modify the patient's own account of his problem.

History

Identifying data which initiate the patient's history include his name, age, gender, and the examination date (Fig. 2.1). Confirming the patient's name prevents mistaken identity from scheduling, referral, or medical record error. Age connotes general developmental status, activity level, and the potential for particular age-related pathologies. Patient age may also suggest certain modes of management, relative to predicted rates of healing and complications of treatment among various age groups. Gender predisposes individuals to certain illnesses, trauma, genetic defects, and occupation-related conditions. Examination date gives perspective to the current state of the patient's condition relative to date of onset as well as developments to come.

A provisional (working) diagnosis, if available, alerts an examiner to likely manifestations of a disorder, but usually requires further exploration into present status, functional implications, and response to manual therapy techniques. For example, a postsurgical or posttrauma patient may present with a clear-cut diagnosis, but the status of the involved tissue may vary according to stage of inflammation, healing, and strength of repair, considerations which carry important management implications. Known or anticipated precautions relative to a disease state, surgical procedure, immobilization, etc. are also critical to planning further examination and treatment. The patient's chief complaint pinpoints his immediate concern, although it may not be representative of his primary condition or underlying pathology. The complaint serves to clue the examiner to what led the patient to seek therapeutic assistance, but should not bias him regarding the source of the patient's problem. Hand dominance portrays functional demands which have been experienced or can be expected, and is relevant to disability assessment. Prior condition of the involved part of the body may help to determine the severity of a condition, or project the outcome of a treatment program.

The examiner next asks the patient to elaborate on his present illness or episode. A body chart and visual

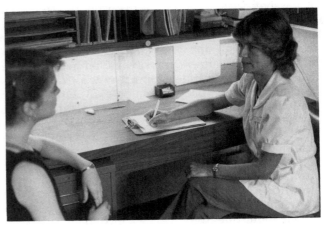

Figure 2.1.   Taking the patient's history.

analog scales facilitate description of symptoms. The patient can detail the exact location of various symptoms, such as pain, paresthesia, and numbness on the diagram, as well as indicate which areas are clear of symptoms. Thoroughly inquiring about all symptoms, and checking off the areas that the patient reports are asymptomatic, is of great value at subsequent sessions. Such thorough questioning and recording avoids the possibility of apparently "new symptoms" arising at a later date. The therapist may assume these symptoms arose from treatment, when they were actually present all along, but were overshadowed during the initial history-taking by more intense symptoms, that were relieved subsequently by treatment. The patient rates the severity of his symptom on a scale from none to worst, which the examiner can compare with future assessment. Likewise, he rates impairment of function from annoying to completely disabling. Description of symptom nature is aided by a checklist of features including aching, burning, tingling, etc.

Symptom behavior is an important aspect of the present episode. It depicts how involved tissues manifest clinically, and assists the examiner in determining the status (e.g., acute vs. chronic inflammatory) and irritability of a condition. Highly irritable lesions are easily aggravated by activity and subside slowly. In contrast, mildly irritable lesions tend to be provoked only by more intense stimuli. Symptoms which are constant and unaffected by activity or rest may not be stemming from a musculoskeletal disorder. They deserve careful attention, and may indicate referral to other specialists.

Most musculoskeletal disorders result in intermittent symptoms, and are aggravated by physical activity. Duration of symptoms and periods of relief characterize certain conditions. For example, osteoarthritis and chondromalacia are disorders which are most painful when movement first occurs after periods of inactivity. Rheumatoid arthritis typically presents morning stiffness lasting up to 2 hours. The stiffness diminishes with activity while the pain increases with activity. The patient may also be able to describe specific activities that bring on, or relieve, symptoms. These not only provide valuable diagnostic information, but also assist in treatment planning. The examiner may characterize these activities according to three qualities: the severity of the symptoms they cause, the intensity of the activities necessary to produce symptoms, and the duration of the symptoms so caused (3). For example, if a mild, transitory pain in the right mid- and lower cervical areas results from sustaining the neck in extreme right rotation while backing the car down a long driveway each morning, the problem would not be very irritable. In contrast, if glancing up at a street light causes a sharp, shooting pain over the shoulder and down the arm, and the resultant ache takes an hour to subside, the problem would be quite irritable.

The examiner next requests that the patient describe how his primary problem behaves over a 24-hour period. Acute disorders often worsen as the day pro-

gresses, but may fluctuate relative to particular activities or postures. If the patient reports that his symptoms are worse at a day's end, one should inquire how long they last and if and how the patient relieves them. The patient should also describe joint characteristics such as catching, locking, giving way, and swelling, and what activities produce them.

Following description of the present episode, the patient elaborates on the episode's background and associated findings. The date of an injury or the onset of an insidious disorder defines the length of involvement. It is important that the patient distinguish the onset of the present episode from the date of original onset. Previous management, including hospitalization and/or other health care, contributes to understanding the condition. Specific information on treatment, particularly physical therapy, and how the patient responded assists in subsequent management. The patient's perception of whether his disorder is better, worse, intermittent, etc. may assist in determining its present status.

If an injury occurred, or if specific events precipitated the episode, the patient describes what happened (Fig. 2.2.). It is necessary for the examiner to explore the mechanism of injury, such as determining exactly what position a shoulder was in when it was struck, or what type of rollers entrapped a hand on an assembly line. These details may elucidate the structures sustaining injury, the depth of tissue damage, and the velocity of force required to disrupt a joint (implications for recurrence), among other things. Understanding the mechanism of injury also allows an examiner to estimate the severity of trauma sustained by a patient. The examiner is able to then compare estimated severity with the degree of disability

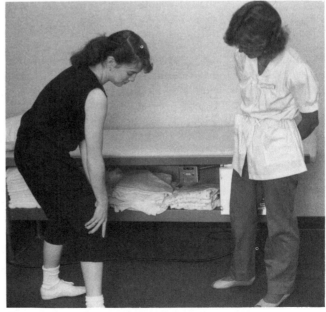

Figure 2.2. The patient describes the mechanism of her injury.

the patient actually appears to have, and how much discomfort the patient reports. Making these comparisons may enable one to estimate the probable degree of movement limitation, what portion of a problem may be due to tissue damage vs. mechanical derangement, and the patient's degree of psychological involvement. If the patient cannot recall an injury, an examiner inquires about any related incidents, unusual activity, or unaccustomed posture which may have incited the current episode. In this way, the injury can be distinguished from a truly insidious condition.

The patient should mention any deformity resulting from an injury, and whether he corrected it. This helps to identify subluxation, dislocation, fracture, locked joint, and perhaps the extent of ligamentous disruption. Any injury-related disability also provides information regarding the nature of the disorder. The patient's perceived cause of disability is equally important; for example, not walking on a leg because of knee pain could implicate certain disorders, whereas not walking on it because of fear the knee will "give way" may implicate others. The patient should also describe specifics of loss of motion or strength, and the chronological order in which they occurred. In order to get a meaningful history, the examiner must ask specifically which motions produce pain, which are unstable, and which are weak (possible neuromuscular involvement). Also, the patient should indicate if and when swelling or bleeding occurred. Swelling within a joint which develops in 3–4 hours indicates hemarthrosis, possibly from an intraarticular fracture or tear of intracapsular ligament such as a cruciate. Swelling arising 24 hours after injury is usually from synovial effusion that occurs, for example, when a joint capsule is damaged.

Once the patient has thoroughly described his present episode, the examiner questions him regarding past and family history. If similar episodes have occurred, he notes their frequency and dates. He should also determine whether the patient completely recovered from the last episode. If there has been a series of episodes, one notes whether a trend in frequency, severity, or status between them exists. Such information helps to put the present episode in proper perspective for setting reasonable goals for treatment, and for predicting the likelihood of recurrence. For a completely new problem, one must concentrate on relieving the present disorder, whereas for a recurrent problem, one may choose to focus less on the immediate symptoms and more on how to help a patient avoid the next episode. Other relevant illnesses or disorders may affect the patient's potential for recovery and level of management. Cardiorespiratory problems, for instance, hamper the patient's aerobic capacity, making some exercise programs impractical or dangerous. Previous injuries which have caused musculoskeletal impairment, joint instability, and other problems alter mechanics and require modification of rehabilitation protocols. Preexisting pain of any type affects the patient both psychologically and physically. There are certain familial patterns which predis-

pose the patient to developing categories of diseases, such as connective tissue disorders. A subsequent section of this chapter covers congenital anomalies, systemic diseases, and other disorders for which manual therapy is contraindicated.

The patient's lifestyle is relevant to management of his present complaint. His occupation and customary daily activities may relate to the etiology of his problem, as well as determine the amount of disability he experiences. For example, a sedentary executive may be able to adapt to stiffness imposed by a "frozen shoulder," whereas a professional golfer cannot. The degree to which the patient voluntarily participates in physical, recreational, and wellness activities may indicate how compliant and motivated he will be in following through with a home exercise program. At the same time, the examiner may note how likely the patient may be to disregard advice to temporarily restrict activity. Knowing the patient's accustomed degree of activity and expectations of treatment helps one to fully understand the degree of disability from his point of view, and to cooperatively set appropriate and attainable long-term treatment goals. It is important to ask for the patient's own opinion of the cause/source of the complaint. At most, one will derive good insight into the true nature of the problem, and at least, one will become aware of misconceptions which need correction.

The last section of the patient's history concerns his current medications and recent radiographs. Medications may mask symptoms or produce a temporary remission. The examiner must discern the effects of medication from the treatment effects. Knowledge of current and past medication is also crucial in determining the risk factors associated with manual therapy treatment. For example, a long course of steroids may induce osteoporosis, so that vigorous manual treatment may pose a risk. Anticoagulant therapy may also make the patient more susceptible to physical trauma from treatment. If radiographs are available, their review is in order. If they are not available, but the examiner believes they are needed, he may request that they be taken before proceeding with treatment. A therapist must recognize the presence of skeletal conditions which contraindicate manual examination and treatment. For example, a fracture generally requires immobilization, whereas an unstable joint may benefit from strengthening or proprioceptive exercises. Extensive osteophytic or mechanical bony blockage indicates the need for treatment other than joint mobilization to increase motion at a joint.

Upon completion of the history, the examiner reviews the information, taking the necessary time to interpret his findings and to formulate a plan for physical examination. Such a plan increases the likelihood of conducting an efficient and appropriate physical examination. The examiner should highlight with asterisks those portions of the history which relate directly to the patient's present episode. He will assess these important findings at the following visit, to note whether they have changed at all, and if so, for better or for worse. He also reviews irritability of the patient's problem, and plans how selective or thorough, gentle or vigorous the physical examination should be (3). He then selects examination procedures that are appropriate for the patient's status and disorder, and which have a high potential for providing baseline or comparative data. Although the data base from the history initially dictates focus and comprehensiveness of the physical examination, the examiner continuously modifies it according to emerging data and the patient's response.

PHYSICAL EXAMINATION

Inspection

Observing the patient's general structural, postural, and functional qualities commences an examination. Gross trunk, extremity, and bilateral comparisons facilitate identification of abnormalities.

The examiner first assesses posture with the patient standing, using a plumb line or posture grid for reference. Viewing the patient from several vantage points is necessary. A posterior view reveals head position in the frontal plane, shoulder level, scapular alignment, arm contour and position, vertebral alignment, pelvic level, gluteal fold symmetry, greater trochanter and fibular head levels, and foot position. Posteriorly, a plumb line should bisect the head, neck, and trunk, and be equidistant from both lower limbs. A lateral view depicts sagittal plane head position, spinal alignment, scapular and pelvic attitude, lower extremity alignment, and foot structure. Sagittally, a plumb line should bisect the ear lobe, acromion, and greater trochanter, and fall just anterior to the knee and ankle joints. An anterior view shows properties similar to a posterior view, and in addition, facial, acromioclavicular, and sternoclavicular joint symmetry, rib cage proportion, patellar position, and toe alignment.

A supine position is best suited for measuring true leg length, that distance between the anterior superior iliac spine and medial malleolus. The supine position may also reveal rotational abnormalities such as femoral neck retroversion if the patient lies with his leg laterally rotated or anteversion if the patient lies with his leg medially rotated. Torsional deformities of the femur manifest as a medially or laterally oriented patella; torsional deformities of the tibia manifest as a medially or laterally rotated shank and foot in relation to a normally positioned patella.

Shoes may provide evidence of structural malalignment and gait deviations by uneven wear patterns, modifications such as supports, and abnormal force distribution. Thus, meticulous shoe inspection plays an important role in a physical examination.

The examiner next assesses shape, i.e., the contour of body parts and general body build. Swelling, atrophy, and changes in relative soft tissue proportions are examples of abnormal shape manifestations. Congenital anomalies, as well as shape alterations acquired from trauma, surgery, or disease processes may pro-

duce relevant changes. The examiner observes use of the body part involved in the primary complaint. He notes if use of the body part is protected, restricted, coordinated, etc. relative to the rest of the body. He also notes general gait and movement characteristics as the patient prepares for the examination. Only a cursory overview commences here, as extensive movement assessment occurs later in the examination.

Skin condition may reveal signs of trauma, state of wound healing, systemic disorders, or past conditions which have healed with scar. Skin color often reflects circulatory status and the presence of inflammation. Cyanosis or purplish discoloration occur when there is inadequate perfusion; redness occurs in areas of vasodilation with increased flow. Trophic changes (shiny, hairless, hyperpigmented areas) signify diminished blood supply, such as that resulting from peripheral vascular disease. Callus or blister formation results from excessive pressure or friction.

Adaptive devices, or aids for enhanced mechanical function, that the patient presently uses contribute to assessment of the nature of a disorder. The examiner describes both the device, and its intended use (Fig. 2.3). The patient may require a sling or cast for protective or immobilization purposes. Splints align body parts, guide, and restrict movement. Orthoses, corsets, and collars stabilize body parts, and by doing so, they may reduce pain and improve function. Assistive devices, such as canes and crutches, substitute for or relieve pressure on weightbearing areas to facilitate ambulation.

Palpation

Palpation of all tissues associated with the area of symptoms discloses both physiologic and structural changes. As the examiner progressively palpates from

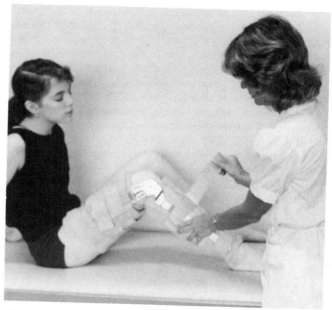

Figure 2.3. Inspecting the type and function of an orthosis.

superficial to deep layers, he notes both the location and nature of any abnormality he may find. He uses the back of his hand to initially discern variations in skin temperature and sweating between symptomatic and nonsymptomatic areas. He then palpates the skin and subcutaneous tissues with his fingertips to identify tension and resistance to gentle displacement in all directions. He progresses to more vigorous displacement (if indicated and tolerated)—possibly even to "skin rolling." Findings could include exquisite tenderness, movement restriction, turgor due to local edema or hemorrhage, "thickening" of these superficial tissues, or "orange peel" effect upon skin rolling. He notes if any of these maneuvers reproduce or relieve the patient's primary complaint.

He next palpates muscles and tendons, to identify areas of tenderness, inflammation, and decreased mobility. He notes bulk and tonus compared with the opposite side, probing simultaneously to the same depth and in corresponding directions. He also observes localized turgor due to inflammation or hemorrhage, localized firm areas, taut bands of muscle fibers, and changes in overall resting length of muscle. Palpation may progress from gentle probing or massaging to grasping or displacing muscle bellies and tendons. Note reproduction or relief of the patient's complaint, and resistance to displacement or stretch, and crepitus or "catching" of soft tissues.

Progressing to tendon sheaths and bursae, the examiner assesses tenderness, temperature, swelling, and crepitus. The synovial lining of these structures may produce effusion or calcium deposits in response to trauma. It is most revealing to palpate the entire extent of a tendon sheath during contraction of its respective muscle. A characteristic vibration, as if the tendon needs lubrication, represents tenosynonitis.

Bone and joint palpation is somewhat restricted to the more superficial parts. Often, probing these areas reveals a source of tenderness, swelling, or mechanical deformation. One may be able to identify degenerative bony changes which occur generally or are concentrated at specific levels, or structural anomalies such as a deviated spinous process. Such changes and anomalies may or may not prove relevant to the source of symptoms or movement restriction.

Arteries and nerves, likewise, are accessible to palpation only where they traverse superficially. Pulses are indicative of arterial patency. Occluding blood flow or compressing nerves by manual pressure may reproduce the symptoms of conditions such as thoracic outlet and carpel tunnel syndromes. Tapping a peripheral nerve that is damaged or regenerating may elicit a Tinel sign which manifests as paresthesias in its particular distribution.

Movement Assessment

Movement assessment, including active, passive, resistive, and special tests, constitutes a major part of a manual examination. It assists the examiner in identifying a lesion by reproducing or altering a patient's

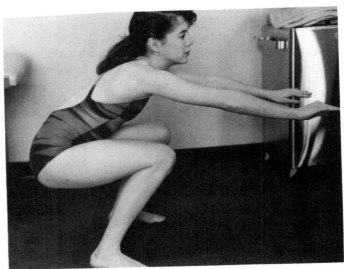

Figure 2.4.   Assessing general functional activity prior to specific tests.

primary complaint. The process is built upon a system of examining function by selective tissue tension, introduced by Cyriax (4). This system allows one to locate a lesion through biomechanical analysis, by selectively applying tension to all tissues which might be a possible source of symptoms. Using this method, the examiner may differentiate inert tissue (bones, joint capsules, ligaments, bursae, dura mater, nerve roots, and fascia) lesions from contractile tissue (muscles and tendons) lesions. Pain arising from inert tissues usually occurs with active (or resistive) and passive movement in the same direction. For example, an inflamed anterior elbow joint capsule is irritated by stretch as the elbow extends, whether the extension is active or passive. Pain from contractile tissue usually occurs with active (or resistive) and passive movement in opposite directions. For example, a strained biceps is irritated by active muscle contraction (elbow flexion) or passive stretch (elbow extension). Movement assessment generally commences at the site of the primary complaint, and works outward as necessary (rather than considering the patient's total body movements and working inward toward the site of symptoms). This approach assumes that local tissues exist and are responsible for a mechanical problem, that they can be discovered by detailed examination, and that specific mechanical procedures (movements) may be found which are effective in reversing the localized disorder. Failure or partial success in relieving symptoms or correcting dysfunction by following this approach warrents taking a more global or holistic view of the patient's entire musculoskeletal system.

Initially, testing functional active movement, a gross test, familiarizes the examiner with what he can expect from the patient (Fig. 2.4). He requests that the patient perform selected functional movements, specific to each joint, and grades them according to a key as follows: C indicates that the patient completes a task; D indicates that he completes it with some difficulty; N indicates that he is not able to complete it.

Specific active movement testing reveals the patient's willingness and ability to complete ROM in the cardinal planes. The therapist assesses range, associated signs and symptoms, and quality of movement, i.e., control, deviations, and adventitious motions. Abnormal movement usually signifies a painful lesion or joint stiffness (3). He asks the patient to perform each active movement, and if this is possible without symptoms, he applies a passive overpressure at the end of range. If the patient remains asymptomatic the examiner may request that he perform several repetitions of a particular active movement, combine it with movement in other planes, or perform it in functional or injuring positions with varied weightbearing forces, traction, and speed. These maneuvers are all an attempt to reproduce the patient's primary complaint. Although active movement may produce symptoms, it will not differentiate between inert and contractile tissue lesions because active joint motion stresses both types of tissues. Therefore, it is necessary to follow through with testing passive and resistive movement.

A painful arc occurs if pain erupts in some central part of the ROM, but disappears as the limb passes this point in either direction (Fig. 2.5). The presence of a painful arc implies that two surfaces are pinching a sensitive structure, e.g., the acromion and greater humeral tuberosity pinch the subacromial bursa. Also, painfully stretching a tissue may produce a compensatory adjustment to relieve it while completing the primary movement.

Passive movement testing discloses a number of qualities of inert tissues, as well as the effects of passive stretch on contractile tissues. A therapist examines physiologic ROM, related signs and symptoms, nature of limitation (end feel), movement patterns, and irritability. It is important that a patient relax completely during passive movement testing, in an attempt to minimize the influence of contractile tissues. A physical therapist can greatly enhance such relaxation by skillful handling.

The examiner performs traditional goniometric joint measurement (Fig. 2.6) (7). In addition, he notes the sensation he feels as a part reaches the end of its ROM as one of the following end feels (Fig. 2.7) (4):

1. Bone-to-bone: an abrupt halt to movement when two hard surfaces meet; e.g., full passive extension of a normal elbow; once this finding emerges, further passive treatment movement will not increase the ROM;
2. Capsular feel: a "hardish" end of movement, with some give to it, like stretching a piece of leather; e.g., full rotation of a normal shoulder;
3. Springy block: a rebound felt at the end of range; e.g., attempted extension of a knee "locked" by internal derangement;
4. Tissue approximation: a gradual, asymptomatic halt to movement as one body part engages another; e.g., thigh pressing into protuberant abdomen (range of motion is full and painless);
5. Empty feel: 1) pain prevents moving farther into the range before a mechanical barrier is reached; 2) movement clearly beyond its anatomical limit, e.g., an acute, complete ligamentous tear.
6. Spasm: 1) a steady resistance produced by involuntary muscle contraction, which persists regardless of how carefully the examiner moves the part; 2) an involuntary flickering of muscle contraction that doesn't vary as one tests movement at different speeds.

The examiner also identifies capsular versus noncapsular movement patterns (4). A capsular pattern is a characteristic, proportional limitation of movement from joint capsule inflammation, such as that occuring in arthritis. Table 2.3 describes the capsular patterns of selected joints.

A noncapsular pattern is limitation of movement not in the proportions of the capsular pattern. Arthritis is generally absent. Lesions capable of selectively restricting the range are responsible, and may be:

1. Ligamentous adhesions: limitation in one plane with full, painless range in the other planes;
2. Internal derangement: partial limitation in one plane, with motion in the opposite direction in that plane,

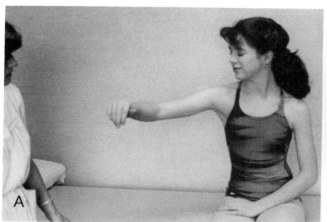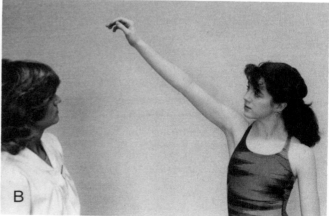

Figure 2.5. The patient demonstrates a painful arc. *A*, Pain occurs at a specific point in the mid-range of motion. *B*, Pain is absent in other parts of the range of motion.

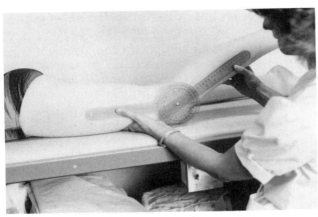

Figure 2.6.   Goniometric measurement of knee range of motion.

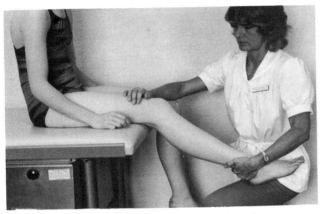

Figure 2.7.   Assessing passive knee extension.

Table 2.3.
Capsular Patterns of Selected Joints[a]

Joint	Pattern of Limitation
Sternoclavicular and acromioclavicular	Pain at the extremes of range
Shoulder	Given a limitation of abduction, there will be a greater percentage loss of external rotation and a lesser percentage loss of internal rotation
Elbow	More limitation of flexion than extension
Wrist	Equal limitation of flexion and extension
Thumb and fingers	More limitation of flexion than extension
Hip	Gross limitation of flexion, abduction, and internal rotation; slight limitation of extension; and little or no limitation of external rotation
Knee	Gross limitation of flexion; slight limitation of extension

[a]From Cyriax J: *Textbook of Orthopaedic Medicine*, ed 6. Baltimore, Williams & Wilkins, 1975, vol 1 and Cookson JC, Kent BE: Orthopedic manual therapy—an overview. Part I: The extremities. *Phys Ther* 59:136–146, 1979.

which is normal and pain-free; the direction of limitation may change due to the movement of the loose fragment; painful arc possible;
3. Extra-articular lesions: limitation usually confined to one plane by painful lesions, adhesions, or soft tissue contracture.

The sequence of pain and limitation (passive resistance to movement) indicates the irritability of a lesion (4), and may occur as follows:

1. Pain before resistance: an acute inflammatory process not suitable for stretching;
2. Pain synchronous with resistance: a semiacute condition which has progressed to some inert tissue fibrosis;
3. Pain after resistance: chronic condition in which contractures have replaced inflammation.

Resistive movement testing primarily reveals the status of contractile elements (Fig. 2.8). Resisting an isometric contraction near midrange minimizes stress or pinching of inert tissues, and may thus produce clinical findings such as pain or weakness stemming from a muscle or tendon lesion. However, since muscle contraction is dependent upon neural control, this test unavoidably reflects the status of the nervous system as well. A more detailed neurologic evaluation described later in this chapter may be required. Keeping possible neurologic involvement in mind, however, the examiner concentrates at this stage on the signs and symptoms as they relate to the contractile tissues themselves. One must also be aware that an isometric contraction may slightly shift joint alignment, or increase intraarticular pressure, producing false-positive tests for contractile tissue lesions.

The therapist evaluates muscle strength, using standard manual muscle testing protocols (8), or instrumented systems such as dynamometers or isokinetic systems. He precisely positions the segment to be tested, instructs the patient, "Don't let me move you," and then gradually presses upon the segment until he feels his own force just exceeding the patient's resistive force. While a patient is holding at this "maximum" force, the examiner should inquire, "Any dis-

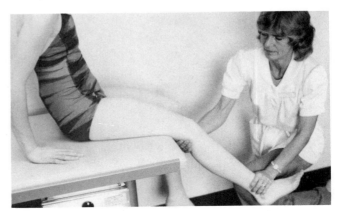

Figure 2.8.   Assessing resistive knee extension.

comfort with this?'' He should then let off the force gradually, and if there was discomfort during the contraction, he should clarify exactly where it was experienced. One must bear in mind the possibility that a contraction may produce pain and may therefore inhibit force production, resulting in a false-positive test for neurological dysfunction.

Cyriax designed a system for differentiating lesions according to isometric strength and symptom combinations as follows (4):

1. Strong and painful: minor lesion of a contractile tissue;
2. Weak and painless: complete rupture of tendon or muscle, or disorder of nervous system;
3. Weak and painful: gross lesion of contractile tissue and/or serious pathology;
4. Strong and painless: normal;
5. Painful on repitition: if a single contraction is strong and painless, but repetition produces pain, possible intermittent claudication of a vascular disorder.

Accessory movement indicates arthrokinematic behavior of a joint, and the status of tissues which control this movement. The therapist evaluates joint mobility on a scale of 0–6, as a previous section of this chapter describes. He also identifies symptoms associated with accessory movement, which include pain, spasm, and passive resistance to movement. He performs traction, compression, and gliding techniques to examine these movements (2). Mennell devised rules for assessory movement testing, which are abbreviated as follows (5,6):

1. A patient must relax; an examiner assures that his joint is supported and protected from unguarded movement.
2. An examiner must relax, and use a firm and protective grasp.
3. One joint is examined at a time.
4. One movement is examined at a time.
5. One articular surface is moved, while the other is stabilized.
6. The extent of accessory movement is evaluated relative to the unaffected side.
7. The examiner must not use forceful or abnormal movements.
8. The examiner must stop if a movement elicits pain.
9. Contraindications for joint mobilization must be respected.

Special tests often contribute to the information that movement assessment provides. They are specific to each joint, and are described in subsequent chapters.

When conducting the numerous procedures described in this section, one must always be aware of a paramount principle of manual examination: it is necessary to correlate the findings of several tests in order to properly interpret the findings of any one test.

Neurologic Evaluation

Results of neurological function tests in an objective examination vary in importance from minor but essen-

tial information, to the most critical information. The physical therapist must be able to accurately and thoroughly determine the presence or absence of central or peripheral neurological deficits in order to be able to closely monitor whether subsequent examination and treatment alter a given patient's neurological status.

For patients not in acute distress with symptoms that are unlikely due to neurological involvement, the neurological examination takes lower priority. Nevertheless, an appropriate screening examination should be performed prior to treatment to confirm normality. Even if a patient's neurological status is found to be completely normal, this information is important to further treatment. If a patient's pain or range of motion worsens—due either to inapproapriate or too vigorous treatment, or to his own activities—the entire neurological examination must be repeated to determine whether the regression in these indicators of function also included changes in neurological function.

For patients in acute distress and whose symptoms raise suspicion of neurological involvement, the examiner may need to perform neurological testing before any other part of the objective examination. Proceeding with caution in this manner may minimize the chances of exacerbating a relatively serious disorder, but may also provide the examiner with the most critically important objective signs to follow as he further examines and treats the patient.

Neurological testing comprises isometric tests of motor function, deep tendon reflexes, sensibility, motor control and coordination, and neural tension tests. An anatomical factor of major importance is that there are overlaps and anomalies of innervation of musculoskeletal structures. Testing selected muscles as representing the motor function of a certain spinal segment, or a specific patch of skin as representing the sensation of a certain dermatome, may be appropriate for general screening purposes. However, cases which appear to present with neurologic involvement require a more detailed assessment of motor function, sensation, etc.

Another important anatomical fact is that nerve root involvement (mechanical irritation) is not required to produce alterations of deep tendon reflexes, paresthesiae, or a ''nerve root'' distribution of pain (9). These neurological signs and symptoms may also result from irritation of tissues innervated by spinal dorsal rami (such as facet joint capsules and interspinous ligaments). Therefore, the only ''hard'' signs of a nerve root involvement are motor weakness and sensory loss. The pattern of such signs assists the examiner in determining the root level involved.

When performing a cursory neurological assessment, the examiner tests the isometric strength of key muscles or movements as representative of nerve root levels as Table 2.4 presents. The examiner should test about three muscles on one side using precise positioning of the patient during the isometric contractions, and should then move to the opposite side of the body to test the same muscles in the same order

Table 2.4.
Key Muscles and Representative Nerve Root Levels

head on neck flexion	C1	finger abduction (dorsal interossei)	T1
head on neck extension	C2	hip flexion (iliopsoas)	L2
cervical side flexion	C3	knee extension (quadriceps)	L3
scapular elevation	C4	ankle dorsiflexion (tibialis anterior)	L4
shoulder abduction (deltoid)	C5	big toe extension (EHL)	L5
elbow flexion (biceps)	C6	ankle plantarflexion (gastroc-soleus)	S1, 2
elbow extension (triceps)	C7		
DIP flexion (FDP)	C8		

using mirror-image positions of the patient and his own body. The results of the patient's right vs. left tests probably provide the best comparison for what are "normal" findings for that patient, in spite of inherent differences due to the patient's (and the examiner's) dominant limbs. If the examiner's findings indicate a more thorough examination, one may employ isometric testing of all muscles, as described previously in the section entitled "Movement Assessment."

Tests of deep tendon reflexes (DTRs) form another area of the neurological exam. Although a DTR can be elicited from many muscles, those commonly tested are biceps (C5-6) (Fig. 2.9), brachioradialis (C6) (Fig. 2.10), triceps (C7) (Fig. 2.11), patellar tendon (L3,4) (Fig. 2.12), and Achilles tendon (S1,2) (Fig. 2.13). While testing these reflexes, the examiner should attempt to produce taps of the same force, in order that any observed variation in response be due to differences in neurologic function rather than unrefined tech-

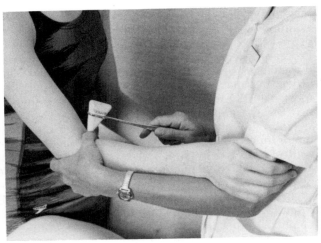

Figure 2.9. Testing the biceps brachii tendon reflex by tapping examiner's thumb which is resting on the tendon just proximal to its insertion.

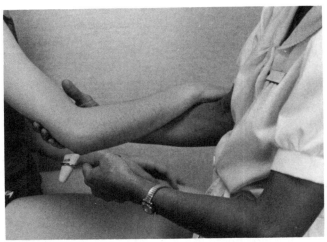

Figure 2.11. Testing the triceps brachii tendon reflex by tapping the tendon just proximal to its insertion.

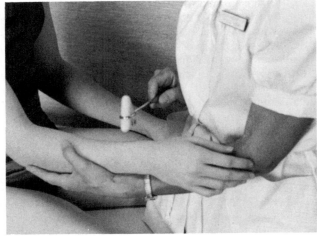

Figure 2.10 Testing the brachioradialis tendon reflex by tapping the tendon just proximal to its insertion.

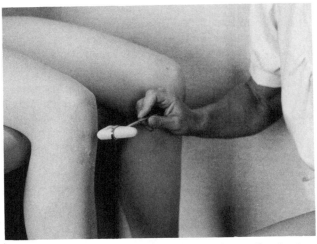

Figure 2.12. Testing the patellar tendon reflex by tapping the tendon just proximal to its insertion.

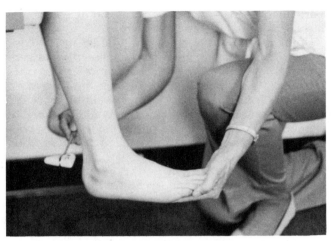

Figure 2.13.   Testing the Achilles tendon reflex by tapping the tendon just proximal to its insertion.

nique. Long-handled (approximately 15 inches) reflex hammers are avaliable which create a consistent and sufficient tap by the examiner's merely letting the rubber weight fall under the influence of gravity. One should repeat the tendon taps at least five times. Assuming an examiner strikes the tendon squarely each time, he may observe whether the amplitude of the reflex decreases with repetition—a subtle sign of abnormality. If a certain upper limb reflex is difficult to elicit, one may make use of a modified Jendrassik maneuver by requesting a patient to twist his legs and squeeze them vigorously together, or to clench his teeth firmly together. When testing the corresponding reflex of the other limb, one must request isometric contractions of the same degree of effort and record the fact that facilitation was used.

The examiner must test plantar reflexes to confirm or rule out suspected spinal cord involvement, and as a precaution prior to performing vigorous spinal manipulation techniques. Babinski's sign is positive if, in response to a curved, firm stroke along the sole of the foot from the heel to the metatarsal heads, the great toe extends and the remaining toes splay. A normal response is toe flexion. Ankle clonus also should be tested by producing a crisp, passive dorsiflexion of the foot. Sustained oscillation numbering three or more beats is an abnormal finding.

Sensibility is another facet of a neurological examination. Having recorded "subjective" disturbances of sensation as symptoms reported by the patient during the history, the examiner at this stage notes what "objective" disturbances of sensation he can identify, and records these signs as distinct from their symptoms. One would expect correspondence between these signs and symptoms, and if correspondence is lacking, should attempt to discover why. One may test light touch by using a piece of tape attached to a dulled pin, which may then be used to test discrimination of "sharp" vs. "dull" stimuli. Pinwheels, two-point discrimination tools, and tuning forks also are useful to quantify sensation. The examiner tests temperature discrimination with vials of water of differing warm-

ness or coolness. He assesses joint proprioception by asking a patient to identify a position in which his limb is placed without visual cues.

A few general guidelines for sensory testing follow. Whenever the examiner introduces a new mode of testing to the patient, he should first demonstrate it on himself and then on the asymptomatic side or limb prior to testing the involved limb. One should commence testing with the distal-most limb segments first, and work toward more proximal segments, testing all aspects (anterior, posterior, medial, and lateral) in whatever detail is warranted. The examiner moves the test instrument perpendicular to the long axis of a limb, in order to cut across dermatomes, thereby providing a patient with a degree of contrast should sensation mediated by a certain segment be abnormal. One must test both sides for comparison against the uninvolved side. If the examiner discovers objective distal numbness or paresthesia, he should consider the possibility that circulatory impairment may be responsible, and should confirm or rule this out by palpating peripheral arterial pulses, noting capillary filling time.

Motor control disorders may manifest as spasticity, flaccidity, rigidity, or clonicity. A patient with such signs may be experiencing brain, upper motor neuron, or long spinal tract dysfunction. Gross coordination tests include reciprocal and isolated movements of involved parts. The examiner grades them according to a key as follows: N indicates that the patient completes the activity witth normal speed and coordination; CD indicates that the patient completes slowly with minimal difficulty; SM indicates that the patient completes with searching movements; and U indicates that the patient is unable to complete. Neural tension tests are essential to determine whether normal neural movement (applied to the spinal dura and nerve roots via tension through the peripheral nerves) is present. Such tests as the passive straight leg-raise, prone knee bend, passive neck flexion, and slump test (see Chapter 3), are used to assess neural and dural mobility. Even for those who respond predictably, these tests can produce symptoms characterized as a deep ache of vague location, so to consider a test "positive," it is important to make bilateral comparisons for range and pain (where possible) and to note if symptoms produced are comparable to the patient's chief complaint in area and quality.

Recommendation of Other Tests

Data arising from the patient's history and physical examination may indicate the need for additional tests in order to make conclusive decisions regarding the patient's disorder. The physical therapist, for example, may find it necessary to refer the patient for radiographic, laboratory, and electrodiagnostic studies, or other consultative opinions.

Interpretation of information gained from informal observation and conversation, a history, and a physical examination should provide an integrated picture of the patient's problem which "fits together." If the examiner is not able to see how some "pieces of the puzzle" fall into place, he should go back through the history and physical examination to fill in omissions or to confirm questioned findings. This approach assumes that at least correlations between findings should be demonstrable, if not logical, cause-effect relationships.

If the examiner still cannot formulate an explanation of the problem that accounts for the key data collected, he may then consider taking any of the following actions. If the examination was limited due to time or irritability of the problem, one may inform the patient that further examination is necessary to select an appropriate course of treatment. If the risk of serious pathology is not apparent, but one questions how genuine the patient himself is, one may choose to provide little or no alternative treatment, and in a day or two may repeat the relevant portions of the subjective and objective examinations to note the degree of consistency with previous findings. If the examiner suspects that a patient's disorder is not of musculoskeletal origin, but only masquerading as a mechanical disorder, then the possibility of serious systemic disease, malignancy, etc. exists, and medical consultation is appropriate.

If the examiner is not able to "make sense" of the findings after further reviewing the case and repeating some tests, then he should question his ability to solve the particular case, and should consider conferring with or referring to a colleague. The possibility also exists that the patient may indeed have a disorder, but not one within the purview of manual examination and treatment. If data remain inconclusive after examination, one must assume this position. Such an outcome in itself may be diagnostic, and by admitting it as soon as it is determined, the examiner expedites the patient to another member of the health care team who may be able to solve the problem.

Otherwise, when the examiner obtains all of the necessary data and finds that they correlate with his hypothesis as to the nature and source of the patient's problem, he is prepared to plan a course of management for the patient.

TREATMENT CONCEPTS

General Treatment Goals and Techniques

The overall aim of treatment is to restore normal, pain-free movement (4). The therapist designing a treatment program selects appropriate procedures and techniques, plans a method of application and schedule of frequency, educates the patient regarding his disorder and treatment goals, coordinates management with other health care professionals, and provides a home program or follow-up care if indicated. Treatment goals may vary from restoring motion, to relieving pain, to compensating instability, or a combination thereof. This section outlines general modalities and procedures that are effective in achieving

particular goals. A subsequent section details guidelines for manual therapy application.

Immobilization remains a traditional method for relieving pain. Local, i.e., limb or segment, and general, i.e., entire body, immobilization techniques include casting, splinting, or placing the patient on bed rest and/or traction. Acutely painful musculoskeletal conditions generally respond favorably to immobilization. However, one must carefully consider the adverse effects of prolonged immobilization when prescribing this treatment modality.

Compression, elevation, and cryotherapy are effective in controlling pain and swelling which accompany many traumatic, inflammatory, and postsurgical disorders. Compression and elevation reduce fluid engorgement of interstitial tissue. Cold application initially causes local vasoconstriction, followed by vasodilatation. Vasodilatation also follows heat application, increasing local circulation, reducing statis and edema, relaxing protective muscle spasm, and reducing pain.

Postural training and exercise alleviate pain by relieving abnormal mechanical stress on tissues. Since movement facilitates synovial fluid circulation, it facilitates articular cartilage nutrition and prevents some types of painful conditions that develop secondary to disuse. Exercise also combats the pain and stiffness which result from adhesions, contractures, and inflexibility. The latter part of this chapter reviews the effects of passive exercise in more detail.

Techniques that decrease or compensate for hypermobility include adhesive strapping, splinting, and bracing. An exercise program which emphasizes strengthening and co-contraction of muscle groups that serve as dynamic joint restraints when primary restraints are damaged may enhance stability and prevent reinjury.

Manual treatment offers a variety of means of increasing mobility. Massage provides relaxation, decongestion, facilitation, and tissue mobilization benefits when administered as various needs dictate. Biofeedback, including active relaxation, produces local and systemic effects which assist a patient in functional control of his body. Sustained passive stretch via positioning, traction, splinting, etc. is thought by some to influence collagen remodelling. Regardless of the specific mechanism involved, these procedures frequently allow tissues to assume desired mobility.

Numerous forms of exercise enhance mobility. Passive exercise maintains or increases the length of both inert and contractile structures (joint and muscle mobility) and may also enhance circulation. The therapist performs passive movement on the patient, using the limbs or trunk as levers to produce a moderate sustained force. Active-assistive exercise maintains or increases inert and contractile structure mobility, in addition to improving muscle function. Techniques use the extremities or body as levers while a patient assists in that part of the range where possible. Active exercise maintains or increases inert or contractile structure mobility, as well as enhances muscle function, coordination, relaxation, circulation, flexibility, posture, and kinesthetic sense. A patient performs active exercise independently, employing active contraction, relaxation, or self-stretching techniques. Resistive exercise improves function of contractile structures, such as strength, endurance, speed, and coordination by requiring the patient to work against a load (Fig. 2.14).

Proprioceptive neuromuscular facilitation, in theory, utilizes Sherrington's principles of successive induction and reciprocal inhibition to reinforce voluntary effort. A "slow reversal hold" technique use isotonic contractions of antagonist muscles, then isometric (hold) contractions of agonist muscles. This most often promotes mobility, strength, and proprioception. If done through decrements, this technique may be used to promote stability. A "rhythmic stabilization" technique employs isometric co-contraction principally for stability, though secondary relaxation may ultimately aid with mobility. (Fig. 2.15). "Muscle energy" techniques use a submaximal isometric contraction, immediately followed by a gentle passive stretch while the muscle is in a refractory state (reduced myotatic reflex opposition), with repetition of this sequence as necessary to increase soft tissue mobility. Aerobic exercise programs enhance local muscle endurance and cardiorespiratory capacity.

One must consider the possible effects of exercise on all tissues: muscle, ligament, articular cartilage, bone, tendon, bursa, etc. One tissue usually forms the "weakest link" that is most easily injured or exacerbated, and it is not always the tissue that was initially involved. For instance, a bone may be adequately healed postfracture to withstand moderately vigorous exercise which also benefits the surrounding muscles; however, prior immobilization of the fracture may have deconditioned the articular cartilage of an adjacent joint, so that it is traumatized by this level of exercise. A general rule of exercise is to avoid any "sharp" pain, but permit a "dull ache" under close supervision, which vanishes upon completion of the exercise, and does not increase in magnitude as a patient repeats the exercise. If effusion is present, a therapist should not allow exercise with enough intensity to increase it.

Manual Therapy

This section deals with the therapeutic use of specific passive accessory movements to relieve pain, decrease muscle guarding, lengthen tissue (especially joint capsule and ligament), and reduce intraarticular derangement.

In addition to mechanical effects, passive joint movement also produces neurophysiological effects. Manual therapy procedures which place tension upon a joint capsule and supporting ligaments activate joint mechanoreceptors. Either unidirectional or traction procedures produce a three-fold effect which incorporates reflexogenic, perceptual, and pain suppression elements. A reflexogenic effect occurs through fusimotor-muscle spindle loop systems, which may exert either facilitatory or inhibitory influences on muscle tone and the excitability of stretch reflexes (10). A perceptual effect occurs through afferent pathways

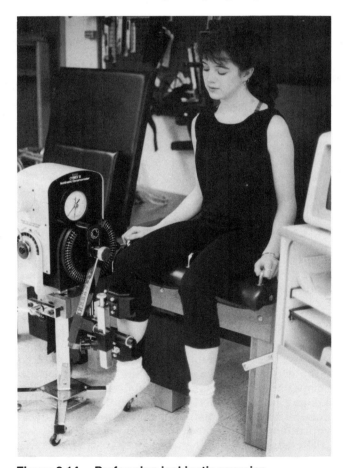

Figure 2.14.   Performing isokinetic exercise.

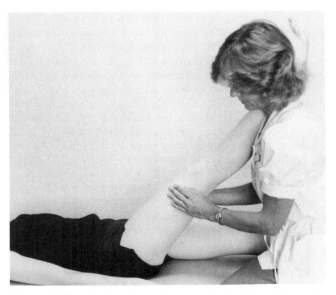

Figure 2.15.   Performing a "contract-relax" technique for increasing hamstring muscle length.

to the cerebral cortex, by which Type I receptors evoke postural and kinesthetic awareness, and Type IV receptors evoke joint pain perception (10). A pain suppression effect occurs through apical spinal interneurons, which produce presynaptic inhibition of nociceptive afferent activity (10). Therefore, applying various stimuli, e.g., massage, compression, and stretching, may influence pain perception.

Recent animal studies indicate that passive oscillatory movement (unlike transcutaneous electrical nerve stimulation) may not be able to selectively excite a significant number of large diameter joint afferent fibers to produce pain relief (11). To produce significant neural output, passive movement must place a joint at or slightly beyond its end ROM. Others have found that a significant proportion of smaller fiber, thinly myelinated and unmyelinated receptors may be excited by non-noxious stimulation (midrange joint mobilization), and that in the presence of joint inflammation, small fiber activity increases substantially (11). Therefore, midrange passive movement of inflamed joints would provoke nociceptor activity, rather than large fiber activity, and would increase, rather than decrease, pain. Thus, although there is agreement that manual therapy produces reflexogenic and kinesthetic influences on the musculoskeletal system, the mechanisms of pain relief remain speculative.

Previous sections of this chapter emphasize the importance of the iterative process of examination, interpretation, and treatment to successful manual therapy. In comparison, the *particular* treatment techniques the therapist chooses to bring about desired results are *relatively* less important. Regardless of the treatment techniques chosen, several important principles govern administration of manual therapy. The therapist should perform a given technique in a controlled, reproducible manner, and in a position and grade appropriate for treating stiffness, pain, spasm, or their combination. Another principle is that one continuously reassess the patient's response to treatment. Chapters 3–9 describe selected manual treatment techniques for the individual joints.

If the therapist determines that results of an initial examination indicate manual therapy, and no contraindications exist, he first administers a "trial treatment." He usually keeps this brief, following what may have been an extensive examination. For example, he may administer several repetitions of joint traction, oscillations short of or up to the point of pain, or graded physiologic movement, in the trial treatment. He warns the patient that this may temporarily exacerbate his symptoms, and instructs him to take careful note of his condition during the 24-hour period after this treatment. He reassesses the patient's irritability, mobility, and functional status the next day, prior to and following any subsequent treatments. Modifying treatment according to clinical response, the therapist builds upon the techniques that prove successful, and discontinues those that produce no, or adverse, affects. The therapist should add new techniques one at a time to avoid confusion as to the

effects of each. A typical treatment of one joint may include 3–4 joint mobilization sessions lasting up to 30 seconds each, 1–3 oscillations per second (3).

The direction of a technique may be that producing the sign most comparable to the patient's primary complaint, e.g., pain or stiffness. For acute, irritable joints, it is usually the direction that relieves pain or spasm. In chronic cases, it is the direction that increases mobility. Often the direction of accessory movement most effective in increasing physiologic movement correlates with kinematic principles covered in Chapter 1. When a concave articular surface moves upon a convex, mobilize in the *same* direction as the osteokinematic (distal limb segment) movement desired. When a convex articular surface moves upon a concave, mobilize in the *opposite* direction as the osteokinematic movement desired (2). If the desired direction of motion increases pain, however, the therapist may apply a technique in the opposite direction until the patient is able to tolerate the desired direction.

The distance a joint is passively moved into its total range is the amplitude, or grade, of mobilization (Table 2.2). Joint irritability (intensity, severity, and duration of symptoms from a particular stimulus), and the relative proportions of pain, spasm, and resistance to movement, dictate the grade of mobilization. The therapist administers Grade I (small amplitude oscillations at the beginning of range) when:

1. Pain exists at rest or is provoked early in the range;
2. Movement elicits spasm early in the range, with pain less dominant;
3. Both pain and spasm limit movement early in the range (3).

One should note that if spasm occurs in response to a technique, performing it more slowly or not so deep may produce better results. Grade II (large amplitude oscillations within the range, but short of resistance) is effective when:

1. Spasm limits movement sooner with a quick oscillation than with a slow one;
2. Slowly rising pain limits movement halfway into the range (3).

Grade III (large amplitude oscillations from mid-to end of restricted range) is indicated when pain and resistance (from spasm, inert tissue tension, or tissue compression) together limit movement near the end of range (3). Grade IV (small amplitude oscillations at the end of the restricted range) is used when resistance limits movement, in the absence of pain and spasm (3). Grade V (sharp thrust at the pathological limitation) is used when minimal resistance limits the end of range. Only properly trained and experienced clinicians should apply Grade V mobilization, due to the skill and judgment necessary to its safe and effective practice. Most therapists can achieve the same effects by prudent application of the other grades.

The same positioning and mechanical principles that govern execution of examination techniques apply to mobilization techniques. Both the patient and the therapist are relaxed and positioned optimally with regard to body mechanics. The therapist specifically mobilizes only one joint at a time. Generally, he stabilizes one articular surface while moving the other with a secure, comfortable grasp as near the joint as possible.

As important as knowing the indications for manual therapy is knowing the contraindications. Some aspects of an examination, or the patient's response to particular procedures, should serve as warning signs that alert the examiner to possible pathology for which manual therapy is contraindicated. These are often relative, so one must consider them in the overall context of the general problem and its many manifestations.

Continuous pain which is unrelated to posture or activity, and not relieved by rest is uncharacteristic of musculoskeletal disorders. A vague, often deep reference of pain may indicate a lesion of visceral or vascular origin. Pain that responds to treatment one day, but returns the next could represent a condition that requires further evaluation or modification of treatment. Pain unaffected by treatment, or gradual, relentless worsening of a condition is definitely not responding appropriately and demands close scrutiny or consultation.

Onset of new symptoms indicates a need for further examination; one should particularly ascertain whether the symptoms are related to the treatment he administered. Having noted at the initial examination both the patient's symptomatic and asymptomatic areas on a body chart proves extremely helpful at this point when it is necessary to evaluate "new" symptoms. The examiner can compare the areas of current symptoms with the initial findings, to note if they are truly new and different.

If the patient presents with a history of any type of malignancy, one should be aware of the possibility of skeletal metastases, and rule out their existence before proceeding with treatment. Pain so intense that it requires morphia may stem from a lesion that is beyond assistance from manual therapy. Systemic signs, e.g., fever, weight loss, malaise, and general weakness, suggest a major disease or inflammatory process which should be diagnosed specifically prior to any form of treatment. Widespread loss of strength represents neurologic involvement, the precise nature of which should be diagnosed before one administers a treatment. Vertebral artery signs include dizziness and visual changes with sustained cervical positions or rapid cervical movements and preclude cervical examination and treatment, as Chapter 3 describes. Rheumatoid arthritis may induce laxity of the alanto-axial cruciate ligament, and is therefore a definite contraindication for manual procedures in the cervical area; ligamentous laxity also presents a relative contraindication for manual therapy in other areas.

In summary, this chapter presents the objectives of manual examination and treatment of musculoskeletal structures. It describes the process of biomechanical and physiological analysis to identify the cause of pain and pathologic joint movement. Finally, it offers information for interpreting examination data, and for providing the appropriate therapeutic measures.

References

1. Salter RB: *Textbook of Disorders and Injuries of the Musculoskeletal System,* ed 2. Baltimore, Williams & Wilkins, 1983.
2. Kaltenborn F: *Mobilization of the Extremity Joints.* Oslo, Norway, Olaf Norlis Bokhandel, 1980.
3. Maitland GD: *Vertebral Manipulation,* ed 5. Kent, England, Butterworth, 1987.
4. Cyriax J: *Textbook of Orthopaedic Medicine,* ed 6. Baltimore, Williams & Wilkins, 1975, vol 1.
5. Mennell J: *Joint Pain.* Boston, Little, Brown & Co, 1964.
6. Cookson JC, Kent BE: Orthopedic manual therapy—an overview. Part I: The extremities. *Phys. Ther.* 59:136–146, 1979.
7. Minor MAD, Minor SD: *Patient Evaluation Methods for the Health Professional.* Reston, VA, Reston Publishing Co, 1985.
8. Daniels L, Worthingham C: *Muscle Testing: Techniques of Manual Examination.* Philadelphia, WB Saunders, 1980.
9. Bogduk N: The innervation of the lumbar spine. *Spine* 8:286–293, 1983.
10. Wyke BD: Articular neurology and manipulative therapy. In Idczak RM (ed): *Aspects of Manipulative Therapy.* Melborne, Lincoln Institute of Health Sciences, 1979, pp 67–72.
11. Zusman M: Reappraisal of a proposed neurophysiological mechanism for the relief of joint pain with passive joint movements. *Physiotherapy Practice* 1:61–70, 1985.

CHAPTER 3

THE SPINE

Carolyn T. Wadsworth, L.P.T., M.S.
Richard P. DiFabio, L.P.T., Ph.D.
David Johnson, L.P.T.

CLINICAL ANATOMY AND MECHANICS OF THE SPINE

EMBRYOLOGY

The human spine comprises neurologic elements encased by a stiff but flexible rod. Following is a brief description of the embryologic development of both the spinal cord and the supporting vertebral column. This section also explains the segmental derivation of the remaining components of the trunk and limbs.

The embryo emerges from germ layers by the 20th day of gestation as a flat oval disc (1). Following the gastrulation stage of development, the disc differentiates into three cell layers: the endoderm, the mesoderm, and the ectoderm. The endoderm produces most of the epithelial lining of the respiratory and alimentary tracts. The mesoderm produces muscle and connective tissue. The ectoderm eventually produces neural tissue, and the epidermis with associated appendages, but first forms an intermediate structure, the neural plate. This plate invaginates along its central axis, and the folds fuse to form the neural tube which becomes the spinal canal. Neural crest tissue from the ectoderm condenses and begins formation of the spinal cord; moreover, it also creates the dorsal

root ganglia at each segmental level, the autonomic nervous system, and the cells responsible for myelination of the peripheral nerves (Fig. 3.1).

During the 3rd week of development, a thick band of tissue, the primitive streak, appears dorsally along the midline of the disc. Cells from the primitive streak condense into a cylinder which extends cephalad and becomes the notochord (Fig. 3.1). The notochord provides the framework around which the mesoderm-derived vertebral column forms (1,2).

By the end of the 3rd week, the columns of mesoderm along both sides of the notochord undergo segmentation. This process produces a column of somites which grows in cranial and caudal directions until 42–45 pairs of somites are present. The somites correspond to regions as follows: 4–5 are associated with the skull; 8 with the cervical area; 12 with the thoracic area; 5 with the lumbar area; 5 with the sacral area; and 8 with the coccygeal area (3). Each somite has three divisions: a sclerotome, a myotome, and a dermatome. The sclerotome produces bone, cartilage, and ligaments. The myotome produces skeletal muscle tissue, and the dermatome produces dermis and loose connective tissue. Each segment of the neural tube produces a nerve for its corresponding somite. Since nerves or nerve branches from a given segment (spinal

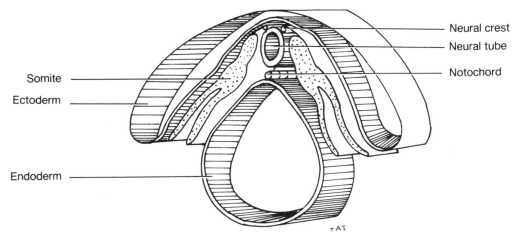

Figure 3.1. Gastrulation and formation of neural tube.

level) supply the bone, ligaments, muscle, blood vessels, and dermal tissue derived from the corresponding somite, sensory input from these tissues is thought to converge on the same spinal neuron, or on spinal neurons which themselves converge on the same pathway to the cerebral cortex. Thus, sensory input arising from these tissues innervated by the same spinal level ultimately may reach the same area of the sensory cortex and be perceived as pain of similar quality and area regardless of the tissue of origin. For example, a noxious stimulus arising from a deep structure (e.g., bone or ligament) which infrequently originates such stimuli may be perceived by the sensory cortex as arising from the skin areas also innervated by that spinal segment (structures which more frequently originate noxious stimuli). Such an error in perception is a proposed mechanism for symptoms being "referred" from one tissue to another, or from one structure to another.

The vertebral column develops in stages to gradually replace the notochord. Each sclerotomic segment divides into cephalic and caudal parts (Fig. 3.2). The cephalic part of one segment fuses with the caudal part of the adjacent segment, and together they form the centrum of a vertebra (4). Additional condensation of the dorsal aspects of sclerotomes forms the neural arches and processes. Chondrification occurring in the 6th week produces a cartilaginous vertebral column. Ossification occurs in primary centers (located in the vertebral bodies) during the second embryonic month, while secondary centers (located in several parts of

the vertebral arch and processes) of ossification are not active until the 15th year. Fusion is not complete until the mid-30s.

It is possible to distinguish the notochord traversing the cartilaginous vertebral column for several months. Eventually the notochord disappears except for vestigial tissue which remains between the vertebral segments. The notochord remnants between the vertebrae expand to form the gelatinous nucleus pulposus of the intervertebral disc. Formation of the disc's anulus fibrosus begins at 10 weeks, when fibroelastic cells of the vertebral bodies differentiate to form fibrocartilage. This tissue remains attached to the vertebral bodies above and below, and makes up the outer layers of the anulus. Thus the intervertebral disc has a dual origin: the notochord and the vertebral bodies (4).

After the 6th month of gestation, the cells derived from the notochord degenerate, and cells from the anulus fibrosus begin replacing them. By the 2nd decade, all notochord cells are gone and only noncellular matrix represents the notochord in the adult (3).

Osteology

Multiple superimposed segments form the vertebral column which constitutes the central axis of the body. It provides static support for the body but also allows movement, protects the spinal cord and nerve roots, and transmits forces.

The ventral (anterior) portion of the column consists of vertebral bodies joined by fibrocartilaginous

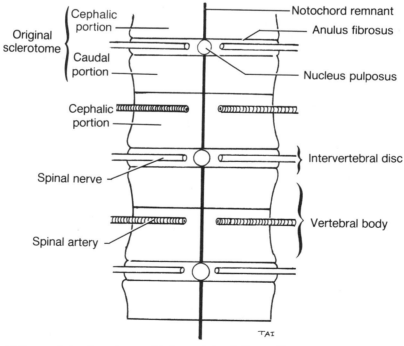

Figure 3.2. Formation of the vertebral centra and intervertebral discs. The cephalic and caudal portions of adjacent sclerotomes fuse to form the vertebral bodies. Notochord remnants form the nucleus pulposus, and cells differentiated from the vertebral bodies form the anulus fibrosus. In early development, the relations of the centra and discs after rearrangement of sclerotomic tissue.

intervertebral discs. The bodies are roughly oval in horizontal cross-section, but in the lumbar region become somewhat concave posteriorly (Fig. 3.3). Their size increases the more caudal their location, reflecting the amount of superincumbent weight borne by the respective segment. They possess a dense cortex surrounding a central spongy area in which trabeculae are aligned parallel to superimposed forces. Trabeculae are thinnest in a triangular area located anteriorly, producing a relatively weakened area which is the site where a "wedge" type of vertebral fracture (6) may occur. Small arterial and venous foramina pierce the vertebral bodies; the larger nutrient foramina occur posteriorly to accommodate the basivertebral veins.

Cartilaginous endplates cover the superior and inferior surfaces of the bodies at birth, but subsequently ossify and fuse with their respective vertebrae by the 2nd decade. These endplates also comprise the cranial and caudal borders of the disc, and provide attachment for the anulus fibrosus. The central portion of the endplate is semipermeable, allowing selective passage of fluids in and out of the disc.

The dorsal (posterior) portion of the column consists of vertebral arches that encase the spinal cord, meninges, and vessels (Fig. 3.3). Two short thick projections, pedicles, attach the arches to the vertebral bodies. Concavities on the superior and inferior borders of the pedicles constitute the vertebral notches; the space between the notches of two adjacent pedicles is the intervertebral foramen.

The right and left laminae are continuous with their respective pedicles, and course posteromedially to join one another at the midline (Fig. 3.3). Failure of such

bony union is spina bifida (of various types); should the failure of closure also include neural tissues, the condition becomes meningomyelocele.

The pedicle-lamina junction, the "pars interarticularis," may lack bony union due to failure of ossification or fracture. This condition is unilateral or bilateral spondylolysis, depending on whether the defect is present on one or both sides. Should the pars interarticularis have a spondylolytic bony defect, or consist of thin bony or relatively weaker cartilaginous or fibrous tissue, it may separate or elongate under the stress of superincumbent weight. It thereby allows the body of the involved vertebral segment to slip anteriorly upon the body of the vertebra below. Such anterior displacement of the superior vertebra (carrying the remainder of the vertebral column with it) is lytic spondylolisthesis. One should note that in this situation the spinous process and laminae of the involved vertebra remain in their normal alignment. For example, an L5 lytic spondylolisthesis (anterior displacement of the body of L5 on S1) may be detected upon palpation by noting the spinous process of L4 positioned more anteriorly than that of L5, which is aligned with that of S1.

Superior and inferior articular processes, arising from the right and left pedicle-lamina junctions, form the facet (zygapophyseal) joints of adjacent vertebrae. The superior facet articular surfaces generally face posteriorly and superiorly and slightly laterally in the cervical region; posteriorly and slightly laterally in the thoracic region; and curve from a posterior to a medial orientation in the lumbar region. The inferior facet articular surfaces of the cervical region generally face anteriorly and inferiorly and slightly medially; those

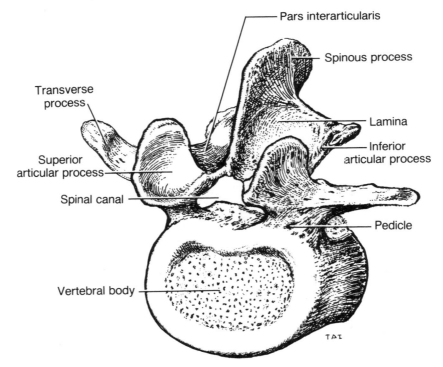

Figure 3.3. Lumbar vertebra.

of the thoracic region face anteriorly and slightly medially, and those of the lumber region curve from an anterior to a lateral orientation.

Transverse processes (projecting laterally from the pedicle-lamina junctions), spinous processes (projecting posteriorly along the midline), and much of the bony surface connecting them, provide attachment for spinal muscles. The leverage afforded by the projecting processes assists the muscles in producing or preventing movement of the vertebral column.

The cervical vertebrae differ from other vertebrae in several general aspects. They are smaller and have short, bifid spinous processes. Their transverse processes are also short; contain transverse foramina which transmit the vertebral arteries, veins, and paravertebral plexi; and terminate in tiny tubercles which provide muscle attachment sites. The cervical facet joints lie in a transverse-frontal plane, with upper segments adopting a more transverse orientation, and lower segments a more frontal one. Unciform processes arise in a superolateral direction from the lateral margins of the upper surfaces of vertebral bodies 3–7. These structures are unique to the cervical region, and articulate with beveled facets of the adjacent vertebral body's lateral margins.

The first cervical vertebra, the atlas, is unique because it has neither a body nor a spinous process. The tissue that might have developed into its body instead forms the dens of the axis (Fig. 3.4). The atlas resembles a ring, and is composed of slender anterior and posterior arches that connect its bulky lateral masses. The anterior arch possesses a facet for articulation with the dens. The lateral masses are thicker laterally than medially, and possess biconcave facets for articulation with the occipital condyles, and flat or slightly convex facets for articulation with C2. The long transverse processes project laterally and are easily palpated in the area between the mandible and mastoid processes. The C1 vertebra is wider than all cervical vertebral

except C7. The odontoid process of the second cervical vertebra differentiates it from the others (Fig. 3.4). This process projects superiorly from the body of the axis and articulates with the atlas, forming a pivot for rotation of the atlas (and thus the head).

Distinguishing features of the lumbar vertebrae include large, kidney-shaped bodies (concave posteriorly) and rectangular spinous processes. As mentioned above, the lumbar facets are curved so that their medial portion lies in a frontal plane, and their lateral portion lies in a sagittal plane, except for the lumbosacral facets which, although variable, may approximate a frontal plane.

The sacrum and coccyx form the most caudal portion of the spinal column. The sacrum forms a wedge between two innominate bones. Irregular convex surfaces of the sacrum articulate with concavities in the ilia. The rest position of the sacrum is slightly rotated forward, placing a stretch on the sacrotuberous ligaments and results in a stabilized pelvic girdle. The keystone effect probably occurs from ligamentous stabilization rather than from the wedge shape of the sacrum (7).

Arthrology

Cervical Spine. Articulations between vertebral bodies in the cervical spine have two forms at each level from C2–C7. The first is a central interbody articulation with an approximate center of rotation at a point within the nucleus pulposus. This central articulation is a symphysis type of joint. The second form, the lateral interbody articulations, occur at the right and left perimeters of the cervical vertebral bodies. Their articular surfaces are the small unciform processes that project from the periphery of the vertebral plateaus (6). These joints, classified as pseudarthroses, are the joints of von Luschka or uncovertebral joints (6). Because their corresponding surfaces approximate each other, the joints of von Luschka

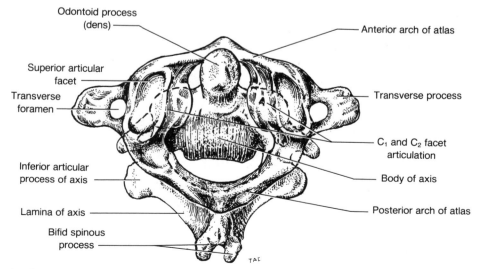

Figure 3.4. Atlas and axis.

guide flexion and extension and provide a stabilizing force during lateral bending. They may degenerate, forming bony spurs, which may impinge on spinal nerves exiting the canal.

Articulations at the facet (zygapophyseal) joints of C2–C7 are synovial joints, and resemble other plane diarthrodial joints in composition. Hyaline cartilage lines their surfaces, and a synovial-lined capsule attaches peripherally to the margins of the articular processes. Tongue-like extensions of the synovial capsular lining, meniscoid inclusions (composed of synovial and cartilage tissue), sometimes project into the cleft between articular surfaces. These structures may become entrapped further into the cleft or extrapped out of their normal position in the cleft, causing pain and reflex muscle spasm due to their basal attachment to the richly innervated synovial capsular lining (8,9). The capsules and ligaments of the facet joints contain pain receptors as well as proprioceptors which monitor vertebral position and capsular stress, and which participate in a feedback loop with muscles spanning the respective joints. Facet joints bear load under conditions of spinal flexion and extension and in the neutral position, and by doing so, serve to guide and limit spinal movements.

The arthrology of the atlanto-axial and atlanto-occipital joints differs from that of other vertebral joints. The occiput articulates with the atlas at paired ellipsoid joints formed by the convex occipital condyles and the concave superior facets of the lateral masses of the atlas (Fig. 3.4). The joints, enveloped by fibrous capsules, allow maximum flexion and extension, and slight side bending and rotation. The atlanto-axial joint comprises three synovial joints: two lateral plane joints between the convex inferior surfaces of the lateral masses of the atlas and the convex superior articular facets of the axis; and a trochoid joint between the odontoid and the osteoligamentous ring formed by the transverse ligament and the anterior arch of the atlas. The primary movement at this joint is rotation. Posterior dislocation of the odontoid secondary to transverse ligament laxity is a rare but potentially dangerous complication of rheumatoid arthritis; passive

movement is, therefore, contraindicated in this condition.

The transverse ligament, a major ligament of the upper cervical region, is a strong band maintaining the odontoid in close contact with the atlas; along with the longitudinal bands (transverso-occipital and transverso-axial), it collectively forms the cruciate ligament (10) (Fig. 3.5). The apical ligament runs from the apex of the odontoid to the lateral margins of the foramen magnum. The anterior and posterior atlanto-occipital ligaments pass between and connect the foramen magnum with the superior border of the atlas (Fig. 3.5).

Other ligaments of the spinal column either originate in the cervical area or are common to cervical, thoracic, and lumbar spines (Fig. 3.6). The anterior longitudinal ligament stretches from the occiput to the sacrum along the anterior part of the spinal column, and attaches to the discs and margins of the vertebral bodies. It limits backward bending. The posterior longitudinal ligament runs the length of the spinal column, posterior to the vertebral bodies and within the vertebral canal. The posterior longitudinal ligament attaches only to the discs and lips of the bodies, and is narrower over the bodies and wider over the discs. It becomes thinner in the lumbar area, but does limit forward bending. The ligamentum flavum is yellow, elastic tissue spanning adjacent lamina. It covers the lamina from the articular capsules laterally to the spinous processes medially. The supraspinous ligament connects the apices of spines C7–L5 or S1. It limits forward bending and rotation. The interspinous and intertransverse ligaments are fibrous bands between the spinous and transverse processes respectively. They limit lateral bending, forward bending, and rotation. The ligamentum nuchae runs from the occiput to C7, where it is continuous with the supraspinous and interspinous ligaments of lower levels. It limits forward bending and rotation of the neck.

Thoracolumbar Spine. The thoracolumbar spine does not have lateral interbody articulations. Instead, a change in the orientation of the facet joints stabilizes lateral spinal movements. The role of the spinal facets

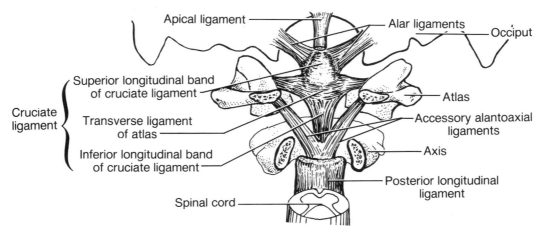

Figure 3.5.   Cervical ligaments.

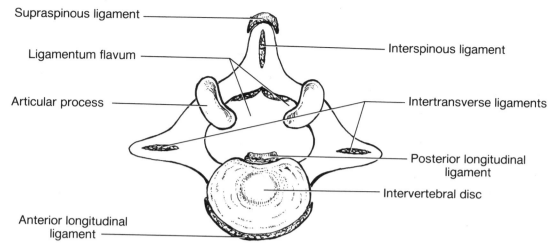

Supraspinous ligament

Ligamentum flavum

Articular process

Anterior longitudinal ligament

Interspinous ligament

Intertransverse ligaments

Posterior longitudinal ligament

Intervertebral disc

Figure 3.6.   Spinal column ligaments.

will be discussed in more detail under "Mechanics." The structure and function of the central interbody articulations and facet joints are similar to the cervical region: the central articulations are the focal point of segmental motion, and the synovial facet joints limit and guide the path of motion. Ligaments of the thoracolumbar region are summarized above.

At the lumbosacral joint, the facets lie closer to the frontal plane. This joint also marks the junction between a mobile chain of vertebrae and the relatively immobile sacrum, becoming the site of abrupt cessation of movement. It is a "weak link" in the system and therefore a common area of disc degeneration. Also, the inferior inclination of the surface of S1 promotes anterior slippage of L5, i.e., spondylolisthesis (11).

Sacral Spine.   The pelvic girdle comprises two sacral-innominate joints, which are classified as combination synovial and fibrous (syndesmosis) articulations, and a public symphysis. Five vertebral bodies fuse together to form the wedge-shaped sacrum, eliminating any

functional central articulations. The only mobile facet articulation is between L5 and S1.

There are several primary pelvic ligaments (Fig. 3.7). The interosseous ligament lies posterior and superior to the synovial portion of the SI joint at the levels of S1 through S3. This ligament, together with other dorsal ligaments, is responsible for the stability of the pelvic girdle. The dorsal ligament begins at the lowest point on the posterior sacrum and attaches diagonally to the posterior iliac spines. Extensions of this ligament also merge with the interosseous ligament. The ventral ligament is comprised of horizontal bands which pass from the superior portion of the iliac fossa and attach to the superior portion of the sacrum. Their function is to stabilize anterior rotation of the ilium on the sacrum. The sacrotuberous ligament attaches diagonally from the lower sacrum to the ischial tuberosity and functions to limit posterior rotation of the ilium. The sacrospinous ligament runs between the ischial spine and the medial lower third

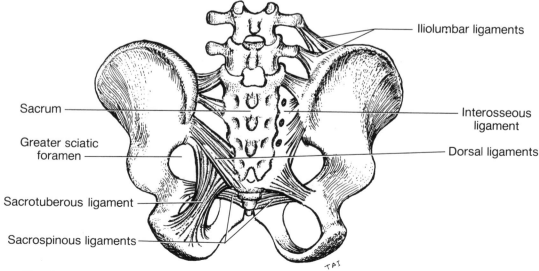

Iliolumbar ligaments

Sacrum

Greater sciatic foramen

Sacrotuberous ligament

Sacrospinous ligaments

Interosseous ligament

Dorsal ligaments

Figure 3.7.   Sacroiliac ligaments.

of the sacrum, and also checks posterior rotation of the ilium. In the standing position, anterior rotary forces on the sacrum stress the sacrotuberous and sacrospinous ligaments. This action pulls the innominate bones closer together on the sacrum and enhances pelvic stability. The pubic symphysis is simultaneously stabilized by the superior pubic and arcuate ligaments.

Mechanics

A thorough review of the paravertebral, suboccipital, abdominal, and thoracic muscles is recommended for a complete understanding of movement of the head and trunk. However, due to extensive coverage elsewhere, (2, 6, 11, 19) muscle origin, insertion, and function will not be elaborated here.

A vertebral segment, for mechanical purposes, is defined as two vertebrae and an intervening disc. Any segment within the spine has the potential of 6° of freedom. In various locations of the spine, mobility is limited by fusion of segments (e.g., the sacrum) or by articulating bony structures (e.g., the rib-thoracic spine junction). In the cervical and lumbar spines, freedom of movement is obtained at the expense of stability. These areas are also at the highest risk for acute spinal pathology. (13)

Movement of the trunk depends on the structure and spatial orientation of the intervertebral disc and the lateral articulations. Normally, the nucleus effectively provides a pivot point for spinal movement. Weightbearing in the upright position is transmitted through the nucleus to the semipermeable cartilaginous membrane and vertebral body. In this manner, the disc acts as a spacer between the shock-absorbing vertebral bodies. Failure of this shock absorbing mechanism may result in Schmorl's nodes, i.e., nuclear protrusion into the intervertebral body through end-plate fractures.

The orientation of the facet joints changes with segmental level, and is largely responsible for differences in spinal range of motion (Fig. 3.8). For example, the cervical spine has a relatively large capacity for axial rotation. In contrast, the lumbar facets block rotation due to their vertical and sagittal position.

Facet orientation also guides the direction of spinal accessory movement much the same way that the shape of knee joint members facilitates accessory glide and spin of the knee. Therefore, spinal motions are not "pure," but consist of several motions coupled together. In the cervical spine, the physiologic movement of side bending is coupled with the accessory movement of rotation in the same direction (Fig. 3.9). Physiologic side bending and accessory rotation are coupled in the opposite direction in the lumbar spine (except during flexion, when they occur in the same direction). Forward bending and simultaneous side bending place a high level of torsion on the disc, and contribute heavily to disc pathology (14).

The direction of physiologic movement will also determine the direction of fluid movement within the disc. Some clinicians use backward bending to influence an anterior shift of the nucleus pulposus and to contain nuclear protrusions (15). Backward bending may also protect the posterior portion of the disc,

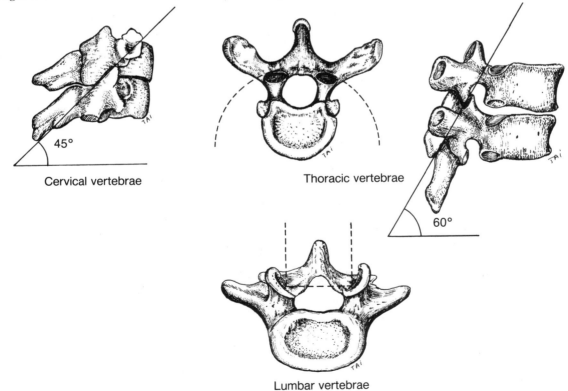

Cervical vertebrae 45°

Thoracic vertebrae

Lumbar vertebrae

60°

Figure 3.8.   Facet joint orientation.

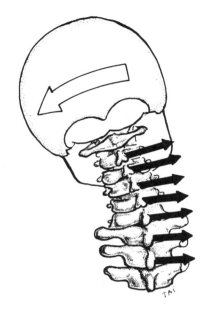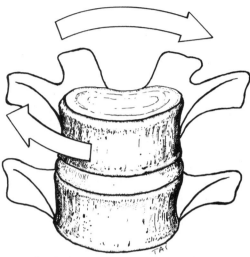

Figure 3.9. Coupled spinal motion. *A,* In the cervical region, vertebral side bending and rotation occur in the same direction. *B,* In the lumbar region, vertebral side bending and rotation occur in opposite directions. (From White AA and Panjabi MM: *Clinical Biomechanics of the Spine.* Philadelphia, JB Lippincott, 1978.)

which is at a greater risk for trauma because the posterior anular fibers are less dense than the anterior anular rings.

Imbibition is a process of fluid accumulation within the disc. The nucleus pulposus contains a mucoprotein gel derived embryologically from the notochord. During childhood it contains about 85% water, but with aging, fibrocartilage gradually replaces the water. Therefore, after the age of 50, a soft pulpy nuclear herniation is rare (9). The gel can imbibe almost nine times its volume of water, so the disc is able to maintain balance between intrinsic fluid pressure and external mechanical pressure (5). In fact, the disc's ability to maintain a self-contained fluid system directly relates to its integrity because: a. it allows the disc to maintain a constant pressure to separate the endplates and transmit force to the anulus, and b. it produces a preloaded state which resists the forces of bending and compression, and permits rocking motion.

Vertical weightbearing activities, such as standing, compress the segment and result in a diffusion process which causes fluid to move across the semipermeable cartilaginous membrane into the spongy bone of the vertebral body. The process of imbibition influences the height of the spinal segment and hence, the articular relationships of approximating facet joints. When the capacity to imbibe fluid is reduced, weightbearing is shifted from the nucleus to the anular rings (16). The negative effects of this shift are seen commonly in older patients who often present with signs and symptoms resulting from a displaced anular fracture (17). In the case of "soft" extrusions of the nucleus pulposus, discal material may expand when outside

the confines of the disc, imbibe fluid, and compress neural structures within the spinal canal.

Disc disease can also interfere with proper mechanical function of the facet joints. When disc degeneration or acute nuclear prolapse compromises the intervertebral space, it also alters the orientation of the facet joints (6, 18). Abnormal compressive forces obtained when the joint members approximate each other, and the eventual loss of joint mobility, can lead to osteophytic spurring (18). In addition to limiting motion, bony spurs can protrude into the intervertebral foramen and cause neurologic deficits.

In relaxed standing position, the spinal curves are essentially maintained by bony and ligamentous support; little or no EMG activity is recorded in paravertebral musculature. However, with forward displacement or addition of heavy loads, these muscles quickly become active. In fact, the forces of the paravertebral muscles alone required to counteract a load of 10 kg lifted with the trunk flexed and arms stretched forward would crush the lumbar discs (6). To avoid this situation, the trunk is utilized as a whole to help stabilize the spine and reduce axial compression. Through the Valsalva maneuver, a closed cavity is converted to a rigid beam, which provides spinal support.

A common finding among patients with primary or secondary paravertebral muscle spasm is a flattened lumbar lordosis (19). The explanation lies in the fact that the lumbar muscle mass serves as a wedge, reducing the normal lordotic curvature (9). This is opposite the normal action of these muscles, whose contraction usually accentuates the lumbar curve.

Neurology

The nervous system contains two divisions: the central, which includes the brain and spinal cord, and the peripheral, which includes the cranial and spinal nerves and autonomic system for descriptive purposes, although it functions as a coordinated network. The central nervous system occupies the cranium and vertebral canal to about L2, after which it tapers into the filum terminale, which attaches to the coccyx. Dorsal and ventral nerve roots emanate from each segment of the cord and join laterally to form the spinal nerves that exit through the intervertebral foramina (Fig. 3.10). At each segmental level junction of a somatic root from the ventral ramus and an autonomic root from the grey ramus communicans form a recurrent meningeal (sinuvertebral) nerve. Each spinal nerve returns its meningeal branch through the intervertebral foramen to supply the ventral aspect of the dural sac, the posterior longitudinal ligament, and the posterior aspect of the anulus fibrosus (8, 9, 12).

The spinal nerves then divide into posterior (dorsal) and anterior (ventral) primary rami. The posterior ramus divides into medial and lateral branches, which supply the skin and axial muscles of the back. The medial branch also sends twigs to the facet joint capsule and supraspinous and interspinous ligaments, and possibly to the ligamentum flavum (Fig. 3.10). The anterior ramus supplies the lateral and anterior trunk and the limbs. Lateral and anterior aspects of the anulus fibrosus and the anterior longitudinal ligament are innervated by nerves derived from the ventral rami and the sympathetic nervous system (8).

Bony and Neurologic Relationships.

The cervical spine protects the lower medulla oblongata and cervical cord. The suboccipital region is a highly mobile and mechanically complex area of the spine, making ligamentous and bony stability critical. An odontoid fracture allows anterior or posterior shear of the atlas on the axis with the potential of medullary compression and death. Likewise, laxity or rupture of the transverse ligament allows anterior displacement of the atlas, but is less common than an odontoid fracture (6). In the lower cervical column, the C5-6 segment is the most mobile, and the most common site of traumatic cord damage.

Osteoarthritis frequently produces neurologic dysfunction in the cervical spine. Osteophytes develop at the uncovertebral and facet joints, where they may compress the nerve roots. Disc lesions are much less common than in the lumbar spine, and are often prevented from impinging upon the nerve roots by the unciform processes (6).

In the cervical spine, the nerve roots emerge horizontally across the discs through the intervertebral foramen above their respective vertebrae, except for C8, which exits below C7. In the thoracic and lumbar regions, the nerve roots slope downward, then exit below their respective vertebrae but above the intervertebral discs. This relationship is significant in determining the level of a disc protrusion that affects a particular nerve root. In all levels of the spine, a protruded disc generally impinges the nerve root one level below it. This results because in the cervical spine, for example, the C6 nerve root directly crosses the C5-6 disc; in the lumbar spine, for example, the L4 nerve root exits just above the L4-5 disc, so a protrusion would affect the L5 nerve root. Posterolateral disc protrusions occur commonly in the lumbar spine and frequently impinge the nerve root as it exits through the intervertebral foramina.

Angiology

The vertebral arteries ascend through the transverse foramen, looping around C1 to course through

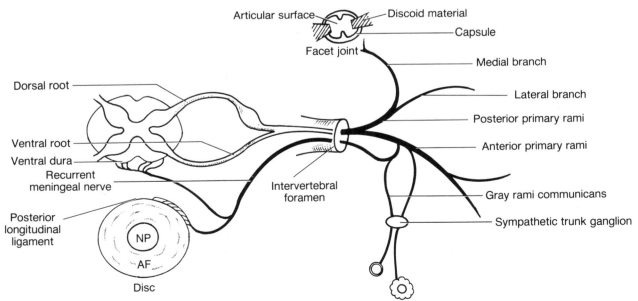

Figure 3.10. Nerve supply of the spine.

the foramen magnum. Position or movement of the cervical spine can affect the patency of these arteries, as can a palpatory examination, which also has the potential of dislodging atherosclerotic plaques.

The anterior spinal artery is formed between the medullary pyramids by union of terminal branches of the vertebral arteries, and descends along the anterior sulcus of the spinal cord. It supplies the cord and may produce sudden paralysis if occluded. The two posterior spinal arteries arise from the posterior inferior cerebellar arteries and descend along the cord medial to the posterior nerve roots. These three spinal arteries are reinforced by spinal branches of the vertebral, deep cervical, intercostal, lumbar, and lateral sacral arteries. These branches form long anastamosing channels and supply the vertebrae, meninges, discs, and spinal cord.

The venous drainage of the spinal column follows the arterial pattern, with longitudinal channels connected by plexuses which anastomose freely and end in the intervertebral veins. These intervertebral veins exit with the spinal nerves and empty into the vertebral, posterior intercostal, lumbar, and lateral sacral veins. The spinal veins have a rich supply of pain receptors, but lack valves; hence congestion of this plexus is a potential cause of back pain (9).

CERVICAL SPINE EXAMINATION

History

At the outset of the examination, the examiner should clarify the identifying data, including the patient's age, gender, and the provisional diagnosis (Fig. 3.11). A patient's age may be a rough indicator of his general activity level, but activity level must be confirmed by questioning later in the exam. Advancing age carries an increased likelihood of osteopenia, osteoporosis, degenerative changes, and the prior occurrence of injury. It also involves a decreased rate of tissue repair and potential for tissue remodelling. Some pathologies correlate with certain age groups, such as lower cervical disc disorders being more frequent among the 25–50-year age group.

Gender may also correlate with certain disorders. Since females generally are more flexible than males, they may demonstrate a higher occurrence of segmental hypermobility and thus may be predisposed to minor intervertebral derangements (considered here as nonspecific regarding involved tissue). Certain pathologies are known to occur more frequently in one gender than another, such as rheumatoid arthritis (RA) being more common among females.

A provisional diagnosis is of obvious importance to the evaluation and treatment of any patient. When the diagnosis is clear-cut, such as a cervical fracture or a documented disc herniation, a protocol developed by a referring physician and a therapist may govern physical therapy management. In addition, a given diagnosis may carry with it rigid precautions to patient management which are expressed by referring prac-

titioners, or that may be assumed by virtue of the diagnosis itself. For example, RA may make the transverse ligament of the atlas insufficient to maintain the dens in alignment. Therefore, even if RA is a secondary diagnosis for a given cervical patient, the practitioner must respect it while managing the primary component of that patient's problem.

For a number of cervical patients, a specific diagnosis is not available. No measurable structural abnormality, disease, or other pathology may be present. The history may be inclusive, yet a patient may have very definite subjective symptoms and objective signs of dysfunction. Such problems, which are relatively difficult to diagnose, may be termed "cervical pain," "cervical syndrome," "cervical spasm," "cervical sprain or strain" (in the absence of trauma), "cervical myofascial syndrome," etc.

The examiner should request a description of the patient's "chief complaint" in terms of specific everyday movements which are restricted or symptomatic. If such a description is possible, it provides a means of determining the ease with which the disorder is exacerbated and also provides a means to assess the effects of subsequent treatment.

The patient's dominant side may be found to bear a relationship (direct or inverse) to the side most affected by his cervical disorder, due to habitual movements affecting the body asymmetrically. Along this line, arrangement of a person's work environment may predispose a person to a cervical disorder, or may perpetuate one already present. For example, a person who habitually holds a telephone handset between his left shoulder and ear while jotting notes, or another who frequently backs up a vehicle while looking over his right shoulder, may create or aggravate a cervical disorder.

Of major importance to guiding the physical examination are the area(s) of symptoms currently experienced. Patients experience symptoms that arise from the cervical region in a variety of areas. The upper division of the cervical segments (0/C1, C1/C2, and C2/C3) may produce symptoms in the upper and middle cervical regions, any area of the cranium, the face, the region of the temporomandibular joint, the anterior and lateral aspects of the neck, the sternoclavicular region, and the suprascapular region. The middle division (C3/C4 and C4/C5) may produce symptoms in the middle and lower cervical regions, the supra- and medial scapular regions, the shoulder, and the lateral aspect of the upper arm. The lower cervical division (C5/C6, C6/C7 and C7/T1) may produce symptoms in the lower cervical region, the supra- and medial scapular regions, and any aspect of the upper limb, except for perhaps the axilla.

The examiner defines the area(s) of symptoms by marking the affected areas on a body chart (Fig. 3.11). He notes asymptomatic areas as well with checkmarks, indicating that they are "clear," and have been confirmed as such. The patient characterizes each area of symptoms by the quality or nature of the symptoms (e.g., sharp, dull, deep, superficial, "pins and nee-

CERVICAL EXAMINATION FORM

A. HISTORY

 1. Identifying Data

 Name _____ Age _____ Gender _____ Date _____

 Provisional diagnosis _____ Precautions _____

 Chief complaint _____

 Dominant side R _____ L _____ Prior condition of involved part _____

 2. Present Episode or Illness

 a. Description of symptoms

 1) location: //// = pain
        ==== = paresthesia
        ○○○○ = numbness
        xxxx = other _____

 2) severity:

 _____
 none   worst

 3) impairment:

 _____
 annoying   completely disabling

 4) nature:

 cramping _____ aching _____

 shooting _____ burning _____

 throbbing _____ tingling _____

 stabbing _____ sore _____

 other _____

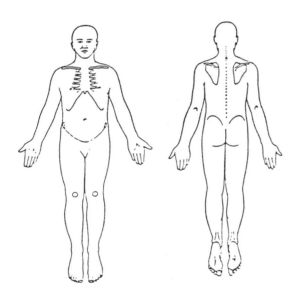

 constant _____ intermittent _____ duration _____

 occurs when _____ elicited by _____

 aggravated by _____ relieved by _____

 24-hour pattern _____

 highly irritable _____ mildly irritable _____ not irritable _____

 6) joint characteristics: catches _____ , locks _____ , swells _____ , gives way _____ , dislocates _____ ,

 other _____

Figure 3.11. Cervical examination form part 1: History.

dles," numb), their severity, and the impairment they impart.

After gathering information concerning the patient's present symptoms, the examiner should also specifically inquire regarding those that are typical of vertebral or basilar artery involvement: dizziness, light-headedness, nausea, giddiness, tinnitus, headache, blurred vision, and facial or tongue paresthesiae. Should symptoms involving any of these qualities occur, one should immediately question whether particular cervical movements or extreme positions (especially rotation, upper cervical extension, and upper cervical flexion) provoke these symptoms. If a patient experiences such symptoms, an examiner should perform specific manual tests of vertebral artery patency prior to manual treatment.

The physical therapist questions if the patient's symptoms are constant or intermittent in duration. If the patient reports constant symptoms, the examiner should clarify whether the intensity of the symptoms varies. Symptoms that are constant in both duration and intensity—in other words, neither rest nor any position or activity affects the symptoms—indicate the possible presence of malignancy or systemic disorders and deserve immediate medical attention.

The examiner should determine what positions or activities aggravate the patient's symptoms, and which ease them. The latter can be a clue to which positions or movements may be effective in treating some disorders. The examiner may next ask how the patient's chief complaint behaves over the course of a 24-hour period. Having asked "what activities bring on your symptoms?" when assessing irritability, one may complete this line of questioning by asking about specific periods of the day and night. If symptoms occur at night, one should ask several follow-up questions. What type of pillow is used? Are there any positions the patient cannot adopt or must adopt to get to sleep? Are the symptoms severe enough to awaken the patient from sleep? What does the patient do to ease the symptoms or to get back to sleep? Answers to these questions may indicate what positions to recommend that the patient adopt or avoid when trying to get to sleep, whether using a cervical pillow or collar would be advisable while sleeping, and what direction(s) of movement may be useful to treatment or which should be avoided. While symptoms occurring at night are typical of acute inflammation from any cause, a disorder that is worst at night may indicate some type of serious pathology out of the scope of physical therapy.

One would expect most mechanical disorders to be less symptomatic after a night's rest. If symptoms occur on waking in the morning, one should differentiate between pain and stiffness. Pain in the morning may reflect mechanical stress accumulated while sleeping, and which may have been masked by medication that induces narcosis. Cervical disc disorders are often worse in the morning, especially if a patient uses a thick, spongy pillow that places the neck in sustained flexion while sleeping supine, or sustained lateral flexion while sleeping side lying. Stiffness in the morning may indicate an arthritic disorder.

The examiner should ask whether symptoms are noted during sitting and specifically during sustained cervical flexion, which typically occurs while reading, doing handwork, or watching television. One may also query the response to resuming erect cervical posture following a period of sustained flexion; on occasion, symptoms are produced or movement is restricted only upon such an attempted return to neutral. If coughing, sneezing, or laughing produces the patient's symptoms, one has additional support for a disc lesion (or other lesion occupying space in the spinal canal) being present. Symptoms produced upon swallowing may occur in the presence of a space-occupying lesion at the anterior aspect of the cervical vertebral column.

An area closely related to the cervical region is the temporomandibular joint or gnathostomatic mechanism. This area is beyond the scope of this chapter, but cervical examination and treatment are incomplete without considering the interaction between these two related areas. In addition, there is interaction between thoracic, lumbar, and pelvic regions and the cervical region, as well as between the shoulder and cervical regions. A final point regarding related areas of the body concerns the patient's hands: A quick look at all patients' hands may save one from forgetting to consider whether a given cervical patient has RA.

Having gathered introductory information concerning the patient's problem, the examiner may now consider the patient's present illness in depth (Fig. 3.12). It is important to note whether the patient's problem was provoked by an injury or began insidiously. One should ask the patient for the details and dates of hospitalization (if applicable) and all treatment rendered for the current episode. Knowing how an emergency room physician or referring physician managed the patient indicates how serious he initially considered the problem to be. Patients who have sustained trauma, or present with considerable spasm and apparent inflammation are often given a cervical orthosis, placed in static traction, or put on bed rest. These treatments are necessary initially to reduce inflammation; however, they are often a cause of cervical stiffness.

If a patient who sustained trauma also experienced a blow to the head during the incident, the examiner must inquire very specifically whether a headache or disturbance of mental function, vision, or hearing ensued. Such an individual should have received immediate medical attention. A physical therapist should not administer treatment to any individual who has sustained trauma and has not undergone medical screening for closed cranial trauma, fracture, dislocation, or subluxation.

Having considered what loss of motion the patient may have incurred, one should also consider what degree of disability (if any) this actually poses for the patient. The patient's own concept of his problem as

b. Background and associated findings

Date of present injury _____ or onset _____ Insidious _____

Dates of hospitalization _____ and/or other health care _____

Treatments; dates; results _____

_____

Status of condition: acute _____ or chronic _____

constant _____ or intermittent _____

better _____ or worse _____

Nature and mechanism of injury or events precipitating present episode _____

_____

Results of injury (if applicable): deformity (describe) _____

corrected _____ disability (type and cause) _____

loss of motion (specify) _____ when occurred _____

loss of strength (specify) _____ when occurred _____

swelling (specify) _____ when occurred _____

bleeding (specify) _____ when occurred _____

3. Relevant Past History and Family History

History of similar condition: dates _____ nature _____

_____

Treatment _____

Other relevant illnesses or disorders _____

General health status _____

Health problems of immediate family _____

4. Life-style

Occupation _____ ADL _____

Regular (3 times/week minimum) physical activities requiring: strength _____ agility _____ endurance _____

flexibility _____ other _____

What patient does to promote wellness _____

Patient's concept of cause of condition _____

Patient's concept of functional and/or cosmetic deficit(s) _____

Anticipated goals _____

5. Other

Current medications _____

Recent radiographs _____

6. Therapist's Interpretation and Plans for Physical Exam _____

Figure 3.12.   Cervical examination form part 2: History, continued.

it affects his life puts the problem in proper perspective for the examiner. It is important for the examiner to clarify if limitations of movement have changed since their onset (for better or worse). Also, he should confirm the initial site and nature (quality) of symptoms experienced, whether they have subsequently changed in area, quality, and intensity, and whether new symptoms have arisen between the initial incident and the present time. Such information indicates whether the patient is generally improving, maintaining, or worsening, and assists the therapist in focusing the examination and treatment on the various components of the patient's problem.

The mechanism of injury may correlate with the pattern of restricted or symptomatic movement observed at the time of examination. A common observation is that the position the neck was in during the injury (e.g., a degree of flexion) may be the last position to be regained, or movement toward this position may be the last to become full and painless. In contrast, the opposite motion (e.g., extension) initially may be used therapeutically to increase overall function of the involved spinal region. Avoiding the injuring movement or position early in the recovery period allows healing to take place, and later an examiner may employ the injuring movement or position (e.g., flexion) to further increase function.

If the patient sustained no injury or specific incident that precipitated the present problem, one should question him regarding the activities performed during the period immediately preceding the onset of symptoms or dysfunction. Some cervical problems do arise gradually over a prolonged period, but it is wise to exhaust all possibilities of a related incident, unusual activity, or unaccustomed posture provoking the current episode.

A deformity occurring at the time of injury or soon after—whether corrected by the time of examination or not—may also reflect the mechanism of injury and will reveal which movements must be restored. A distinction should be made between an injuring movement (e.g., flexion) that results in a flexion deformity (i.e., loss of extension) and an injury that results in an extension deformity (i.e., loss of flexion). The point is that the same mechanism of injury may result in different limitations.

A loss of strength specific to the muscles innervated by a spinal segment may indicate nerve root involvement. More widespread loss of strength (affecting an entire upper quarter, parts of both upper quarters, or any lower quarter involvement) could indicate possible spinal cord involvement and obviously deserves the immediate attention of a physician. Swelling that develops in the first few hours after an injury most likely is extravasated blood, while swelling that is not present until 24 hours after a traumatic incident, is due to inflammation. Knowing these data, one may then estimate the relevance of tissue damage, inflammation, or fibrosis to the patient's problem as it presents at the time of examination.

The examiner should determine if episodes similar to the present problem have occurred in the past. If so, it is important to note how long ago, and if more than one episode of the same problem has occurred. If the patient has experienced a previous episode, one should note if he was completely or only partially better during the time since the most recent exacerbation. Noting what treatment the patient has received for past episodes, and whether it has been effective over the short term, may help one to select or rule out possibilities for the present problem. Familial disorders or diseases may also be very relevant to the onset or management of the patient's present problem. If the disorder involves ligamentous insufficiency or bony anomaly, it may well pose a contraindication to a manual approach to treatment.

Next, the patient describes any history of recent, related, or major diseases, illnesses, or surgeries. One should inquire whether the patient has experienced an unexplained change in weight, as often occurs due to a malignancy. One should specifically inquire whether the patient experiences any numbness or tingling in both hands or both feet, as this often results from involvement of the cervical spinal cord itself, rather than from two separate nerve root lesions. A large central disc protrusion or other central space-occupying lesion could produce such spinal cord symptoms.

A final section of the subjective examination concerns the lifestyle of the patient. His social, physical, and recreational involvements are important to providing a holistic program of care. The examiner should have clarified the patient's occupation by this stage; the most relevant information concerns the positions and activities the head and neck assume during work, rather than the occupational title itself.

Final considerations concern medications and x-rays. It is useful to note what medications were prescribed for the patient, and whether the patient actually took them, or continues to take them (one cannot assume all patients comply with physicians' orders). The examiner should also inquire whether recent cervical x-rays have been taken, and if so, when and by whom. Although x-rays are of limited value in guiding treatment of the cervical problems most often referred for physical therapy, they do indicate the presence of serious bony involvement (tumor, fracture, structural anomalies, etc.) Therefore, many physical therapists insist that an x-ray screening be performed prior to administering manual therapy.

Planning the Physical Examination

Once the physical therapist has completed the history, he should take a few minutes to summarize the most important findings and collect his thoughts prior to commencing the physical examination. He should review the findings from the "special questions" and the nature and area of symptoms reported by the patient to note whether caution, for any reason, should be observed upon examination. Absolute and relative

B. PHYSICAL EXAMINATION

	frontal plane			sagittal plane		
1. Inspection	standing	sup-ported sitting	unsup-ported sitting	standing	sup-ported sitting	unsup-ported sitting
a. Posture head						
cervical spine						
shoulders						
thoracic spine						
lumbar spine						
pelvis						
lower limbs						
deformity actively correctable						

b. Shape: ectomorph _____ , mesomorph _____ , endomorph _____

  deformity (describe) _____

  deformity actively correctable: yes _____ no _____ ; effect on symptoms _____

  deformity passively correctable: yes _____ no _____ ; effect on symptoms _____

  asymmetry _____ , swelling or masses _____ , atrophy _____

c. Use

  handles clothing: independently _____ minimum assistance _____

        maximum assistance _____

  movement: jerky _____ stiff _____ uncoordinated _____ limited by pain _____

d. Skin: color _____ condition _____ lesions _____ scars _____

e. Aids: hard collar _____ soft collar _____ other _____

2. Palpation (note location and nature of abnormality)

  a. Skin and subcutaneous tissue: tenderness _____ temperature _____ sweating _____ swelling _____

    decreased mobility _____ trigger points _____ other _____

  b. Muscles and tendons: tenderness _____ temperature _____ spasm _____ loss of continuity _____

    decreased mobility _____ other _____

  c. Bones and joints: tenderness _____ temperature _____ swelling _____ bony prominences _____ other _____

  d. Arteries and nerves: brachial artery _____ radial artery _____ peripheral nerves _____

Figure 3.13.   Cervical examination form part 3: Inspection and palpation.

contraindications to consider at this point are RA, symptoms of cervical spinal cord involvement, symptoms of vertebral artery involvement, symptoms of any serious pathology, including malignancy, acute bony disorders, and recent severe trauma such as an acceleration injury (whiplash). One should also determine the areas of the upper quarter that warrant examination, due to symptoms either occurring in a given area, or possibly being referred from an area.

Physical Examination

Inspection. Inspection begins prior to the subjective examination with observation of the patient while he/she is speaking casually. It is necessary to adequately expose the upper half of the body during the subjective examination as well as the objective; therefore, a patient should remove his shirt or her blouse, and women should wear bathing suit tops, etc. Spontaneous cervical movements (such as turning the entire trunk in one direction rather than just the head) can provide valuable insight into the actual effect of a problem on function.

The examiner may assess postural alignment in standing, sitting unsupported, and sitting supported in order to note postural habits which may be responsible for or contribute to the patient's symptoms (Fig. 3.13).

If the head, neck, shoulders, or upper thoracic area presents a deviation (deformity) at rest, the therapist should request the patient to correct the deviation without assistance. He notes production or relief of symptoms and how much of the deviation is correctable actively. Then, the therapist should attempt to passively correct this deviation to note whether the restriction is correctable, the quality of endfeel, and whether resting symptoms are altered (for better or worse). The goal here is to determine whether the apparent abnormality is directly related to the patient's complaint. Sustaining the corrected position, or exaggerating the apparent abnormality and sustaining it for a few minutes may in fact be necessary to establish relevance.

Palpation. Prior to examining movements, one may wish to palpate (using the backs of the fingers or hands) for variation in skin temperature or sweating between symptomatic areas vs. asymptomatic areas, thereby appreciating these qualities prior to inducing further changes due to anxiety or overexamination. Having examined skin temperature and sweating, one should then perform a thorough assessment of the soft tissues within the area(s) of symptoms. The examiner should perform soft tissue palpation of the posterior aspect of the neck and shoulders with the patient lying prone with the forehead resting in the palms of the hands (Fig. 3.14). The therapist may palpate each side of the neck and shoulders simultaneously by using the fingertips of each hand. These areas may be examined layer by layer, proceeding from superficial to deep and noting the following: skin tension and mobility; subcutaneous tissue tension/thickness; areas

of tonus, tenderness, and firmness of superficial muscles; the same qualities in deeper muscles; and bony changes at the facet joints.

A final aspect concerns palpation of the course of peripheral nerves, with special attention paid to common sites of entrapment. Proximal entrapments or compressions can occur as the cervical trunks and divisions emerge between the scalene muscles, as the brachial plexus courses between the first rib and clavicle, and as the neurovascular bundle passes along the thorax under the coracoid process and deep to the pectoralis minor tendon. Peripheral nerve entrapments most commonly occur as follows: greater occipital nerve in the suboccipital area or between the insertions of the upper trapezius and sternocleidomastoid muscle, suprascapular nerve at the suprascapular notch, radial nerve along the spiral groove of a formerly fractured humerus, posterior interosseous nerve as it passes

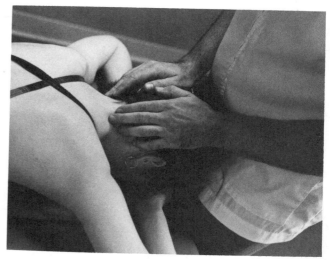

Figure 3.14.   Soft tissue palpation.
Indications: Recommended as one of the initial evaluative techniques for virtually all patients.

Patient position: Lying prone with the forehead resting in the palms of the hands, with arms relaxed and not propping up the head, neck, and shoulders. The top of the patient's head should be at the edge of the table. A pillow under the chest should be avoided, and a table with an opening for breathing is ideal.

Therapist position: The therapist stands facing the head of the patient, with the pads of the fingers resting on the area of interest. The hands should be relaxed.

Procedure: Starting with the most gentle contact, the therapist displaces the superficial soft tissues to examine mobility in all directions, and gradually applies more pressure to sense the mobility of deeper soft tissue layers. In this manner, areas that feel firm, thickened, or cord-like may be discovered.

Comments: As one gains experience, he may be able to differentiate recent soft tissue changes (softer, more tender, more spongy) from longstanding soft tissue changes (harder, more leathery, more stringy). He may also discover the former superimposed on the latter. Such discrimination aids in prioritizing the segments in relationship to the patient's present disorder.

3. Movement Assessment

a/b/c. Physiologic movement

	ACTIVE		PASSIVE PHYSIOLOGICAL INTERVERTEBRAL MOVEMENT			RESISTIVE	
	ROM	Symptoms	Quality	Mobility	Symptoms	Strength	Symptoms
Flexion							
Extension							
Right side bending							
Left side bending							
Right side gliding							
Left side gliding							
Right rotation							
Left rotation							
Protraction							
Retraction							

d. Accessory movement

	Central PA glide		Unilaterial PA glide		Transverse glide	
	mobility	symptoms	mobility	symptoms	mobility	symptoms
Occiput-C1						
C1–C2						
C2–C3						
C3–C4						
C4–C5						
C5–C6						
C6–C7						
C7–T1						

e. Special passive tests

	Mobility	Symptoms	Comments
Cervical traction			
Cervical compression			
Cervical traction in rotation			
Vertebral artery test head moving			
body moving			
passive position			

Figure 3.15. Cervical examination form part 4: Movement assessment.

through the supinator muscle, median nerve at the anterior aspect of the elbow, ulnar nerve at the medial humeral condyle, median nerve at the carpal tunnel, and ulnar nerve at the tunnel of Guyon (hook of hamate). Palpation along the course of peripheral nerves, or Tinel's sign, may reveal a site of irritation or entrapment by producing acute local tenderness or paresthesiae generally reported distal to the site of entrapment. Such disorders of peripheral nerves must be differentiated from cervical disorders producing symptoms of similar quality and location.

The examiner must also consider circulatory insufficiency as a possible cause of upper quarter disorders which produce symptoms of tingling, numbness, heaviness, or coldness. If sustained palpation or positions of the upper limb reproduce symptoms comparable to those reported by the patient, the examiner should simultaneously monitor the strength of the brachial or radial pulse. If production and relief of such symptoms coincide with variations in arterial pulse strength, then the symptoms may be due to vascular compromise. Since vascular and neural structures often travel together in the upper quarter, one must differentiate between them as well. Applying mechanical tension to cervical nerve roots by lateral flexion of the head and neck away from the side under consideration, is one way to further stress neural tissue without stressing brachial vascular structures.

Movement Assessment. Prior to commencing active movements (Fig. 3.15), the therapist should consider whether caution is warranted due to the presence of any of the following findings from the subjective examination: rheumatoid arthritis, acute nerve root symptoms, vertebral artery symptoms, pain constant in duration and unvarying in intensity, bilateral limb symptoms (upper or lower), a recent long course of steroid medications, current use of anticoagulant medications, and a recent unexplained change in weight.

The patient first performs active rotation, flexion, extension, side flexion, and head protraction and retraction in the sitting position. The examiner may lightly guide active movements to assure that the patient performs them correctly. He may also apply overpressure at the end of the range (Figs. 3.16–3.18). The purpose of examining active cervical movements is to begin confirming or altering one's estimation of the problem's irritability, and to get a general overview of the pattern of motion restriction or production of symptoms. Such an overview indicates where to focus further assessment of the problem, by examining passive movements (accessory, physiologic, or combined), repeated movements, sustained positions, or isometric contractions in specific directions while maintaining a specific position.

Accessory Movements. A therapist next tests accessory movements (Fig. 3.15). To improve manual contact with bony prominences, he may displace overlying soft tissues medially or laterally. This portion of the examination is aimed at discovering two main findings: if movement of an appropriate spinal seg-

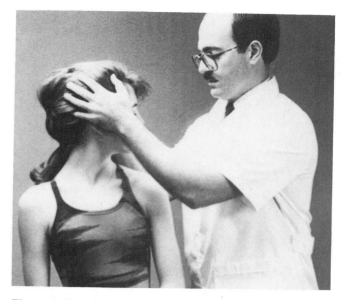

Figure 3.16. Active cervical rotation with passive overpressure.
Indications: Active rotation is requested for all patients, but some should proceed only to the onset of pain and others may proceed to the limit. For the latter group (those with a nonirritable cervical disorder whose rotation is limited by stiffness rather than pain), overpressure may be added at the limit of the active movement. Therefore, only for the latter group may the therapist assess endfeel and the pain response upon application of light, moderate, or firm overpressure.

Patient position: Sitting erect at the end of a table.

Therapist position: Standing close beside the patient with one hand applying overpressure at the temporal region (above the TMJ) and the other hand (not visible) applying a counterforce on the opposite side of the head more posteriorly at the occipital region. The elbow of the latter arm is applied against the back of the patient's scapula, in order to stabilize the trunk and localize the overpressure to the cervical region.

Procedure: If the patient has reached his limit of active rotation, the therapist may apply overpressure further into rotation. One proceeds from light to moderate to firm overpressure as necessary to elicit a pain response at the limit. If the motion is full range and painless upon firm overpressure, then that motion is considered normal.

Comments: Overpressure should not be applied to patients who have an irritable or predominantly painful cervical disorder. They should perform only the active movement to the onset or increase of pain, rather than to the limit.

ment reproduces the patient's chief complaint, and which segments may be restricted in various accessory motions.

The therapist should examine accessory movements with the patient lying prone with his forehead resting in the palms of his hands, preferably without a pillow under the chest or chin. This position relaxes the tension in the scapular elevators, and is usually quite tolerable if the treatment table has an opening for breathing and if the patient does not have a shoulder disorder. In general, the therapist produces move-

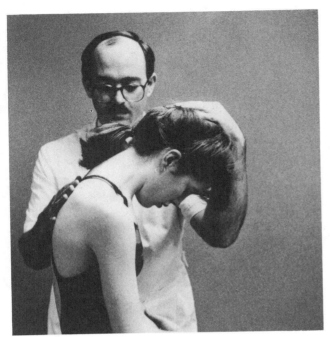

Figure 3.17.   Active cervical flexion with overpressure.

Indications: Upon reaching a resistance limit to active cervical flexion, overpressure may be applied to determine the endfeel and pain response at the limit. Only the active movement is performed by patients with irritable or predominantly painful disorders.

Patient position: Sitting erect at the end of a table.

Therapist position: Standing at the patient's side with one hand over the upper thoracic area to monitor that trunk movement does not occur. The palm of the other hand is placed on the crown of the patient's head, with the forearm aligned with the median sagittal plane.

Procedure: At the limit of active flexion, apply overpressure further into flexion of the entire cervical region, ensuring that flexion occurs primarily in the cervical region, rather than in lower regions of the spine.

Comments: The therapist determines whether the patient will flex to the point of pain, or to the limit of the range. Overpressure should be applied only if movement is taken to the limit, and the degree of overpressure applied is the minimum necessary to characterize a pain response at the limit.

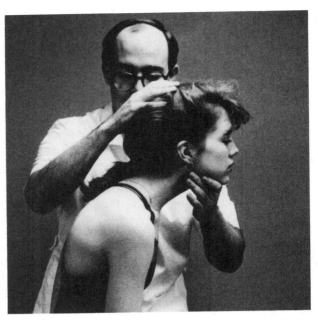

Figure 3.18.   Active head protraction in sitting, with overpressure.

Indications: A means to differentiate involvement of upper vs. lower divisions of the cervical region, by comparison with cervical flexion, extension, and head retraction.

Patient position: Sitting erect at the end of a table.

Therapist position: Standing beside the patient, with one hand on the crown of the patient's head, and the other under the patient's chin. Both forearms should be aligned in the median sagittal plane.

Procedure: Have the patient shift the head forward, keeping the face aligned with the vertical. Overpressure may be applied to further flex the lower cervical division, and to further extend the upper.

Comments: Note that the end position of this movement could be reached from that depicted in Figure 3.17 by having the patient extend the head on neck while keeping the neck flexed on the thorax.

ment by the tips or pads of his thumbs (Fig. 3.19). The thumbs should be placed side by side, making contact with each other but not overriding one another. Movement of the thumbs in respect to the hands should not occur (one should not be able to see contraction of the therapist's intrinsic muscles while oscillating a segment). Instead, the therapist produces the oscillations by movement of the upper arms or shoulders. The digits and hands should remain in an isometric position so that these distal limb components are focused primarily on sensing a segment's response to motion, while one's proximal limb segments produce the motion.

The therapist should examine accessory movement in stages, observing the following points:

1. Examine first for bony alignment (position) with a very gentle touch of the index or long fingers of each hand on the sides of the spinous processes and laminae. Note the alignment of the spinous processes, and confirm any apparent vertebral rotational malpositions by comparing the relative positions of the right and left facets. For example, a spinous process deviated to the patient's right could indicate any of several possibilities: the vertebra itself could be fixed in a position of left rotation; the spinous process could merely be bent to the right; or the left fork of the bifid spinous process could be missing, giving the impression that the tip is located to the right of midline. In a true case of left rotational fixation, one may palpate the articular pillars of the involved segment and note

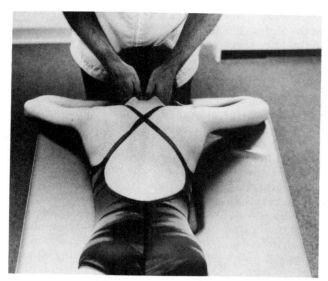

Figure 3.19. Central posterior-anterior (PA) oscillations.

Indications: Usually, central PA's are the first accessory movement examined. They may be selected as a general pain-relieving treatment technique when they are performed at grades I or II with the cervical spine in neutral or a pain-relieving position. They may be used to decrease stiffness when performed at grades III or IV with the cervical spine in neutral or at the end of a motion limited by stiffness. They may be found more effective than unilateral techniques for patients whose symptoms or movement restrictions are symmetrical with the midline.

Patient position: Lying prone with the forehead resting in the palms of the hands, with arms relaxed and not propping up the head, neck, and shoulders. The top of the patient's head should be at the edge of the table. A pillow under the chest should be avoided, and a table with an opening for breathing is ideal.

Therapist position: He stands at the patient's head, leaning slightly forward so that his shoulders are directly over the cervical segment of interest. His thumbs are placed thumbnail-to-thumbnail (not overlapped) with the tips of their pads over the tip of the spinous process of the segment of interest. Contact by the tips of the thumbs makes a more precise technique, but contact with the pads of the thumbs may be necessary for patient comfort. His fingers are oriented toward the floor, making comfortable contact with the sides of the patient's neck.

Procedure: He begins a small amplitude oscillation produced by movement of his hands, rather than by movement of his thumbs in respect to his hands. This movement is imparted by the action of his arms and trunk. The oscillations are gradually increased in depth while assessing the pain, stiffness, and spasm responses.

Comments: During the course of treatment of a given patient, the grade may be increased or the treatment position progressed from the neutral position to a position within the range of an involved physiologic motion, as allowed by a painful disorder, or as necessary to provide sufficient vigor for treatment of a stiffness disorder (see Figure 3.34).

that the left one is more prominent posteriorly. In the two misleading possibilities mentioned above, no such facet involvement may be detected.

2. Gain a brief overall appraisal of the cervical segments by performing grades I–II central posterior-anterior (PA) oscillations (Fig. 3.19). Such oscillations may be performed by contacting each spinous process with the tips of both thumbs. As the name implies, central PA pressures are oscillatory movements applied to the posterior aspect of a vertebra and directed anteriorly. The therapist produces an anterior movement, and the elastic recoil of the soft tissues about the vertebra provides a force, which tends to return it to the starting position. The therapist controls the amplitude of the oscillations and the rhythm of both the anterior displacement and the posterior recoil.

At the first appraisal, the examiner should tell the patient not to report whether oscillation of a given segment is painful (unless severe), so that he can concentrate on the quality of movement through the initial part of this PA movement. In addition, this very gentle, preliminary examination helps one to avoid performing too vigorous an examination, as well as acquaints the patient with the overall procedure.

3. Central PA oscillations are then repeated progressively farther and farther into the range to ascertain the behavior of pain, inert tissue resistance, and muscle spasm in terms of the location of their onset within this range; their rate of increase with greater displacement of the segment; which of these three factors is responsible for limiting this accessory motion; and the significance (amount) of the other two factors at the limit of motion.

4. Further examination of accessory motion may be undertaken using unilateral PA oscillations with contact at each level of the right and left articular (facet) pillars (Fig. 3.20). As was advised for central PAs, initial assessment should be done at a grade I or II depth, followed by a more detailed assessment of the behavior of pain, inert tissue resistance, and muscle spasm through the range of this accessory motion.

5. Other accessory motions that may be assessed are transverse (right to left or left to right) pressures on the spinous processes of C2, the lower three cervical segments, and the upper thoracic segments. The midcervical segments are usually difficult to contact.

The examiner should assess the spinal levels which lie under the area(s) of symptoms, those which could refer symptoms to any of the symptomatic areas, and those joints "above and below" the region of concern. For the cervical region, the latter might include the TMJ, shoulder girdle, thoracic outlet/inlet, first rib, and glenohumeral joint. Areas more remote than those mentioned (such as the lower limb or pelvic girdle) may also ultimately be found to be responsible for or contribute to a given patient's problem.

Passive Physiologic Movements. Passive physiologic movement testing localized to each vertebral segment is among the most difficult cervical examination skills. In brief, the purpose of examining passive physiologic movement is to derive an appreciation of the degree of mobility (whether hypomobile, normal, or hypermobile) of each segment in flexion, extension, rotation, and side flexion.

The following discussion will concern only nonspecific passive physiological movement testing which involves the cervical and upper thoracic areas as a whole. For this purpose, the cervical spine is considered in three divisions: upper: 0/C1, C1/C2, and C2/C3; middle: C3/C4 and C4/C5; and lower: C5/C6, C6/C7, and C7/T1. A clinically useful concept of biomechanics is to note the effects of given movements in terms of stretch and compression. For example, side flexion of the head and neck to the right appears to

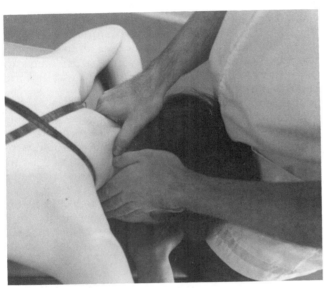

Figure 3.20.   Unilateral posterior-anterior (PA) oscillations.

Indications: Used for examination and treatment of disorders which result in symptoms asymmetrical with respect to the midline, or which cause unequal limitations of right vs. left rotation or side flexion. Such cases often respond more readily to a unilateral technique. Unilateral PAs may be employed to treat pain or to treat stiffness, as described for Central PA's.

Patient position: Lying prone as for central PAs.

Therapist position: Standing as for central PAs, with arms oriented in a similar manner. However, contact is made with the tips of the thumbs over the articular pillar of the segment of interest. The thumb of the more medially located hand should displace the soft tissue over the facet joint medially toward the spinous process. The interphalangeal joint of the thumb should remain flexed and should maintain contact over the medial aspect of the facet joint of interest. The thumb of the more laterally located hand should be positioned thumbnail-to-thumbnail, making contact over the lateral aspect of the facet joint. The fingers rest confidently along the sides of the neck.

Procedure: Same as for central PAs.

Comments: Although the technique is described as a straight anterior movement, the direction may be varied. One variation is depicted by Figure 3.33. Some therapists prefer to align the direction of movement with the presumed plane of the facet joint.

involve the following effects: compression of tissues on the right aspect of the neck, and stretch of tissues on the left aspect.

General differentiation for rotation may be estimated roughly by noting the angle of restriction or production of symptoms. Upon commencing rotation, upper segments generally move before lower, so that findings early in the range of rotation may indicate upper division involvement, while findings late in the range of rotation may implicate more caudal segments. One should qualify this guideline by noting that acute disorders of the lower segments may also produce findings early in the range, and that minor disorders of upper segments may not produce symptoms unless overpressure at the end range is applied.

Following is a somewhat more complex example which may assist in differentiating involvement of upper vs. lower cervical divisions. In testing sagittal plane movements, the examiner should include flexion, extension, head protraction, and head retraction. If the entire cervical region is flexed (Fig. 3.17), and this movement is found to be restricted or reproduces the patient's symptoms, further examination is necessary to determine the cervical division responsible for the observed limitation or pain. The reason for this lack of clarity is that the movement of overall head and neck flexion involves flexion of all cervical divisions. Head protraction (Fig. 3.18) may also clarify the situation. It appears to involve the following effects: a localized stretch of the anterior aspect of the upper cervical division, a localized compression of the posterior aspect of the upper cervical division, a localized compression of the anterior aspect of the lower cervical division, a localized stretch of the posterior aspect of the lower cervical division, and no stretch or slackening of the tissues that span all cervical divisions. Upon further examination, if head protraction is also restricted or symptomatic, then the problem probably does not lie in the upper division and may be found to lie in the lower division.

This hypothesis may be tested further by examining head retraction (which involves upper cervical flexion and lower cervical extension). If head retraction is not found to be restricted or does not reproduce the same symptoms, the hypothesis is further supported that a segment (or segments) in the lower cervical division is responsible for the symptoms or restriction noted on testing overall cervical flexion.

A similar line of thinking may be applied to differentiating extension of the entire cervical region. After noting the response to overall extension, head retraction (lower cervical extension) and head protraction (upper cervical extension) may be employed to note which division may have been responsible for the symptoms or restriction noted upon overall extension.

It is entirely possible that a given patient may have restrictions or symptoms upon both flexion and extension of any cervical division, thereby making this differentiation process more challenging. For example, at the limit of overall cervical flexion, a person might report a stretching sensation at the right aspect of the midcervical area (a finding noted as symptom "A" occurring upon overpressure at the limit of overall flexion). Upon examination of overall cervical extension, this patient might also experience a sharp pain at the right midcervical area, which limits extension to half the expected range. Although the areas of these symptoms are the same, their qualities are quite different. Therefore, the latter symptom must be considered as being different from "A," and might be recorded as symptom "B," causing overall extension to be limited to half-range. The use of different letters to distinguish between symptoms of different quality, nature, or location is important to accurate examination and treatment.

Continuing with this example, the therapist should examine both head protraction and retraction. If protraction were found to produce symptom "B," but retraction did not, then the upper cervical division probably contains the source of the patient's problem. If neither head protraction nor head retraction were found to produce symptom "A," it still is unclear which division contains the source of this problem. It may be that not enough overpressure was applied to these movements to elicit symptom "A." However, rather than assuming that the source of symptom "A" must be confined to one cervical segment, one must remain open to the possibility that a tissue which spans the entire cervical region may contain the source of symptom "A"—thus explaining why only a movement that would stretch such a tissue reproduced symptom "A."

These concepts may be incorporated into the examination process in the following way: one may examine the physiologic movements that occur in one plane, and then note which movements provoke similar responses in terms of symptom reproduction or movement restriction. One may then determine if one aspect of a certain cervical division was consistently placed on either stretch or compression by the provoking movements. If so, one may then expect this division to contain the source of the patient's problem. Thus, in the above examples, further examination would be necessary—such as accessory movement testing to localize the segment producing the symptoms or restriction noted upon examining rotation.

Physiologic movements in a second plane—the frontal—may also be used to determine the cervical division containing the patient's problem. Passive movements which should be tested include overall left and right side-flexion of the head on neck and neck on trunk (Fig. 3.21), and a lateral shift of the head to either side of the midline while maintaining its alignment with the long axis of the body (Fig. 3.22). Differentiation in this plane follows a line of thinking similar to that described for sagittal plane movements.

Resistive Tests. The author is biased in stating that use of isometric resistive tests to differentiate "contractile" from "noncontractile" lesions has limited application to the vertebral column. The reasons for this bias are: spinal muscles that resist a given movement are not confined to one aspect of the ver-

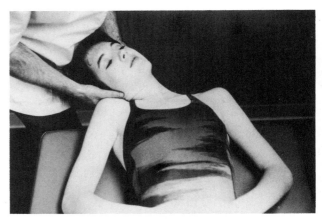

Figure 3.21. Passive side flexion of entire cervical region.

Indications: An examination movement to place all cervical divisions in side flexion toward the same direction. It also stretches structures that span the entire cervical region on the side opposite the movement.

Patient position: Lying supine with the head and neck extending beyond the end of the treatment table.

Therapist position: Standing at the patient's head, cradling the mastoid processes in the palms of his hands.

Procedure: Starting with the head and neck in neutral flexion/extension and rotation, tilt the head on the neck and the neck on the trunk fully to the same side.

Comments: The range of motion and pain response of this movement may be compared with side gliding to the same side and to the opposite side, in order to implicate a specific cervical division as containing a movement dysfunction.

tebral column (such as anterior, posterior, left, or right), and a given muscle contracts while resisting a number of movements. The method of "selective tissue tension testing" depends on the examiner's being able to selectively stress individual contractile units, and is assisted by the patient's being able to differentiate the locations of symptoms upon muscular contraction resisting forces applied in various directions. Because the former requirement is virtually impossible to meet, and the latter is quite difficult for most patients, it is doubtful whether this method is applicable to spinal disorders. Also, isometric contraction of nearly any cervical muscle appears to exert a significant compressive effect upon the mobile segments it spans. Such an effect may result in the production of symptoms due to compression of an intervertebral disc or facet joint. In addition, muscular contraction may tilt or shift vertebral segments. In this manner, muscular contractions which cause a vertebral compression, tilt, or shift, increasing deformation of pain-sensitive joint (disc, facet, or LIAs) structures, may mimic a "contractile lesion" by producing symptoms upon contraction.

The above paragraph is not intended to imply that because isometric tests or techniques appear unable to differentiate the tissue at fault as they appear to do for peripheral disorders, they are not useful to exam-

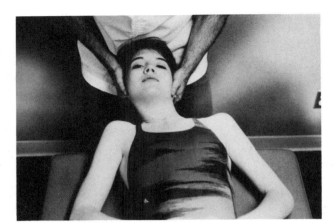

Figure 3.22.   Passive side gliding of the head.

Indications: An examination movement to be compared with overall cervical side flexion. It places the upper and lower cervical divisions in side flexion to opposite sides, with the middle division serving as a transition zone.

Patient position: Lying supine with the head and neck extending beyond the end of the treatment table.

Therapist position: Standing at the patient's head, cradling the mastoid processes in the palms of his hands.

Procedure: Starting with the head and neck in neutral flexion/extension and rotation, shift the head to one side, maintaining its orientation with the long axis of the body. The shifting movement may be restricted by either production of symptoms or stiffness.

Comments: Comparison of the pain response of this procedure with that of overall cervical side flexion aids in differentiating between upper and lower cervical disorders.

ination and treatment. Positioning the head and neck in specific positions and then asking for sustained or repeated brief isometric resistance to forces in specific directions may be very informative, useful, gentle, and effective. In addition, one should assess whether symptoms change with repeated contractions. If they are found to decrease in intensity or size of area, this direction of contraction may be used as a treatment technique. In contrast, muscular contractions may also be found to cause a vertebral tilt or shift, which reduces deformation of pain-sensitive joint structures—such that a position that was painful while the patient was relaxed is found to be painless during contraction. A contraction in such a direction may also be employed as a treatment technique, and upon repetition, may be found to result in increase in range of motion and relief of symptoms associated with movement.

Special Tests.   One set of "special tests" of cervical structures includes manual traction and compression (Fig. 3.23).

Testing the effects of manual traction is useful for several reasons, one being the assessment of the response of symptoms characteristic of an acute nerve root disorder (pain, numbness, or tingling running distally down an upper limb, with perhaps a deep ache noted at the base of the neck or top of shoulder). If the patient has symptoms at rest, manual traction

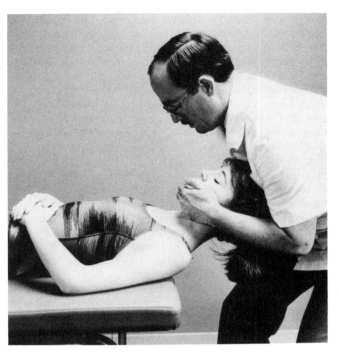

Figure 3.23.   Manual traction in neutral rotation.

Indications: Both an evaluative and a treatment technique, it is especially useful if distal (upper limb) symptoms predominate. The neutral position is usually selected for the initial application of traction, although if another position (perhaps involving a degree of rotation) is more comfortable, it may be used initially instead (see Figure 3.24). Cervical traction may affect spinal segments from C1 to the midthoracic region.

Patient position: Lying supine with the head lying beyond the end of the table. His hands should rest comfortably on his abdomen. For patients whose cervical disorder is especially acute or irritable, the head instead may rest on a small pillow at the end of the table. The security (and subsequent relaxation) afforded by contact with a pillow, as opposed to the head extending into space beyond the table, is well worth the minor inconvenience to the therapist.

Therapist position: The therapist stands facing the patient's head, in a slight crouch and with one foot placed in front of the other, so as to allow controlled weight shifting during the application of the traction force. One hand cradles the occiput, and the other the chin. The forearms are parallel to the long axis of the patient, and the elbows are bent to position the patient's head gently in contact with the therapist's abdomen.

Procedure: Throughout the procedure, the therapist's arms and the patient's head move as a unit, with no slippage between them. The traction force is produced by precise weight shifting from the front foot to the back foot.

Comments: For patients with irritable disorders, the primary guide to selecting the appropriate initial amount of force is any change in the patient's symptoms while the force is on. In lieu of an alteration of symptoms, a secondary guide is the minimal force necessary to produce barely palpable separation of the cervical joint of interest.

may be found to decrease or increase them. If manual traction decreases them, it may be selected as the treatment technique, or may be incorporated into another technique. The minimum amount of force necessary to decrease (but not abolish) symptoms at rest may then be selected for use at the initial treatment. If one were inclined to use sufficient traction to abolish symptoms, he should bear in mind the possibility that rather than completely removing the source of irritation to a nerve, he may in fact have increased the irritation enough to prevent transmission of any sensation at all—thus, the reported abolition of symptoms. In addition, the patient who receives traction of this magnitude is relieved to have his pain abolished while the traction is on, but sometimes the traction cannot be removed (or even decreased) without a significant return or increase of his symptoms. The therapist may avoid this difficult situation by initially employing only enough traction force to produce a slight decrease in resting pain, or to produce minimal separation of the involved cervical segment (as indicated by palpation) for cases not involving resting pain.

As implied above, traction may be found to increase symptoms at rest, or reproduce symptoms that were not present at rest. If such an increase or onset of symptoms does not immediately subside with release of the traction movement, then no further assessment of traction should be made, and traction may be ruled out as a possible treatment choice. If such an increase or onset of symptoms is found to disappear immediately on release of the traction movement, one may further assess the effect of repeating this degree of movement. Repetition of gentle traction (of a degree just necessary to reproduce symptoms) may be found to result in several possible outcomes. If repetition results in a decrease in the intensity of symptoms or in their centralization, then intermittent traction of this degree of pull may be an appropriate treatment. On the other hand, repetition of gentle traction may result in three outcomes indicating that traction is not an appropriate treatment: if symptoms take longer and longer to subside between each traction cycle, and if the intensity of symptoms is progressively greater with each cycle, and if the area of symptoms spreads with each cycle.

While a test of cervical traction should be applied initially with the head and neck in a neutral (Fig. 3.23), pain-free, or pain-minimized position, one may also test the effects of traction in varying degrees of flexion in an attempt to concentrate the effects of the traction force at the cervical segment responsible for the patient's symptoms. A rule of thumb is that the occipitoatlantal joint is best affected with about zero° of flexion, and each subjacent joint is best affected by adding about 5° of flexion, such that the effects of traction are concentrated at the C7-T1 joint with the cervical spine at about 35° of flexion. By concentrating the traction at the segment of interest, the traction force is then applied most efficiently, and the amount of pull necessary to affect the symptoms will be at a minimum.

In addition to assessing the effect of sagittal plane movement on the response to traction, one may also find informative an assessment of traction with the head rotated (Fig. 3.24) or side-flexed toward or away from the side of unilateral symptoms.

The examiner should perform screening tests for vertebral artery involvement prior to performing cervical treatment techniques at the limit of the patient's range of motion. Accidental injury to the vertebrobasilar artery system (possibly leading to brainstem ischemia), although rare, has been known to occur following cervical manipulation and following mobilization of the upper cervical region, even among patients who have been screened by tests such as those described here. Thus, vertebral artery tests may be positive for some conditions, but they are not completely reliable. For example, compromise of a vertebral artery may be imminent due to an osteophyte, but physical tests still may be negative.

Upon initial vertebral artery testing, the patient may not possess full cervical range of motion into rotation

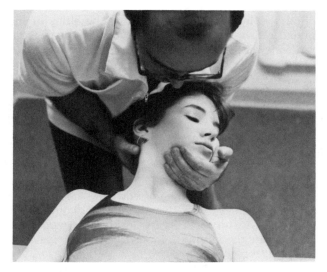

Figure 3.24.   Manual traction in rotation.

Indications: 1. To employ traction to treat pain by first placing the neck at the most comfortable angle, whether it involves rotation toward or away from the side of symptoms, or 2. To rotate the head to the onset of nonirritable pain or resistance prior to applying traction, in an attempt to more aggressively affect the tissues causing the symptoms or movement restriction.

Patient position: Same as in Figure 3.23.

Therapist position: Same as in Figure 3.23, or he may stand slightly to one side, as depicted.

Procedure: Same as for Figure 3.23.

Comments: One may vary the degree of cervical flexion to attempt to focus the effect of traction on the segment of interest. Instead of varying rotation, side flexion may be varied instead, although it may be more difficult to control. Thus, a specific three-dimensional position may be adopted prior to applying traction. Once the starting position is determined, the traction pull should produce longitudinal movement which does not raise, lower, or alter the orientation of the head or neck.

and extension, as required by the tests. The tests should be performed as far into the range as tolerable, but the examiner should bear in mind that screening must be repeated as a patient gains greater range of motion. A general rule is that one must have performed vertebral artery tests into or beyond the range of motion selected for performing a treatment technique.

The vertebral artery tests themselves are of two types: motion tests and static tests. If symptoms characteristic of vertebral artery involvement (see page 39) are associated with movement rather than position, they may instead be due to a middle ear disorder. To differentiate middle ear involvement from vertebral artery involvement, one should perform the following motion tests:

1. Stand behind a patient, grasp his shoulders and prevent his body from moving (Fig. 3.25). Ask him to turn his head quickly from side to side for approximately ten seconds (while you prevent his body from moving), and to report what, if any, symptoms this motion produces. Note that this test involves both neck and middle ear movement.
2. Stand behind the patient, grasp the sides of his head above the ears, and prevent his head from moving (Fig. 2.26). Ask him to turn his body quickly from side to side for approximately 10 seconds (while you prevent his head from moving), and to report what, if any, symptoms this motion produces. Note that this test involves neck movement, but not middle ear movement.

An interpretation of these tests is that "vertebral artery symptoms" produced by the first test, but not by the second, are due to middle ear involvement. "Vertebral artery symptoms" produced by the second test must be assumed to be of vertebral artery origin until a physician provides an alternative diagnosis. In such a case, the physical therapist should immediately communicate the findings of these tests to the patient's physician.

Static tests for vertebral artery involvement are indicated if the patient reports that vertebral artery symptoms result from assuming specific positions of the head and neck. These tests involve sustaining each of five positions of the head and neck for 10 seconds, observing the patient's pupillary diameters during each test, inquiring whether he experiences his reported symptoms during each test, and pausing 10 seconds between each test to observe for latent adverse responses. The five test positions are: maximum head and neck rotation to each side, maximum head and neck extension, and a combination of maximum extension and rotation to each side (Fig. 3.27).

These five test positions may be tested with a patient in either a sitting position or while supine. For some patients, the sitting position may be more likely to provide true positive results for vertbral artery involvement, because while sitting, vertebral arterial blood must flow against gravity in addition to overcoming the restriction to its passage. However, for other patients, the increased maximum range of

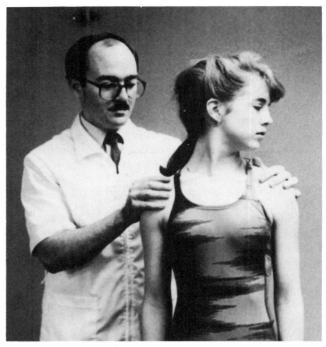

Figure 3.25.   Vertebral artery motion test (head moving).

Indications: To determine if "vertebral artery symptoms" reported during the subjective exam are provoked by movement which stresses the vertebral arteries.

Patient position: Standing with feet apart to provide a base of support adequate to allow rapid body movements side to side.

Therapist position: Standing facing the patient, with hands firmly grasping the shoulders to prevent the body from moving (the opposite position, as illustrated by Figure 3.25, was adopted only to provide a good view of the patient).

Procedure: While stabilizing the patient's body, ask him to quickly turn his head from side to side, keeping his eyes open. He should continue for 10 seconds or until positive symptoms arise, whichever comes sooner, and should then stand quietly for another 10 seconds, in case latent effects occur. The therapist should observe facial expression and compare pupil diameters throughout the test.

Comments: This test stresses the vertebral arteries throughout all divisions of the cervical region, and also affects the cervical proprioceptors and middle ear (semicircular canals). Should short-term provocation of "vertebral artery symptoms" occur, this test may be followed up with that depicted by Figure 3.26. Alteration of pupil diameters may indicate decreased vertebral artery blood flow, but may be caused by exposure to a bright light while turning to one side.

extension and rotation allowed by a supine position, may result in more valid testing by allowing the restriction of blood flow to have greater effect. Because there is rationale for both test positions, and because for a given patient it is unknown which position might provide more valid test results, the thorough or cautious examiner employs both test positions. In addi-

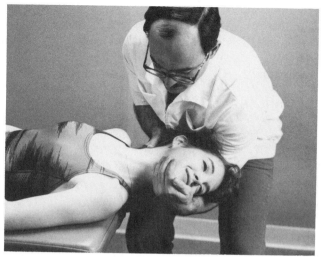

Figure 3.27.   Vertebral artery position test (rotation plus extension).

Indications: To test if sustained positional stress to the vertebral artery provokes "vertebral artery symptoms" reported during the subjective exam. Similar tests involving rotation alone and extension alone should be performed prior to testing this combined position. All positional tests should be performed while sitting and while supine.

Patient position: Supine with head, neck, and uppermost thoracic segments beyond the end of the table, with his side at the edge of the table at which the therapist stands.

Therapist position: Standing at the patient's head, facing the direction of cervical rotation, with the hand cradling the occiput, and the other cradling the chin.

Procedure: Rotate the head and neck fully to one side (as far as allowed by pain), and while maintaining the rotated position, fully extend the head on neck, and then the neck on thorax. Instruct the patient to keep the eyes open, sustain the position for 10 seconds, and observe his facial expression and compare pupil diameters. Instruct him to inform you of any vertebral artery symptoms that arise. Observe for 10 seconds after returning to a neutral position, in case latent responses occur.

Comments: 1. Should a unilateral or bilateral pretest vs. during-test difference in pupil diameters occur, consider variation in the relative position of a bright light as a possible cause, in addition to a true positive vertebral artery test. 2. The test positions adopted are limited by how much pain can be produced during the test, and how much range of motion is present at the time of the test. A patient may have vertebral artery involvement, but the tests may not provoke symptoms at the time. Therefore, as a patient improves in range of motion, the tests should be repeated prior to each treatment involving end-range techniques, especially those affecting the upper cervical division.

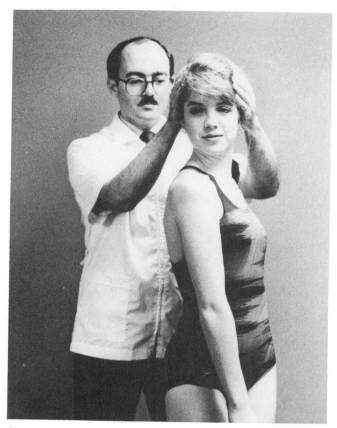

Figure 3.26.   Vertebral artery motion test (body moving).

Indications: To differentiate between the middle ear vs. the cervical region as the source of "vertebral artery symptoms" arising from the vertebral artery motion test (head moving).

Patient position: Standing with feat apart.

Therapist position: Standing facing the patient (the opposite position, as illustrated by Figure 3.26, was adopted only to provide a good view of the patient). Hands on sides of the patient's head, not sealing ear openings. Observe the patient's facial expressing and compare pupil diameters.

Procedure: Tell patient you will fix his head in one place while he quickly rotates his body from side to side underneath his stationary head. He should continue for 10 seconds or until positive symptoms arise, whichever comes sooner, and should then stand quietly for another 10 seconds, in case latent effects occur.

Comments: By maintaining the head motionless, motion of the middle ear is eliminated, but motion of the cervical region occurs as in movement of the head on the body. Symptoms provoked by this test may arise due to vertebral artery or cervical spine proprioceptive disordes, but not due to middle ear disorders.

tion, head and neck motions other than those mentioned (such as maximum flexion combined with rotation) may also be found to produce vertebral artery symptoms. A patient may be aware of what position tends to reproduce the reported symptoms, and sustaining an extreme of this position would be appro-

priate for further testing prior to commencing treatment.

Neurologic Evaluation.   Resistive tests of the musculature of the upper quarter play a part in the neurologic assessment of cervical segments. The examiner tests key muscles to identify lesions of the C1–C8

4. Neurologic Evaluation
    a. Key muscles (strength grade 0–5)

    R ___ L ___ C1,2 = head on neck
    flexion & extension

    R ___ L ___ C2,3,4 = upper trapezius
    & levator scapula muscles

    R ___ L ___ C5 = deltoid muscle

    R ___ L ___ C5 = biceps brachii muscle

    R ___ L ___ C7 = triceps muscle

    R ___ L ___ C8 = FDS muscle & FDP muscle

    b. Key reflexes (graded +1 through +3)

    R ___ L ___ C5,6 = biceps brachii
    muscle

    R ___ L ___ C6 = brachioradialis muscle

    R ___ L ___ C7 = triceps muscle

    c. Sensibility

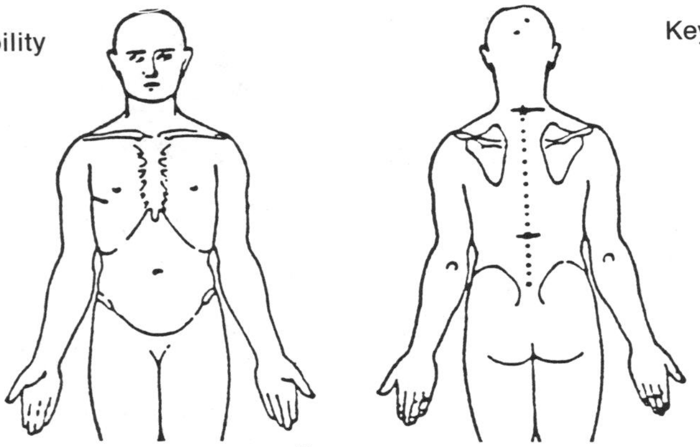

    Key: lacking   A = light touch sensation
                      B = sharp/dull discrimination
                      C = temperature discrimination
                      D = proprioception

    d. Motoric (central vs. peripheral)

	muscle tone	location
spastic		
flaccid		
rigid		
clonic		
spasm		
Babinski		
ankle clonus		

    e. Coordination

    Index finger to nose _____

    Reciprocal supination/pronation _____

    key: C = completes task
            D = completes task with
                difficulty or discomfort
            N = not able to complete
                task

5. Recommendation of Other Tests

    a. Radiology _____

    b. Laboratory _____

    c. Electrodiagnostic _____

    d. Punctures _____

    e. Myelogram _____

    f. Other _____

Figure 3.28.   Cervical examination form part 5: Neurologic evaluation and recommendation of other tests.

nerve roots (Fig. 3.28). He also completes reflex and sensory testing, as Chapter 2 describes.

If the patient experiences numbness or tingling in both hands or both feet, one must consider him to have cervical spinal cord involvement (perhaps due to some type of space-occupying lesion), until proven otherwise. One should immediately test the plantar reflexes (Babinski and clonus), which would indicate involvement of the long tracts of the spinal cord or upper motor neurons serving the lower limbs. Babinski's sign is positive if, in response to a firm stroke along the sole of the foot from the heel to the metatarsal heads, the great toe extends and the remaining toes splay. A normal response is toe flexion. Ankle clonus should also be tested by producing a sharp, passive dorsiflexion of the foot. Three or more sustained oscillations are an abnormal finding. Prior to performing any vigorous cervical technique (such as a manipulation or end-range mobilization), one also should assess plantar reflexes as a precautionary measure.

CERVICAL SPINE MOBILIZATION

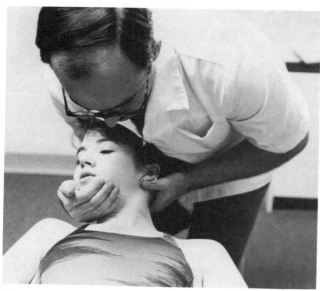

Figure 3.29. Cervical rotation, grade II or III.

Indications: A treatment technique generally used for disorders presenting an asymmetrical distribution of symptoms or movement restriction. May be used 1. to "treat pain" when performed painlessly (or nearly so) toward the side of limited rotation (grade II), 2. to "treat pain" that is irritable when performed away from the side of limited rotation (grade II), or 3. to "treat stiffness" respecting pain, when taken just to the onset of resistance or to the limit of rotation (grade III).

Patient position: Supine with head and neck positioned beyond the end of the treatment table, lying along the table edge opposite to the side toward which the neck is rotated. The upper cervical region is maintained in flexion (chin tucked in).

Therapist position: Crouched at the patient's head with one foot ahead of the other, facing more transversely to the patient the further into the range the technique is performed. One hand cradles the patient's chin primarily with the ring and little fingers (so as not to choke the patient), with the forearm applied along the side of the patient's head. The other hand cradles the occiput by the tips of the thumb and long finger contacting the mastoid processes. Keeping the crown of the patient's head against the therapist's upper pectoral area provides an additional point of contact which ensures a more precise rotational motion and which creates in the patient a feeling of security.

Procedure: The rotational motion is produced by a coordinated movement of the therapist's arms, with the therapist's body remaining motionless. He should attempt to move the patient's head precisely about an axis passing through the crown of the head, without its wobbling about other axes. He should be sure not to pull the head into extension during the rotational movement.

Comments: If the head is moving in pure rotation, the patient's crown should only pivot (not shift in position) at its point of contact on the therapist's upper pectoral area, and the patient's body should not sway from side to side. The effect of the technique may be focussed at a particular cervical segment by placing this segment at its midposition of flexion extension. In doing so, one is in effect placing the entire cervical region in more flexion the lower the segment of interest.

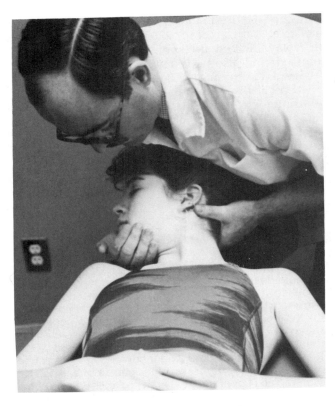

Figure 3.30. Cervical rotation, grade IV.

Indications: To treat cervical rotation stiffness at the onset of resistance or at the limit.

Patient position: Same as in Figure 3.29.

Therapist position: Same as in Figure 3.29. Note that he would be facing transversely to the patient if the range of rotation is close to full.

Procedure: Same as Figure 3.29, with the technique performed as a small amplitude movement at the onset of resistance or the limit of motion.

Comments: With the same grip, the therapist could maintain the neck at the onset of resistance or the limit of motion and resist isometric contractions of the antagonistic muscles. If the neck is rotated to an angle that produces discomfort, repeated isometric contractions may be found to decrease the discomfort or to result in increased range.

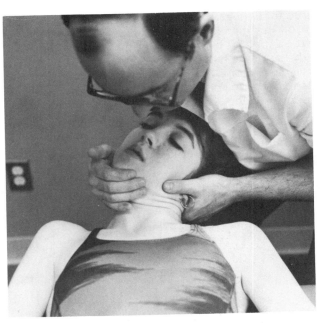

Figure 3.31. Cervical side flexion, grade IV.

Indications: To treat cervical side flexion stiffness at the onset of resistance or at the limit. Which side of the neck the patient perceives such resistance may not matter if the technique is performed as a passive movement (see Comments).

Patient position: Same as in Figure 3.29.

Therapist position: Same as in Figure 3.29, except that his feet should be placed facing outward along an imaginary arc with its center aligned with the patient's nose. This foot position allows the therapist to move his body and the patient's head as a unit while producing side flexion.

Procedure: The therapist's body and the patient's head move as a unit, with the patient's nose at the center of the side flexion motion. The technique is performed as a small amplitude motion at the onset of resistance or limit of side flexion.

Comments: The patient's upper cervical region should be maintained in flexion while performing the technique. The effect of the technique may be focussed by placing the segment of interest at its midposition of flexion/extension prior to performing the technique. The same grip and therapist position may be used to perform a technique involving isometric contractions toward any direction. If the patient perceives resistance to side flexion on the side opposite the motion, isometric contraction of the antagonists to the motion (performed at the limit) may be more effective than passive stretching.

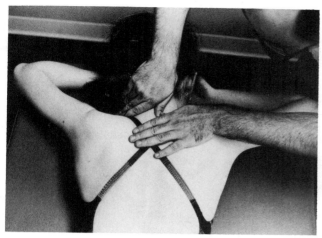

Figure 3.32.   Transverse pressures on spinous process.

Indications: An examining technique to note accessory movement restrictions which may be related to restriction of cervical side flexion. As a treatment technique performed with the neck in neutral, transverse pressures may be used to relieve unilateral symptoms on either side or to decrease asymmetrical stiffness. When the neck is first rotated or side flexed toward the side of thumb contact, transverse pressures may be used to more aggressively decrease asymmetrical stiffness. Most commonly this treatment is performed at C2, C5, and below (the spinous processes of C3 and C4 are relatively inaccessible).

Patient position: Lying prone with the forehead resting in the palms of the hands, with arms relaxed and not propping up the head, neck, and shoulders. The top of the patient's head should be at the edge of the table. A pillow under the chest should be avoided, and a table with an opening for breathing is ideal.

Therapist position: He stands to the side of the patient's shoulder with one foot in front of the other. One thumb is aligned with the patient's midline, with the thumb tip making firm contact with the side of the spinous process. The fingers of this hand rest gently over the neck. The respective forearm is aligned with the patient's midline and somewhat vertically, to apply enough downward pressure to prevent the thumb from slipping off the spinous process. The other thumb is oriented transversely with the tip making contact with the other thumbnail. The respective forearm is oriented horizontally and transversely so that it is aligned with the direction of movement.

Procedure: One thumb functions to make firm contact with the spinous process of interest, and the other provides the transverse movement, which is produced by its respective forearm. The spinous process, thumbs, hands, and forearms should move as a unit throughout the technique.

Comments: The relative hand placement depicted may be most suitable for a technique performing at C2, such that the thumb in contact with the spinous process is the one closer to the patient's head. For lower cervical and upper thoracic segments, the therapist may prefer to use the thumb farthest from the patient's head for contact with the spinous process.

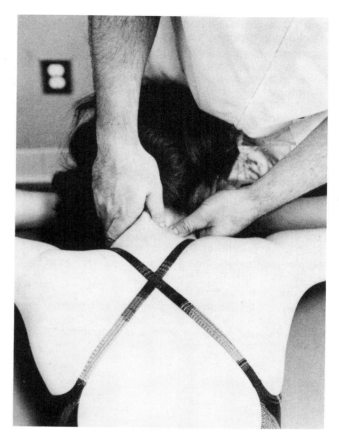

Figure 3.33.   Unilateral posterior-anterior (PA) oscillation, angled medially.

Indications: An example of a variation used in examination to make precise note of the direction of movement restriction or symptom reproduction. May be used in treatment to increase movement such as rotation or side flexion toward the side on which the technique is performed. The technique may also be used to improve cervical extension by performing it on the same side as the responsible stiffness or nonirritable pain.

Patient position: Same as in Figure 3.32.

Therapist position: The therapist stands a bit more to the side than for unilateral PAs. Contact is made by the tips of the thumbs over the articular pillar of the segment of interest. The thumb of the more medially located hand should displace the soft tissue over the facet joint medially toward the spinous process. Its interphalangeal joint should remain flexed and should maintain contact over the medial aspect of the facet joint of interest. The thumb of the more laterally located hand should be positioned thumbnail-to-thumbnail, making contact over the lateral aspect of the facet joint. The fingers rest confidently along the sides of the neck. The therapist's body should be facing the direction of movement.

Procedure: He begins a small amplitude oscillation produced by movement of his hands, rather than by movement of his thumbs in respect to his hands. This movement is imparted by the action of his arms and trunk. The oscillations are gradually increased in depth while assessing the pain, stiffness, and spasm responses.

Comments: This is an example of the many possible variations on a basic technique. The direction may also be angled laterally, caudally, or cephaladly, or the neck may be first positioned in a degree of any physiologic movement prior to performing the technique.

Figure 3.34.   Unilateral posterior-anterior (PA) oscillations in cervical rotation.

Indications: May be used to determine which segment is responsible for symptoms produced at the limit of cervical rotation. In doing so, thumb contact should be on the side of symptoms. May be used to aggressively treat stiffness restricting cervical rotation. The technique would be most effective if the side of symptoms happened to be the same as the direction of limited rotation. For patients whose side of symptoms is opposite to the limited rotation, a similar technique may be performed with the patient supine and head rotated toward the limit. In such a case, the supine position may make the involved facet more accessible to an accessory technique.

Patient position: Same as in Figure 3.33, but with the head turned to one side. The degree of rotation selected may be the limit of motion, the onset of resistance to rotation, or the maximum rotation that can be assumed painlessly.

Therapist position: Same as for unilateral PAs, as in Figure 3.20.

Procedure: Same as for Figure 3.33.

Comments: This is another variation on basic techniques, illustrating how physiologic and accessory movements may be combined in examination and treatment.

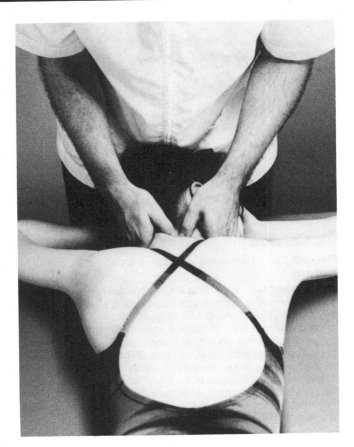

THORACOLUMBAR SPINE EXAMINATION

Considerable variability in the course of syndromes associated with thoracolumbar disorders requires an organized and reliable approach to assessment of back dysfunction. One, or a combination of the following primary components comprises the pathogenesis of most mechanical back disorders (20).

1. Disc protrusion irritating or compressing nerve tissue and causing pain and/or muscle spasm;
2. Deformation of the articular surfaces, ''binding'' movement; i.e., osteophytic formations (at the interbody and facet articulations) or facet joint subluxation;
3. Scarring and soft tissue injury, limiting movement; i.e., between the lamellae of the intervertebral disc, within the joint capsule of the facet articulations, or within muscles controlling spinal motion (i.e., contractures).

A clinical examination of both subjective and objective factors evaluates the role of these components in back dysfunction.

History

The patient's history initiates an examination (Fig. 3.35). Age is a critical variable because it provides one cue to the type of underlying pathology. Acute episodes of back pain or stiffness in a patient 25–50 years of age often involve nuclear prolapse. In contrast, older patients suffering back disorders more frequently have a pathogenesis related to a fracture of the anular rings (17). The age variable is also important because the subsequent treatment for the old and young varies. The effects of spinal traction, for example, would differ according to the patient's age. Since fibrocartilage replaces the nucleus pulposus in the aged, the suction provided by traction would have less effect in drawing the nucleus pulposus back into the intervertebral disc (9). Spinal traction may, however, provide physiologic effects which would contribute to pain relief in the elderly. Osteoarthritis of the lumbar spine in the elderly can lead to a narrowing of the intervertebral space, osteophytic spurring, and associated nerve root irritation or compression (18). In this case, positional distraction and posturing may be most efficient for enhancing the effects of rest. Gentle oscillations may also be of benefit in relieving pain.

The examiner asks the patient to describe his present episode or illness (Fig. 3.35). He uses a body chart to indicate the location of symptoms, and a checklist to denote the impairment, severity, and nature of symptoms. Muscle spasm frequently accompanies back dysfunction as a primary *source* of pain or as a secondary *response* to pain. Subsequently treatment should

THORACOLUMBAR EXAMINATION FORM

A. HISTORY

1. Identifying Data

   Name _____ Age _____ Gender _____ Date _____

   Provisional diagnosis _____ Precautions _____

   Chief complaint _____

   Dominant side R _____ L _____ Prior condition of involved part _____

2. Present Episode or Illness

   a. Description of symptoms

      1) location: //// = pain
                    ==== = paresthesia
                    ∘∘∘∘ = numbness
                    xxxx = other _____

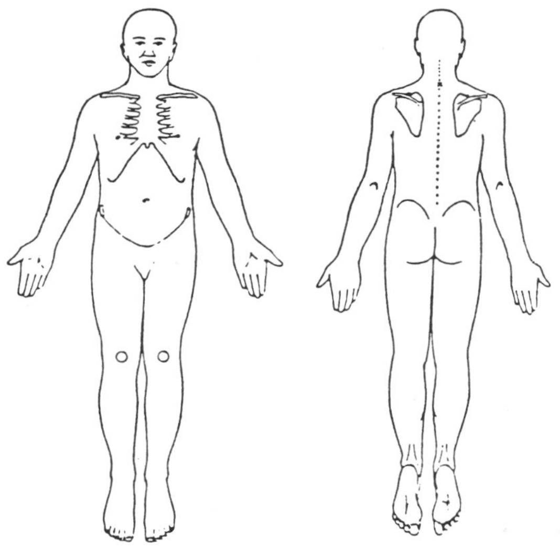

      2) severity:

         _____
         none   worst

      3) impairment:

         _____
         annoying   completely disabling

      4) nature:

         cramping _____ aching _____

         shooting _____ burning _____

         throbbing _____ tingling _____

         stabbing _____ sore _____

         other _____

   5) behavior:

      constant _____ intermittent _____ duration _____

      occurs when _____ elicited by _____

      aggravated by _____ relieved by _____

      24-hour pattern _____

      highly irritable _____ mildly irritable _____ not irritable _____

   6) joint characteristics: catches _____ , locks _____ , swells _____ , gives way _____ , dislocates _____ ,

      other _____

Figure 3.35. Thoracolumbar examination form part 1: History.

b. Background and associated findings

Date of present injury _____ or onset _____ Insidious _____

Dates of hospitalization _____ and/or other health care _____

Treatments; dates; results _____

_____

Status of condition: acute _____ or chronic _____

constant _____ or intermittent _____

better _____ or worse _____

Nature and mechanism of injury or events precipitating present episode _____

_____

Results of injury (if applicable): deformity (describe) _____

corrected _____ disability (type and cause) _____

loss of motion (specify) _____ when occurred _____

loss of strength (specify) _____ when occurred _____

swelling (specify) _____ when occurred _____

bleeding (specify) _____ when occurred _____

3. Relevant Past History and Family History

History of similar condition: dates _____ nature _____

_____

Treatment _____

Other relevant illnesses or disorders _____

General health status _____

Health problems of immediate family _____

4. Life-style

Occupation _____ ADL _____

Regular (3 times/week minimum) physical activities requiring: strength _____ agility _____ endurance _____

flexibility _____ other _____

What patient does to promote wellness _____

Patient's concept of cause of condition _____

Patient's concept of functional and/or cosmetic deficit(s) _____

Anticipated goals _____

5. Other

Current medications _____

Recent radiographs _____

6. Therapist's Interpretation and Plans for Physical Exam _____

_____

Figure 3.36.   Thoracolumbar examination form part 2: History, continued.

B. PHYSICAL EXAMINATION

  1. Inspection

    a. Posture (standing):   frontal plane   sagittal plane

                                  (from back)   (from side)

       head forward or back _____ _____

       thoracic spine _____ _____

       lumbar spine _____ _____

       pelvis _____ _____

       hip joint _____ _____

       knee joint _____ _____

       ankle joint _____ _____

       patient listing   (R) _____ (L) _____

       patient flexed during standing (level) _____

       leg length: ASIS to medial malleolus   (R) _____ (L) _____

    b. Shape: ectomorph _____ , mesomorph _____ , endomorph _____

       deformity (describe) _____ asymmetry _____

       swelling or masses _____ atrophy _____

    c. Use

       handles clothing: independently _____ minimum assistance _____

                         maximum assistance _____

       transfers: normal _____ guarded _____ painful _____ impossible _____

       lift 25 lbs: normal _____ guarded _____ painful _____ impossible _____

    d. Skin: color _____ temperature _____ lesions _____ scars _____

    e. Aids: brace _____ corset _____ shoe life _____ assistive devices _____

  2. Palpation (note location and nature of abnormality)

    a. Skin and subcutaneous tissue: tenderness _____ temperature _____ sweating _____ swelling _____

       decreased mobility _____trigger points _____ other _____

    b. Muscles and tendons: tenderness _____ temperature _____ spasm _____ loss of continuity _____

       decreased mobility _____ other _____

    c. Bones and joints: tenderness _____ temperature _____ swelling _____ bony prominences _____ other _____

Figure 3.37. Thoracolumbar examination form part 3: Inspection and palpation.

reveal its true relationship to the disorder. Usually, the symptoms from both muscle and joint lesions improve with rest and are exacerbated by exercise. Also, movement of the trunk may be associated with pain in the lower extremity (sciatica). An examination of the extremities will be necessary to distinguish vertebral from peripheral origin of symptoms. The sensation of vertebral locking or grating may indicate facet pathology.

The examiner next questions the patient about the background of his condition (Fig. 3.36). The patient frequently reports the date of injury or onset incorrectly. Back disease is most typically insidious, and the patient often forgets the long history of intermittent back pain during the interview, with deference to the primary acute episode. For example, a patient who stocks large cartons in a warehouse may have a two-year course of intermittent back pain exacerbated during forward bending. Then he suddenly experiences an acute onset of radiating pain following an unguarded lift; this may signal an acute primary disc protrusion, the culmination of several years of degeneration. Thus, the examiner must note and record the onset of pathology two years ago as well as the onset of the acute incident.

A description of the position of the body at the time of injury, and the type of force which may have caused the lesion, help the examiner to determine the mechanism of injury. After direct trauma, one must suspect fractures, whereas inability to stand after bending might indicate an acute facet block or disc herniation. By considering loss of strength and motion, together with the type of disability and resulting postural deformity, the results of the injury become apparent. For example, a patient with a disc protrusion may complain of loss of strength (e.g., weak great toe extension), list to one side (deformity), and may be unable to stand fully (disability and loss of motion).

In other cases, loss of motion or strength or may be delayed after injury for 24–48 hours. A gardener may just begin to experience stiffness two days after he "twisted" his back pulling weeds. This delayed onset of limited motion could be a sequela to an initial period of "instability" caused by a severe combined compression and torsion force on the vertebral segment (14). An inflammatory process may present initially as vascular swelling, then progress over a period of several days or weeks to scarring of joint support structures, such as the facet joint capsules. In addition, some neurologic signs (e.g., radiating pain, numbness, tingling) may be latent as a result of gradual swelling of the vessels surrounding irritated nerve roots. Bowel and bladder dysfunction can occur if the sacral nerves are involved.

Previous history of similar back disorders is not unusual (Fig. 3.36). Recurrence of signs and symptoms is four times greater after an initial onset of backache (21). The type of work environment may place the patient in a higher risk category for back injury if poor lifting mechanics, prolonged sitting, or frequent, awkward bending is required. An executive who spends long hours at a desk for example, is in a high risk environment because sedentary employment has been associated with a greater incidence of acute nuclear prolapse (22). Recent literature also suggests that long-term employment involving heavy lifting poses a greater risk for disc degeneration (22). A summary of patient responsibilities and goals for participating in the rehabilitation program, amount and type of analgesics, and the findings of recent radiographs or other spine studies completes the patient's history.

Physical Examination

Inspection. Inspection is the initial component of a physical examination (Fig. 3.37). The examiner first inspects standing posture from the back and then from the side. He notes the position of the patient's head in relation to his trunk to determine if his head rests forward of the base of lower extremity support. He assesses the thoracic and lumbar spine for scoliosis, which may also result in winged scapula and/or asymmetrical shoulder height.

If a disc protrusion is present, a patient may list toward or away from the side of symptoms. The orientation of the protrusion to the nerve root is considered by some to determine the direction of the list (Fig. 3.38). However, Porter and Miller reported findings from 20 patients requiring surgical excision of the disc (23). At the time of operation, they noted the relative position of the disc and nerve root was not invariably associated with a specific direction of list (23). Posture of the lower extremity joints will also indicate the patient's willingness to bear weight on that limb. Inability to assume a fully upright position could indicate a bony block or a protrusion irritating some neural structure. True leg length discrepancies can also cause a postural abnormality and should be checked with the patient supine in addition to standing. A previous history of polio or hip fracture that crossed an epiphyseal plate may be the source of asymmetrical leg length.

As a therapist observes a patient removing clothing for the examination, transferring onto or off of a plinth, and walking back to the reception area, he can record the amount of assistance and assistive device(s) needed for these activities. Neurovascular responses sometimes manifest as unilateral skin discoloration and as a change in local skin temperature (24). Hair patches on the skin covering the spine may indicate underlying pathology, such as a spina bifida.

Palpation. The examiner palpates the thoracolumbar spine in a prone position, or a sidelying position if a patient cannot tolerate lying prone. He can record features such as tenderness, changes in temperature and sweating, swelling, spasm, etc. (Fig. 3.37). The spinous processes of the vertebrae are the most easily palpated bony structures. The alignment of each spinous process may give some clues to positional faults of the segment, such as a rotational deficit, kissing spines, or spondylolisthesis (Fig. 3.40). One

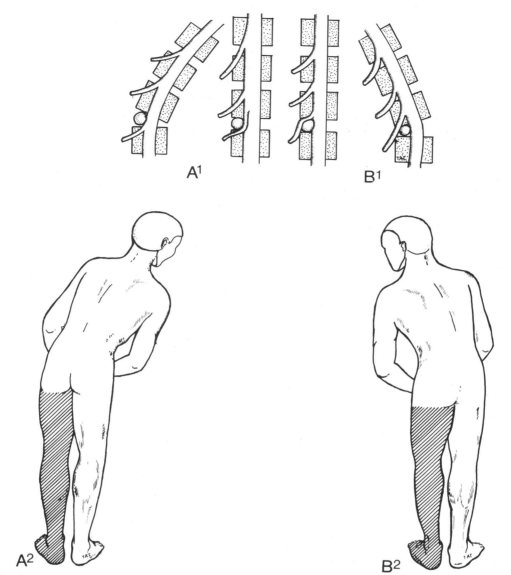

Figure 3.38.   Patient listing as a result of medial and lateral disc protrusions. *A,* protrusion lateral to the nerve root causes the patient to list away from the painful lower extremity. *B,* protrusion medial to the nerve root causes the patient to list toward the painful lower extremity. (From McNab I: *Backache.* Baltimore, Williams & Wilkins, 1977.)

should use caution in the interpretation of palpation. There may be a defect which does not extend as superficially as the spinous process, or a segmental malalignment may not be the actual cause of symptoms (18). For these reasons, positional faults may be only apparent faults.

Movement Assessment.   Active movement of the trunk tests the patient's willingness to move as well as his general extent of motion (Fig. 3.39). The sequence of pain and resistance to movement, the presence of a painful arc, and deviations in the path of movement will provide additional clues to the existing pathology. One method of measuring spinal ROM is to determine the baseline distances while the patient stands from: C6 to L5; the middle finger to the floor; and the xiphoid process to the L5 spinous process. Then, the examiner

again measures the distances while the patient bends forward and backward; bends sideways; and rotates. The differences between the measurements indicate the amount of flexion, extension, side-bending, and rotation respectively.

Passive movement tests the integrity of all tissues spanning a functional spinal unit including muscles, blood vessels, spinal ligaments, facet joint capsules, and the intervertebral disc. Passive motion of the trunk can also be used to stress lesions of the contractile tissues (e.g., the erector spinae) when the examiner moves a part opposite to the direction of muscle action (e.g., flexion) (17). Unlike at most other joints, the examiner does not perform passive physiologic movement testing of the thoracolumbar spine in the same position that he performs active physiological move-

	ACTIVE		PASSIVE PHYSIOLOGICAL INTERVERTEBRAL MOVEMENT			RESISTIVE	
	ROM	Symptoms	Quality	(§) Mobility	Symptoms	Strength	Symptoms
Standing:							
forward bending (*)							
backward bending							
right side bending (+)							
left side bending							
rotation right (#)							
rotation left							
Sitting: Thoracic							
forward bending							
backward bending							
right side bending							
left side bending							
right rotation							
left rotation							
Side lying: Lumbar							
forward bending							
backward bending							
right side bending							
left side bending							
Prone:							
right rotation							
left rotation							
backward bending							
Supine:							
forward bending							
right rotation							
left rotation							

(*)difference in distance between C6 and L5 from standing to bending.
(+)difference in distance between middle finger and floor from standing to bending.
(#)difference in distance between xiphoid process and L5 from standing to rotation.
(§)passive mobility graded as normal, hyper, or hypo.

Figure 3.39.   Thoracolumbar examination form part 4: Physiologic movement.

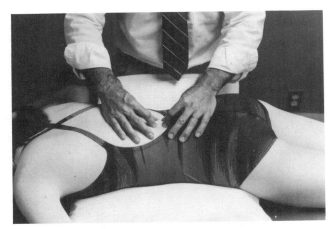

Figure 3.40. Spinous process palpation: if an examiner palpates significant deviation between adjacent spinous processes, the test is positive, implicating the possibility of a displaced segment.

ment testing. The body weight and awkwardness of moving the trunk passively with the patient standing necessitate alternate testing positions, i.e., sitting for the thoracic spine and lying for the lumbar spine. Also, instead of measuring and recording passive physiologic movement in degrees, it is more clinically relevant to use gross passive spinal movement to produce intervertebral movement that is then recorded as hypermobile, or hypomobile (Fig. 3.39). The examiner moves the spine, and with it the intervertebral segment, through the desired range while palpating intervertebral movement. He may compare the amount of intervertebral movement present with the movement at joints above and below, the opposite side, or the expected normal range for a particular patient (25). Figures 3.41–3.45 illustrate the techniques the examiner uses in testing passive physiologic intervertebral movement.

Resisting physiologic motions tests the ability of the erector spinae and abdominal muscles to generate

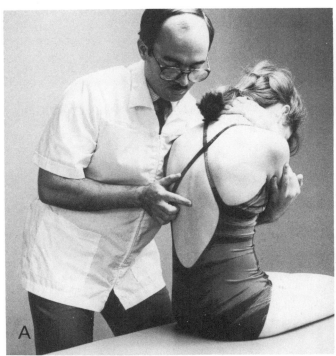

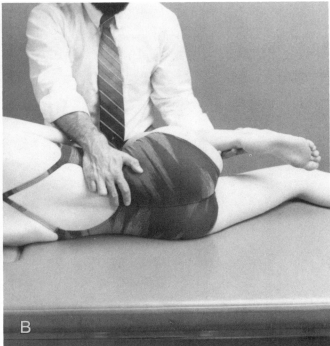

Figure 3.41. Passive physiologic forward bending.

A, Thoracic spine.

Patient position: Sitting with arms crossed in front of chest.

Therapist position: Standing to one side of patient, therapist places arm under patient's crossed arms. Therapist palpates the interspinous space utilizing the index or middle finger.

Technique: Passively guide the shoulders downward to test forward bending. (Reverse the direction of movement to test backward bending.)

B, Lumbar spine.

Patient position: Side lying facing therapist with pillow supporting head.

Therapist position: Standing facing patient; S (stabilizing) finger rests between adjacent spinous processes; M (mobilizing) hand supports uppermost leg (may hold both legs, not shown) with patient's knee against therapist's lateral abdomen.

Technique: Sway hips to produce spinal flexion through leg motion, while palpating relative intervertebral movement.

Comment: Used as a test for passive physiologic intervertebral forward bending.

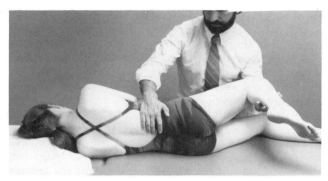

Figure 3.42.   Passive physiologic backward bending (lumbar spine).

Patient position: Side lying facing therapist with pillow supporting head.

Therapist position: Standing facing patient; S finger rests between adjacent spinous processes; M hand supports uppermost leg (may hold both legs, not shown) with patient's knee against therapist's lateral abdomen.

Technique: Sway hips to produce spinal extension through leg motion, while palpating relative intervertebral movement.

Comment: Used as a test for passive physiologic intervertebral backward bending.

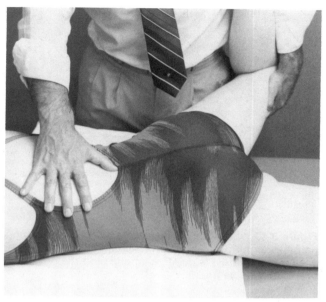

Figure 3.44.   Passive physiologic lumbar side bending (prone).

Patient position: Prone with pillow supporting lower abdomen; knee flexed 90°.

Therapist position: Standing at patient's side, S thumb rests between adjacent spinous process; M hand cradles thigh.

Comments: Used as a test for passive physiologic intervertebral side bending.

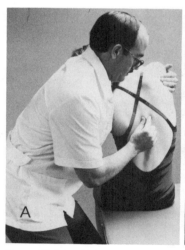
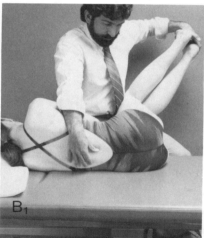
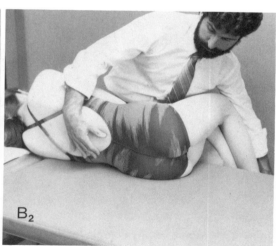

Figure 3.43.   Passive physiologic side bending.

A, Thoracic spine.

Patient position: Sitting with arms crossed in front of chest.

Therapist position: Standing to one side of patient. Therapist places arm under patient's crossed arms. Therapist palpates lateral to the interspinous space utilizing his thumb and index finger.

Technique: Move patient into side bending.

Comment: Therapist will need to switch sides in order to palpate side bending in both right and left directions.

B, Lumbar spine.

Patient position: Side lying facing therapist with head supported by pillow; hips and knees are flexed to 90°.

Therapist position: Standing facing patient; may use thigh to support patient's knees; S thumb rests on spinous process of the cranial member of segment; M hand grasps both feet.

Technique: Raise (1) or lower (2) patient's legs to side bend in appropriate direction; maintain thumb as fulcrum for movement.

Comment: Used as a test for passive physiologic intervertebral side bending.

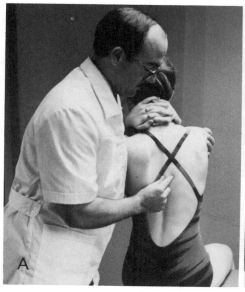
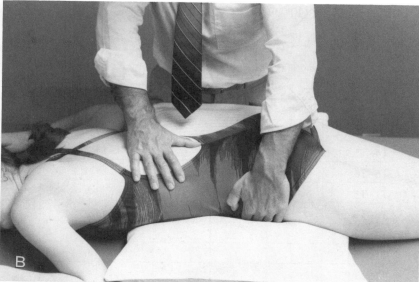

Figure 3.45.   Passive physiologic rotation.

A, Thoracic spine.

Patient position: Sitting with arms crossed in front of chest.

Therapist position: Standing to one side of patient. Therapist places arm under patient's crossed arms. Therapist palpates just lateral to the interspinous space, utilizing his thumb and index finger.

Technique: Rotate patient's shoulders to the right or left.

Comment: Therapist will need to switch sides in order to fully palpate rotation in right and left directions.

B, Lumbar spine (thumb fulcrum).

Patient position: Prone with pillow under lower abdomen.

Therapist position: Standing at patient's side; S hand rests on back with thumb adjacent to spinous process, on side nearest therapist; M hand cradles patient's iliac crest.

Technique: Lift patient's hip and rotate lower spine away from therapist while S thumb fixates upper spine.

Comment: Used as a test for passive physiologic intervertebral rotation.

tension. The examiner tests trunk flexion and rotation by having the patient attempt to sit up, and sit up with rotation respectively, from supine. Trunk extension is tested by having the patient attempt to raise his trunk from a prone position. He tests side-bending by having a patient attempt to raise his trunk from a sidelying position. While resisting movements of the trunk, the examiner should caution the patient to avoid a Valsalva maneuver because pain corresponding to a change in intrathecal pressure might incorrectly mimic a contractile lesion. Also, when testing resisted movement, the examiner should be aware that these techniques will compress the intervertebral joints, so resulting symptoms may not emanate only from contractile structures.

Accessory Movement.   The examiner tests the accessory movement of the thoracolumbar spine (Fig. 3.46). He notes the grade of accessory movement and any associated symptoms. He may use the mobilization techniques described later in this chapter to test accessory movement.

Special Tests.   The examiner performs special tests to help localize the pathology. A Lasègue test (straight leg raise) places a stretch on the sciatic nerve and is considered positive for a disc protrusion if 30–60° of

hip flexion reproduce symptoms (Fig. 3.47). This is the range most likely to press the sciatic nerve on the bulging disc (6). The mere presence of sciatica does not necessarily indicate a disc protrusion. If a patient complains of sciatica, but a Lasègue test is negative, it is possible that damaged spinal ligaments, muscles, and other tissues may refer pain in a sciatic nerve distribution (18). Although injury of these supporting tissues innervated by the dorsal rami could cause sciatica, muscle weakness should not be present unless there actually is sciatic nerve involvement (8).

The lower lumber segments (L4-5 and L5-S1) are the most common locations for back dysfunction (13). However, upper lumbar pathology can also produce radiating pain and paresthesias. An Ely test (prone hip extension) places a stretch on the upper lumbar nerve roots in the presence of disc protrusion between L2 and L4 because the femoral nerve exits the pelvic cavity anterior to the hip joint (Fig. 3.48). The test is positive when stretch reproduces signs and symptoms in the distribution of the femoral nerve. (To rule out a quadriceps muscle lesion, resist isometric knee extension just short of the precise angle of pain onset. By allowing no further movement, this isometric contraction, if symptomatic, should implicate the quad-

d. Accessory Movement

	PA Glide		SBR		SBL		RR		RL	
	mobility	symptoms	mobility	symptoms	mobility	symptoms	mobility	symptoms	mobility	symptoms
T1–T2										
T2–T3										
T3–T4										
T4–T5										
T5–T6										
T7–T8										
T8–T9										
T9–T10										
T10–T11										
T11–T12										
T12–L1										
L1–L2										
L2–L3										
L4–L5										
L5–S1										

e. Special Passive Tests

	Mobility	Symptoms	Comments
Lasèque test			
Ely test			
Kernig test			
Slump test			
Prone press up test			
Segmental instability			
Ant. gap (pelvic rock)			
Post. gap			
Fabere test			
Pinch test			
Manual thoracolumbar traction (sitting)			

Figure 3.46.   Thoracolumbar examination form part 5: Accessory movement and special passive tests.

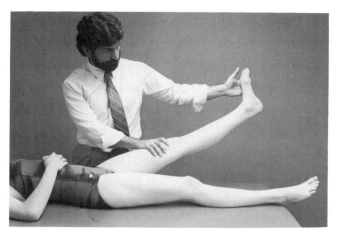

Figure 3.47. Laségue test (straight leg raise): if raising the leg until the point of pain or symptoms is reached, then lowering it slightly and applying a dorsiflexion stretch to the ankle reproduces pain or symptoms between 30–60° of hip flexion, the test is positive, implicating impingement from disc protrusion between the L4 to S3 nerve root levels.

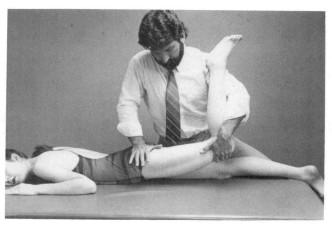

Figure 3.48. Ely test (prone hip extension): if passive hip extension with the patient prone and knee flexed reproduces pain or symptoms, the test is positive, implicating impingement between the L2 to L4 nerve root levels, i.e., femoral nerve. This test may be also stress contractile and noncontractile elements crossing the anterior hip joint, or may stress the SI joint by rotating the innominate bone, so the examiner must differentiate the location and type of symptoms.

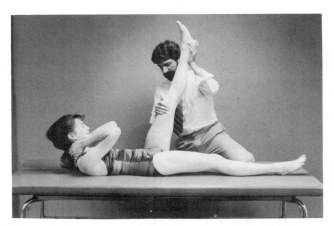

Figure 3.49. Kernig test (supine dural stretch): if flexing the neck and/or performing a straight leg raise while holding the neck flexed reproduces pain or symptoms, the test is positive, implicating impingement upon the dura and spinal cord or nerve roots.

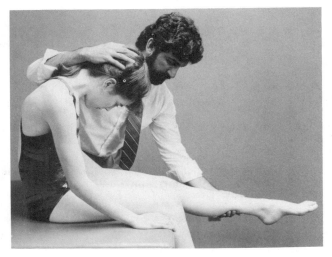

Figure 3.50. Slump test (sitting dural stretch): if extending the knee while the patient is sitting with head and upper thorax flexed reproduces the pain or symptoms, the test is positive, implicating impingement on the dura and spinal cord or nerve roots.

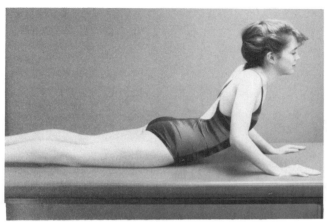

Figure 3.51.   Prone press-up: if pressing up from prone position on extended elbows produces pain localized over the spine, the test shows that pain is centralized and further back extension activities are indicated; if pain radiates to lower limb(s) then back extension is contraindicated.

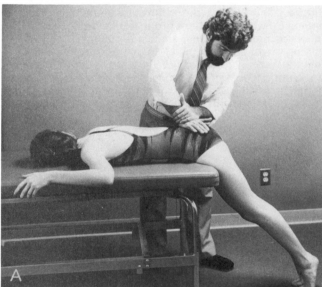
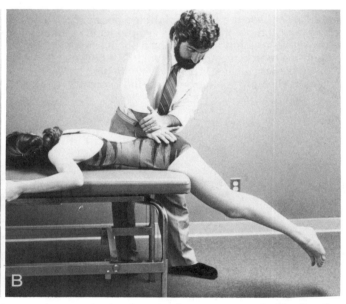

Figure 3.52.   Segmental instability test: if vertebral PA glide produces pain *A,* when the feet are supported by the floor and the paraspinal muscles relaxed, *B,* but not when the hips are actively extended and the paraspinal muscles contracted, the test is positive, implicating segmental instability.

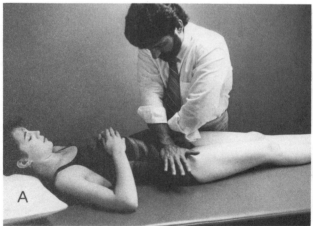
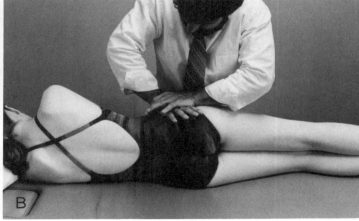

Figure 3.53.   *A,* Anterior SI joint distraction (pelvic rock) test: if forcing the anterior superior iliac spines apart produces pain or symptoms of the SI joint, the test is positive, implicating SI joint dysfunction, such as anterior ligament pathology. *B,* Posterior SI joint distraction test (compression): if a compression force on the innominate while the patient is side lying reproduces pain or symptoms of the SI joint, the test is positive, implicating SI joint dysfunction, such as posterior ligament pathology.

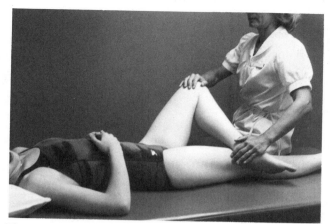

Figure 3.54. Patrick (Fabere) test: if a patient cannot abduct, externally rotate, then extend his hip to allow placement of his lateral malleolus on the opposite knee, the test is positive, implicating hip disease if it reproduces inguinal pain, or sacroiliac joint dysfunction if it reproduces posterior sacral pain.

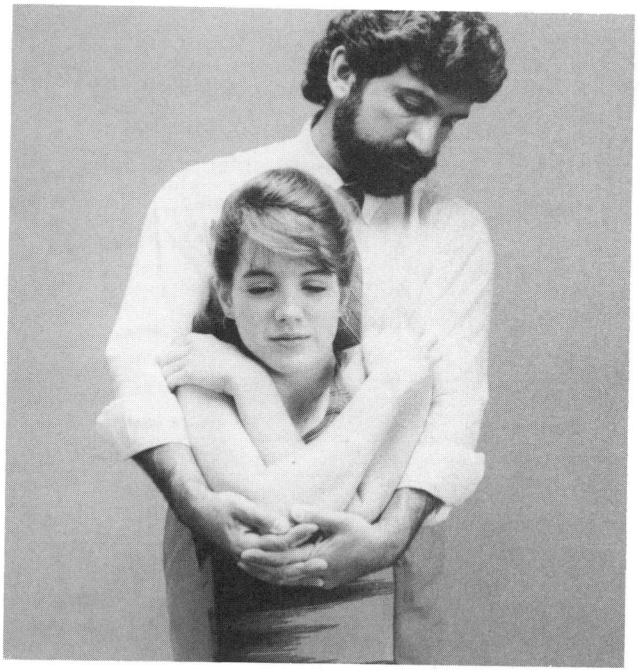

Figure 3.55. Manual thoracolumbar traction: if the therapist applies traction by holding the patient's upper limbs and leaning back while the patient relaxes his trunk, and pain or symptoms decreases, the test is positive, indicating that traction may be used to decrease symptoms.

riceps mechanism.) A disc bulging into the spinal canal can also irritate the dura. A Kernig test will reproduce neurologic symptoms when a stretch to the spinal cord during neck flexion pulls the dura over a protrusion (Fig. 3.49). If results of the neck flexion test are ambiguous, a simultaneous straight leg raise can be added to provide additional tension on the spinal cord. The examiner may also use a slump test to create a dural stretch (Fig. 3.50). He tests the patient in the sitting position, slumped forward, by placing moderate pressure on the head to encourage full cervical flexion; he then gradually extends the knee to complete the dural stretch.

A prone press-up assists the examiner in determining whether repeated extension exercises produce progressively more central or more peripheral symptoms (Fig. 3.51). During this maneuver, if pain is localized over the spine (centralized), then press-up extension exercises are indicated to maintain or increase flexibility and possibly to influence disc position; active and resistive back extension exercises are also recommended to strengthen the trunk. In contrast, if repeated prone press-ups intensify the symptoms or cause peripheral radiation of symptoms to the lower extremities, then activities such as this that increase lumbar lordosis may be contraindicated.

A segmental instability test identifies vertebral instability (Fig. 3.52). The patient lies prone with his legs over the edge of the table and resting on the floor.

The therapist applies pressure on the spinous processes while the patient relaxes. Then the patient contracts the paraspinal and hip extensor muscles and holds his legs above the floor, while the therapist again applies pressure on the spinous processes. Pain present during compression only in the rest position indicates that muscle action is masking an unstable segment.

Special tests for the sacroiliac (SI) and hip joints further enhance localization of pathology. Because the lumbar spine can refer pain to both of these areas, testing each specifically can help identify the source of the lesion. Anterior or posterior gapping of the SI joint (Fig. 3.53) may reproduce symptoms if the sacroiliac joint is at fault whereas a Fabere (Patrick) test (Fig. 3.54) may reproduce pain originating from the hip. If either test is positive, the examiner should perform further testing of the SI and hip joints to localize the problem.

Manual thoracolumbar traction serves as both an assessment tool to observe changes in signs and symptoms, and as a trial treatment (Fig. 3.55). Techniques are available which also apply mechanical traction in various positions (i.e., prone, supine, medial, and lateral tilts). A description of each of these techniques is beyond the scope of this text; the reader may obtain more procedural detail from Saunders (26). Relief of symptoms with traction may indicate a reduction in the size of a disc protrusion or movement of a sensitive structure away from the point of pressure.

4. Neurological evaluation

    a. Key muscles (graded 0–5)

        R __ L __ L2 = iliopsoas muscle

        R __ L __ L3 = quadriceps muscle

        R __ L __ L4 = tibialis anterior muscle

        R __ L __ L5 = extensor hallicus longus muscle

        R __ L __ S1,2 = gastrocsoleus muscle

    b. Key reflexes (graded +1 through +3)

        R __ L __ L4 = quadriceps muscles

        R __ L __ S1,2 = Achilles' tendon

    c. Nerve root signs (enter a check)

	Irritation	Combined Stage	Compression
Pain	Increased	Present but not severe	None
Reflexes	Increased	May be increased	Decreased
Muscle tone	Increased	May be decreased	Decreased
Myotome	Normal	Mixed	Weakness
Sensation	Increased	Mixed	Decreased

    d. Sensibility

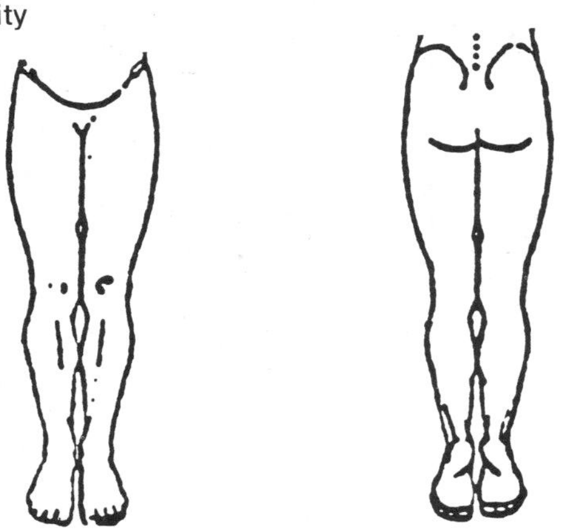

Key: lacking A = light touch sensation
                B = sharp/dull discrimination
                C = temperature discrimination
                D = proprioception

    e. Motor control: spastic _____ flaccid _____ rigid _____ clonic _____

    f. Coordination

        Heel of foot to contralateral knee _____

        Stepping in place _____

        Walking, crossing one foot in front of the other _____

key: C = completes task
        D = completes task with difficulty or discomfort
        N = not able to complete task

5. Recommendation of other tests

    a. Radiography _____

    b. Laboratory _____

    c. Electrodiagnostic _____

    d. Arthroscopy _____

    e. CAT Scan _____

    f. Myelogram _____

    g. Punctures _____

    h. Other _____

Figure 3.56.   Thoracolumbar examination form part 6: Neurologic evaluation and recommendation of other tests.

Table 3.1.
Summary of Differential Diagnosis and Treatment of Common Spinal Disorders

Disorder	Chief Complaint	Onset	Symptom Characteristics	Static Physical Changes	Dynamic Physical Changes	Special Tests	Treatment
Ankylosing, spondylitis	General stiffness and pain	Insidious, nontraumatic	Increasing pain and stiffness; first caudal, then more cranial segments	Fixed spinal deformity	Limited physiologic and segmental mobility	X-ray (+) for ankylosed SI joints, bamboo spine appearance	Maintain appropriate posture, body mechanics, and general fitness
Disc protrusion a. Contained b. Noncontained	Uni- or bilateral flank pain; sciatica; limb weakness or numbness	Unguarded movement; occasionally unidentifiable	Symptoms may increase with flexion, extension, or increased intrathecal pressure; may be asymptomatic; motor or sensory loss	Sciatic scoliosis; unable to stand fully erect	Physiologic and segmental mobility may be decreased	Myelogram/CT (+) for protrusion into canal or foramen. SLR produces radiating symptoms.	Surgical excision or decompression. Rehabilitation: Acute—rest, appropriate graded mobilization, pain relief Subacute—traction, cont. mobilization Chronic—improve function and body mechanics
Disc degeneration a. Cervical b. Lumbar	a. Headache, neck pain, paresthesia in arm, stiffness b. Backache paresthesias in leg, stiffness	Insidious, aging process, or sequela to disc herniation	Pain, reduced mobility, motor or sensory changes	Adaptive posture	Limited physiologic and segmental mobility	X-ray (+) decreased interverterbral space; Osteophytic spurs	Exercise for flexibility and strengthening, body mechanics, temporary support with collar or corset
a. Acute facet lock b. Facet osteoarthritis	Uni- or bilateral localized pain; stiffness or blocking of specific motion	a. Unguarded movement, abnormal mechanics or posture b. Insidious	a. Pain and blocked motion in characteristic pattern b. Symptoms at extreme range and with over-pressure, or when position favors neural irritation	Adaptive posture	Motion blocked, muscle spasm	X-ray, CT (+) for osteophytes if present	Traction; graded mobilization; anesthetic injection or percutaneous nerve block
Sprain or strain	Acute pain	Trauma or unguarded movement	Pain and guarded motion	Muscle guarding secondary to instability and pain	Motion guarded and painful	Tissue tension tests	Rest, splinting while acute; flexibility and strengthening exercises later
Sacroiliac ligamentous laxity	"Slipping" or "clunking" of SI joint	May be related to pregnancy or trauma; insidious	May have episodes of instability or joint locking	SI joint may sublux or lock, fixating in an anterior or posterior torsion	Increased or decreased SI joint mobility	Sacral glide, pelvic gap, and compression	Sacral binder, rest, mobilization to reduce transient locking, sclerosant therapy for severe cases
Spinal stenosis	Pain and paresthesia in legs	Insidious	Symptoms usually worse with extension and prolonged walking	May assume flexed posture to alleviate symptoms	Extension guarded	X-ray; CT (+) for narrowed canal	Possible surgical removal if caused by tumor, osteophytes or disc protrusion; activity modification to accommodate
Spondylolisthesis	Lumbosacral pain; limb weakness or numbness	Insidious; congenital; traumatic	Pain, motor, and sensory changes; may be asymptomatic	Step-off between L4 and L5 spinous processes	May have instability of involved segments	X-ray	Avoid extension exercises; emphasize abdominal strengthening and anterior pelvic tilt; bracing; surgical correction

THORACOLUMBAR SPINE MOBILIZATION

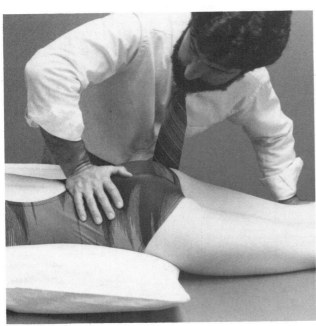

Figure 3.57. Posterior-anterior vertebral glide (pisiform contact).

Patient position: Prone with pillow under lower abdomen.

Therapist position: Standing at patient's side; M hand rests on spine with forearm perpendicular to spine; pisiform contact on spinous process.

Technique: Apply downward pressure over spinous process utilizing pisiform contact.

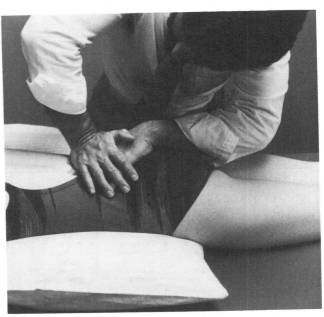

Figure 3.58. Posterior-anterior vertebral glide (finger contact).

Patient position: Prone with pillow under lower abdomen.

Therapist position: Standing at patient's side; S hand and forearm parallel to and resting on spine with distal phalanx of index and middle finger adjacent to the lumbar transverse processes; M hand rests on S hand with forearm perpendicular to spine; hypothenar contact on fingers.

Technique: Apply downward pressure over transverse processes utilizing the hypothenar contact.

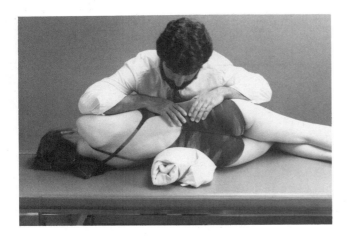

Figure 3.59. Side bending (lateral distraction).

Patient position: Initially sitting while therapist positions bolster adjacent to hip, then side lying over bolster; therapist flexes patient's uppermost knee until he palpate gapping of the appropriate interspinal space; therapist then pulls the patient's lowermost arm forward until rotation of the thoracic and upper lumbar segments reach a close-packed position.

Therapist position: Standing facing patient; one forearm rests on patient's hip; the other forearm rests on patient's ribs; hands cup paraspinal muscles.

Technique: Press forearms down to maximize lateral distraction, and pull up with fingers to produce a fulcrum for bending.

Comment: Massage or modalities may be administered during distraction.

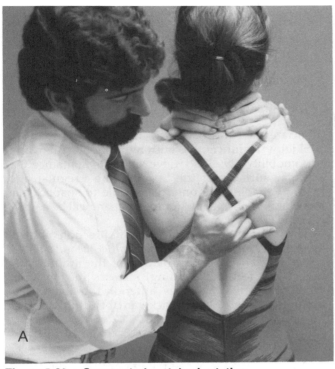

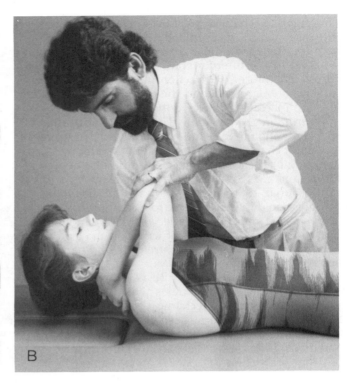

Figure 3.60.   Segmented vertebral rotation.

Patient position: *A,* Initially sitting with hands folded behind neck, elbows pointing forward; *B,* Then supine with arms remaining in same position.

Therapist position: *A,* Standing at patient's side; S hand over involved segments utilizing the thenar contact adjacent to the lower segment and flexed middle and ring finger contacts adjacent to the upper segment; *B,* Therapist maintains S hand contact while patient reclines; M hand rests on patient's elbows.

Technique: Push on patient's elbows by leaning body weight onto M hand, thereby facilitating rotation between adjacent segments.

Comments: This technique is particularly effective for thoracic rotations.

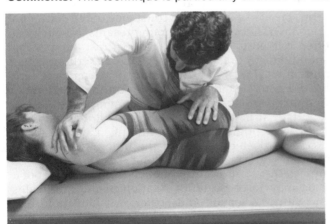

Figure 3.61.   General vertebral rotation (side lying).

Patient position: Side lying facing therapist; head on pillow for comfort.

Therapist position: Standing facing patient; one hand grasps patient's shoulder, the other grasps buttock and thigh of uppermost leg.

Technique: Push patient's shoulder posteriorly and pull patient's hip anteriorly.

Comments: Use body weight to complete end range distraction; may also use oscillations or contract-relax to facilitate maximum range of motion.

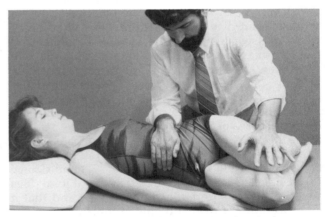

Figure 3.62.   General vertebral rotation (supine).

Patient position: Supine with knees flexed to 160° and hips flexed to 90°.

Therapist position: Standing at patient's side; S hand and forearm rests across patient's lower rib cage; M hand rests on patient's knees.

Technique: Push knees away from therapist to rotate lower spine, while maintaining upper spine relatively stationary.

Comment: Effective for restoring vertebral rotation and paraspinal muscle relaxation.

Prolonged mechanical traction is contraindicated in the case of an acute episode of back dysfunction, because damaged anular rings can no longer contain swelling in the intervertebral space caused by imbibition. Therefore, the traction may allow a disc protrusion to enlarge beyond the confines of the anulus fibrosis, increasing the severity of symptoms.

Neurologic Evaluation. The neurologic portion of an examination reveals the spinal root level of strength and reflex changes associated with the syndrome. Also, neurologic assessment may determine the degree of the lesion, i.e., sensory and motor changes will be proportional to the degree of neural irritation or compression (Fig. 3.56). Nerve root compression results in decreased reflexes, muscle weakness, and numbness. In contrast, nerve root irritation may produce hyperactive reflexes, normal strength, and parasthesias.

Recommendation of Other Tests. Other tests (Fig. 3.56) may unmask pathologies which result in complaints resembling mechanical back dysfunction. Radiography and CT scans can depict Paget's disease, tumors, fractures, or osteoporosis. Electromyography and myelograms also assist in confirming the presence of a disc protrusion.

Following interpretation of data, a therapist is prepared to proceed with treatment planning. Table 3.1 includes a summary of the differential diagnosis and treatment of common spinal disorders.

SACROILIAC EXAMINATION

Clinical examination of the sacroiliac (SI) joint is complicated because many of the objective tests for sacroiliac joint dysfunction also involve other joints. Special passive tests like the Fabere, Lasègue, and Gaenslen may elicit signs and symptoms of SI joint origin, as well as from the hip and lumbar spine (19). While no single passive test alone is adequate to determine the origin of sacroiliac pathology, the examiner uses a combination of tests to identify or rule out suspected cases of SI joint dysfunction.

The literature provides considerable debate regarding the frequency of SI joint dysfunction (for a comprehensive review see Bellamy et al. (27) and Grieve (28)). Clinicians generally agree that the SI joint does move (in persons under 40 years of age) and that it can be a source of pain and limited function (29). The right and left SI joints and the symphysis pubis form an osteoarticular ring which cannot be affected at just one site (28). The anatomical configuration of a closed pelvic girdle requies that simultaneous lesions occur, and may involve two SI joints or one SI joint and the symphysis pubis. Because the sacrum and L5 articulate, a dysfunction of one can directly alter the function of the other; consequently, signs and symptoms arising from one may also be manifested by the other, and treatment directed to one may actually affect either or both.

The primary causes of SI joint dysfunction include:

1. Mechanical—trauma (30), unequal leg length (31), fusion of spinal or hip joints (17), excessive lordosis (32);
2. Hormonal—ligamentous laxity due to pregnancy (33,34);
3. Inflammatory—ankylosing spondylitis (35).

Clinicians have attributed the underlying mechanism of SI joint dysfunction to both hypermobility (36) and hypomobility (29, 37). Grieve suggests that since the articular surfaces of the SI joints are irregular and highly variable, it is only reasonable to suspect that movement of the SI joint for each patient will be equally variable (28).

Throughout this text, movement direction of the SI joint will be referred to as *movement of the innominates on the sacrum.* Posterior rotation of the innominates (e.g., with forward bending) stresses the posterior sacral ligaments, whereas anterior rotation of the innominates (e.g., with backward bending) stresses the anterior sacral ligaments.

History

Age and gender of the patient are important considerations. There is general agreement in the literature that degenerative changes in the SI joint are more common in males. Also, degeneration begins earlier in males (around 40 years) compared with onset of degenerative changes in females (which begins at approximately 50 years) (38).

After obtaining the identifying data, the examiner records the symptoms of the present disorder with the assistance of a body chart on the examination form. He also explores the constancy of the condition (Fig. 3.63). Acute SI joint sprain presents as pain most often related to activity (37). In contrast, ankylosing spondylitis is present irrespective of exertion. Intermittent locking and dislocation may be common with ligamentous instability occurring during pregnancy. Certain positions may also increase symptoms. Grieve reports that in some cases, sitting will increase pain of SI joint origin (10). This finding may be due to excessive posterior glide of the innominates on the sacrum. Information regarding sexual activity is important because during intercourse the weight of a male may force posterior rotation of the innomates and "lock" a female in a posterior subluxation (39). This position would stress the posterior SI ligaments, and chronic stretching may lead to eventual instability.

The examiner determines the acute or chronic status of the condition, as well as nature of the injury or onset (Fig. 3.64). Date of the injury and its time course may help differentiate a ligament sprain from arthritis. Acute cases of SI joint sprain result from an identifiable injury and cause immediate disability, whereas arthritis, such as ankylosing spondylitis, is more insidious in character. If ligamentous instability is present, the innominate bones may "rock" forward

SACROILIAC EXAMINATION FORM

A. HISTORY

1. Identifying Data

Name _____ Age _____ Gender _____ Date _____

Provisional diagnosis _____ Precautions _____

Chief complaint _____

Dominant side R _____ L _____ Prior condition of involved part _____

2. Present Episode or Illness

a. Description of symptoms

1) location: / / / / = pain
$=$ $=$ $=$ $=$ = paresthesia
° ° ° ° = numbness
xxxx = other _____

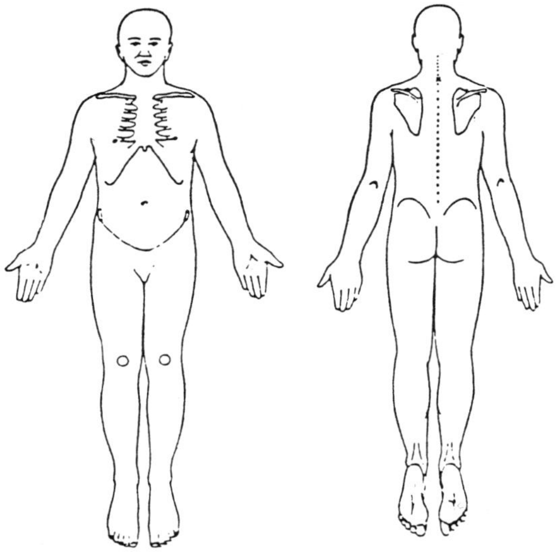

2) severity:

_____
none   worst

3) impairment:

_____
annoying   completely disabling

4) nature:

cramping _____ aching _____

shooting _____ burning _____

throbbing _____ tingling _____

stabbing _____ sore _____

other _____

5) behavior:

constant _____ intermittent _____ duration _____

occurs when _____ elicited by _____

aggravated by _____ relieved by _____

24-hour pattern _____

highly irritable _____ mildly irritable _____ not irritable _____

6) joint characteristics: catches _____ , locks _____ , swells _____ , gives way _____ , dislocates _____ ,

other _____

Figure 3.63. SI examination form part 1: History.

b. Background and associated findings

Date of present injury _____ or onset _____ Insidious _____

Dates of hospitalization _____ and/or other health care _____

Treatments; dates; results _____

_____

Status of condition: acute _____ or chronic _____

constant _____ or intermittent _____

better _____ or worse _____

Nature and mechanism of injury or events precipitating present episode _____

_____

Results of injury (if applicable): deformity (describe) _____

corrected _____ disability (type and cause) _____

loss of motion (specify) _____ when occurred _____

loss of strength (specify) _____ when occurred _____

swelling (specify) _____ when occurred _____

bleeding (specify) _____ when occurred _____

3. Relevant Past History and Family History

History of similar condition: dates _____ nature _____

_____

Treatment _____

Other relevant illnesses or disorders _____

General health status _____

Health problems of immediate family _____

4. Life-style

Occupation _____ ADL _____

Regular (3 times/week minimum) physical activities requiring: strength _____ agility _____ endurance _____

flexibility _____ other _____

What patient does to promote wellness _____

Patient's concept of cause of condition _____

Patient's concept of functional and/or cosmetic deficit(s) _____

Anticipated goals _____

5. Other

Current medications _____

Recent radiographs _____

6. Therapist's Interpretation and Plans for Physical Exam _____

_____

Figure 3.64. SI examination form part 2: History, continued.

and sublux on the sacrum (40), creating an audible "clunk" at the time of injury. Disability associated with the injury may involve the sacral nerves. If the sacral nerves are compromised, sensation around the anus may be absent or hypoaesthetic.

During pregnancy, the onset of SI joint dysfunction may correspond with elevated levels of pregnanediol and oestriol. Hormonal elevations beginning at approximately the 12th week of gestation stimulate softening of SI joint ligaments (34). When the pelvic ligaments are stressed, they may refer pain which follows their relevant dermatomes, and the patient can document these patterns in Figure 3.63. Trauma associated with childbirth can cause sprain of the pelvic ligaments and can lead to postpartum backache (41). A unilateral posterior rotation of an innominate on the sacrum which has locked in place is one cause of postpartum backache. Therefore, recent births should be noted as a possible mechanism of injury.

The past history associated with ankylosing spondylitis begins with sacral pain and stiffness which may progress to the lumbar, thoracic, and cervical spines (15). Relevant past history will provide information necessary to understand this progressive pathology (Fig. 3.64). General stiffness of the trunk due to arthritis is considered a permanent disability and such a patient may require vocational as well as physical rehabilitation. The patient has the opportunity to identify perceptions of his disability as well as his functional goals (Fig. 3.64). Some practitioners speculate that the condition of "false pregnancy" created while taking birth control pills may cause lax ligaments (39), so a patient's taking birth control pills should be noted under the "medications" portion of the evaluation.

Physical Examination

Inspection. A general postural inspection viewing head position, shoulder alignment, spinal curves, and pelvic levels is important because SI joint dysfunction may originate from postural faults which include leg length discrpancy and excessive lordosis (Fig. 3.65).

The direction of innominate displacement on the sacrum will determine the direction of dysfunction. When unilateral anterior dysfunction is present, the posterior superior iliac spine (PSIS) is higher on the affected side compared with the contralateral spine during standing. This means that the anterior superior iliac spine (ASIS) on the affected side would be lower than its contralateral spine. To test for anterior or posterior rotation of the innominate on the sacrum, the examiner inspects the PSIS levels from behind with the patient standing (Fig. 3.66A). He then asks the patient to bend forward (Fig. 3.66B). During forward bending, the hypomobile joint causes a more simultaneous movement of the innominate and sacrum, and consequently raises the crest on the involved side. If unilateral hypomobility exists, the PSIS on the affected side would be higher (with anterior SI joint

dysfunction) or lower (with posterior SI joint dysfynction) compared with the opposite side.

The examiner reviews the PSIS levels from behind in the sitting position and in sitting with the trunk in forward flexion (Fig. 3.67). Movement of the sacrum can now be tested with the innominates relatively stabilized, and with any lower limb length discrepancy removed. As with standing, if unilateral hypomobility exists, the PSIS would be higher for anterior SI joint dysfunction and lower for posterior SI joint dysfunction compared with the opposite side. The examiner should also consider the possibility of unilateral SI hypermobility. In other words, a change in the height of one PSIS may be due to either ipsilateral SI hypomobility or hypermobility, or a seemingly altered PSIS height relative to a contralateral hypomobility or hypermobility. The therapist verifies a simultaneous lesion of the pubic symphysis by palpating the levels of each pubic tubercle.

In a supine position, anterior dysfunction can cause the affected limb to appear longer than the contralateral limb because it brings the acetabulum closer to the plane of the bed, and reduces angulation at the hip (Fig. 3.68A). In sitting, with unilateral anterior dysfunction, the leg on the affected side may appear shorter because the acetabulum moves posteriorly relative to the SI joint (Fig. 3.68B). A measurement taken from the trochanters to the medial malleoli will verify the presence or absence of a true leg length discrepancy. The patient's shape, use, skin, and aids are assessed and documented, as Chapter 2 describes.

Palpation. The skin, subcutaneous tissue, and some muscles in the pelvic region are easily palpated. Most tendon sheaths, bursae, arteries, and nerves are not accessible to palpation in this area. Palpation of the SI joint itself is somewhat difficult because of the dense fascial support and the inherent closed-packed nature of the articulation. Even so, manual pressure in a cranial-caudal direction while a patient is prone may produce muscle spasm which can be correlated with SI dysfunction (Fig. 3.69). This method of palpating the SI joint is also used to mobilize for vertical sacral mobility (with reference to the standing position).

Movement Assessment. Active, passive, and resistive physiologic movement will test the range and quality of movement, and help identify the source of pathology (Fig. 3.70). Active forward and backward bending will place torsion on the SI joint and may possibly indicate posterior or anterior SI dysfunction respectively. The examiner should correlate the direction of each movement with any change in symptoms. Resisted situps and back extension activity will test a patient's strength and willingness to move his trunk against a load. Poor trunk strength may develop from poor posture, resulting in excessive lordosis and a high degree of SI stress.

Passive movement, in addition to stretching contractile and soft tissue structures, tests the integrity of a joint. For example, passive straight leg raise (SLR)

B. PHYSICAL EXAMINATION

    1. Inspection   frontal plane   sagittal plane

                            (from back)   (from side)

    a. Posture

        head forward or back   _____   _____

        thoracic spine   _____   _____

        lumbar spine   _____   _____

        shoulders level   _____   _____

        pelvis   _____   _____

        hip joint   _____   _____

        knee joint   _____   _____

        ankle joint   _____   _____

        patient listing   (R) _____   (L) _____

        standing: PSIS to floor   R _____   L _____

                   ASIS to floor   R _____   L _____

        pelvic alignment standing & standing FB _____

        pelvic alignment sitting & sitting FB _____

        leg length reversal: supine R _____ L _____   sitting R _____ L _____

        leg length: ASIS to medial malleolus   R _____ L _____

    b. Shape: ectomorph _____ , mesomorph _____ , endomorph _____

        deformity (describe) _____ asymmetry _____

        swelling or masses _____ atrophy _____

    c. Use

        removes clothing: independently _____ minimum assistance _____

                   maximum assistance _____

        transfers: normal _____ guarded _____ painful _____ impossible _____

        lift 25 lbs: normal _____ guarded _____ painful _____ impossible _____

    d. Skin: color _____ temperature _____ lesions _____ scars _____

    e. Aids: brace _____ corset _____ shoe lift _____ assistive devices _____

Figure 3.65.   SI examination form part 3: Inspection.

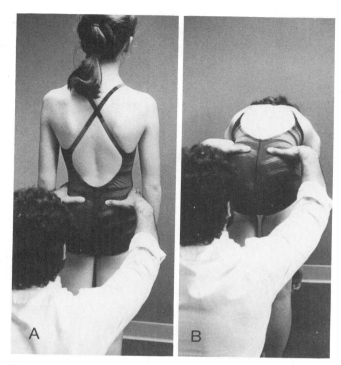

Figure 3.66.   PSIS levels in standing and standing for-ward bend: if the PSIS levels are equal when *A,* standing, but unequal with *B,* forward bending, the test is positive, implicating unilateral hypomobility with either anterior SID on the higher side or posterior SID on the lower side.

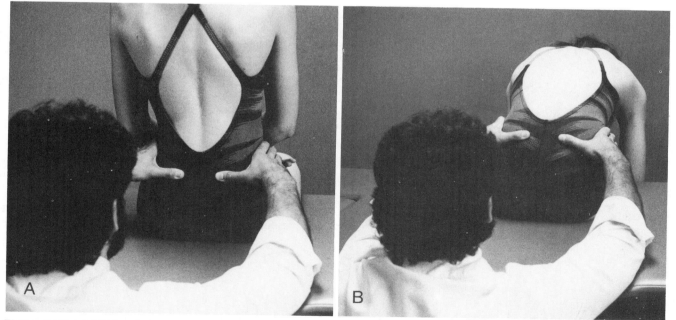

Figure 3.67.   PSIS levels in sitting and sitting forward bend: if the PSIS's are level when *A,* sitting but unequal with *B,* forward bending, the test is positive, implicating unilateral hypomobility with either anterior SID on the higher side or posterior SID on the lower side.

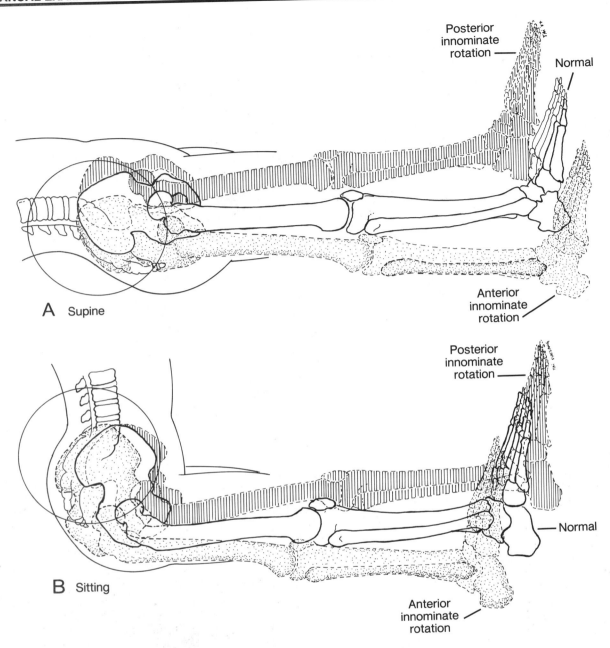

Figure 3.68. Leg length reversal: Supine vs. sitting. If the lower limb on the affected side appears longer when a patient lies supine, but shorter when sitting, the test is positive, implicating anterior innomination rotation on the affected side.

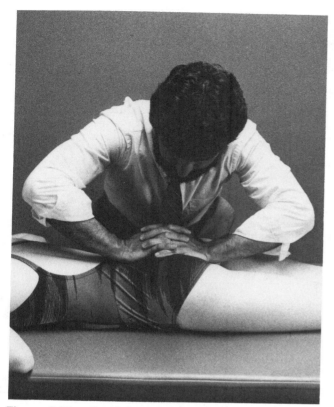

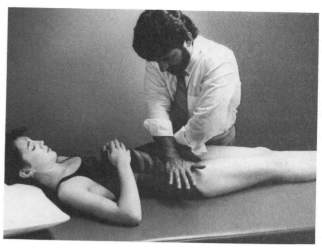

Figure 3.72. Anterior SI joint distraction (pelvic rock) test: if forcing the anterior superior iliac spines apart produces pain or symptoms of the SI joint, the test is positive, implicating SI joint dysfunction, such as anterior ligament tear.

Figure 3.69. Cranial/caudal sacral glide: if cranial or caudal glide of the sacrum through palmar contacts on the superior and inferior aspects of the sacrum reproduces a patient's SI joint symptoms, the test is positive, implicating SI joint dysfunction that is aggravated by cranial/caudal stress.

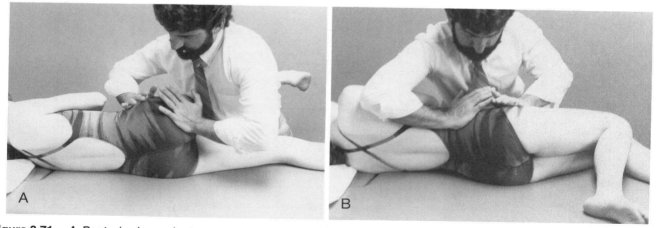

Figure 3.71. *A,* Posterior innominate rotary stress test: if posterior innominate rotation through palmar contacts on the anterior iliac crest and ischial tuberosity reproduces a patient's SI joint symptoms, the test is positive, implicating SI joint dysfunction irritated by posterior stress. *B,* Anterior innominate rotary stress test: if anterior innominate rotation through palmar contacts on the posterior iliac crest and groin reproduce a patient's SI joint symptoms, the test is positive, implicating SI joint dysfunction, which is aggravated by anterior stress.

2. Palpation (note location and nature of abnormality)

 a. Skin and subcutaneous tissue: tenderness ____ temperature ____ swelling ____ decreased mobility ____

  trigger points ____ other _____

 b. Muscles and tendons: tenderness ____ temperature ____ spasm ____ loss of continuity ____

  decreased mobility ____ other _____

 c. Bones and joints: tenderness ____ temperature ____ swelling ____ bony prominences ____ other ____

3. Movement Assessment

 a/b/c. Physiologic movement

	ACTIVE			PASSIVE			RESISTIVE	
	ROM	Symptoms	Quality	ROM	Symptoms	End-feel	Strength	Symptoms
Standing:* Forward trunk bending								
Backward trunk bending								
Side lying: Post. pelvis rotation								
Ant. pelvis rotation								
Prone: Leg lift								
Backward bending								
Supine: Straight leg raise++								
Forward bending								

*Range measured as the change in cm between C6 and L5 as described in the thoracolumbar examination.
++Range measured in cm from the calcaneal tuberosity to the examining table.

 d. Accessory movement and special tests

	Mobility	Symptoms	Comments
Anterior Dystraction supine (pelvic rock)			
prone (central PA)			
prone (lateral (PA)			
Posterior Dystraction (side lying compression)			
Caudal glide			

Figure 3.70.   SI examination form part 4: Palpation, movement assessment, and accessory movement.

places a stretch on the hamstrings and consequently rotates the innominate bone in a posterior direction. The relative rotation of the contralateral innominate is anterior because the resting leg remains on the table. Therefore, buttock pain during SLR of the *contralateral* limb may indicate anterior SID (37). Conversely, relief of anterior SI dysfunction pain may occur with SLR of the limb on the affected side. However, in this instance, if there is an increase in localized symptoms associated with SLR in the tested limb, a possible posterior SI dysfunction exists because the involved innominate is moving in the posterior direction. As with any SLR maneuver, the examiner must differentiate the induced symptoms from lumbar or hip pathology. An increase in symptoms during neck flexion accompanying a straight leg raise would be attributed to a dural stretch

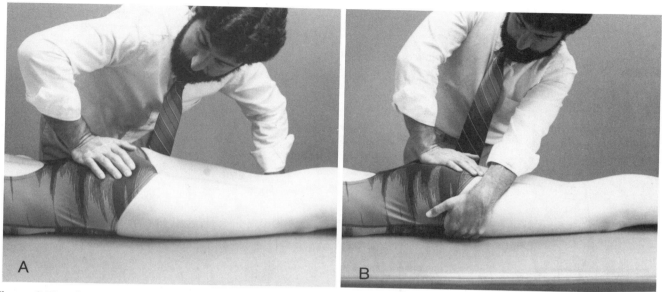

Figure 3.73. Posterior-anterior sacral glide: if anterior pressure over the sacrum and/or the recoil after pressure is released reproduces a patient's SI joint symptoms, the test is positive, implicating SI joint dysfunction which is aggravated by posterior/anterior glide. *A,* Demonstrates stress over upper sacrum. *B,* Demonstrates stress over lower sacrum with stabilization at anterior hip.

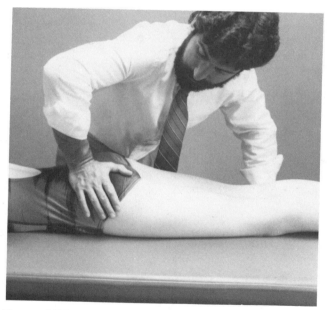

Figure 3.74. Posterior-anterior lateral sacral glide: if anterior pressure over the lateral aspect of the sacrum and/or recoil after pressure is released reproduces a patient's SI joint symptoms, the test is positive, implicating SI joint dysfunction which is aggravated by lateral stress.

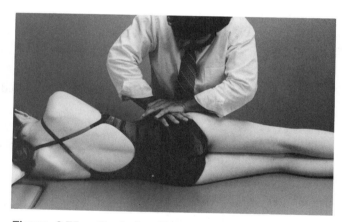

Figure 3.75. Posterior SI joint distraction test: if a compression force on the innominate while the patient is side lying reproduces pain or sumptoms of the SI joint, the test is positive, implicating SI joint dysfunction such as posterior ligament tear.

4. Neurological Evaluation

   a. Key muscle (strength graded 0–5)

   R ___ L ___ L5 = extensor hallicus longus muscle

   R ___ L ___ S1,2 = gastrocsoleus muscle

   b. Key reflexes (graded +1 through +3)

   R ___ L ___ S1 = Achilles' tendon

   c. Sensibility

   Key: lacking A = light touch sensation
                     B = sharp/dull discrimination
                     C = temperature discrimination
                     D = proprioception

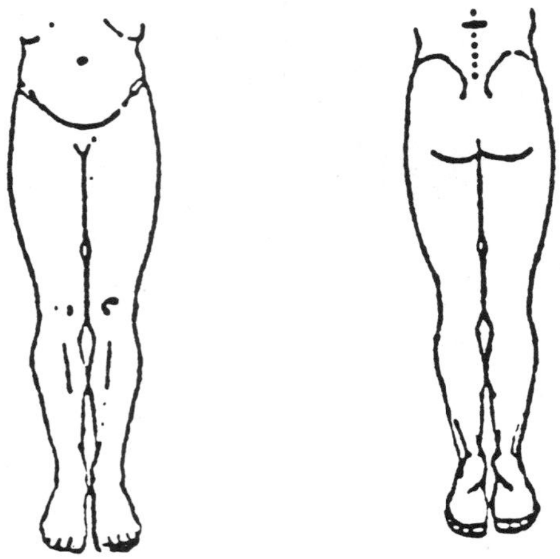

   d. Motor control: spastic _____ flaccid _____ rigid _____ clonic _____

   e. Coordination

   Heel of foot to contralateral knee _____

   Stepping in place _____

   Walking, crossing one foot in front of the other

   key: C = completes task
                completes task with
           D = difficulty or discomfort
                Not able to complete
           N = task

5. Recommendation of other tests

   a. Radiology _____

   b. Laboratory _____

   c. Electrodiagnostic _____

   d. Arthroscopy _____

   e. CAT Scan _____

   f. Myelogram _____

   g. Punctures _____

   h. Other _____

Figure 3.76. SI examination form part 5: Neurologic evaluation and recommendation of other tests.

rather than to the SI joint. The use of hip flexion with knee flexion will affect the SI joint but will not involve the lower lumbar nerve roots. Placing the patient in side-lying position and turning the pelvis with palmar contacts on the ASIS and ischium will allow movement of the SI joint without affecting the hip (Fig. 3.71).

Accessory Movement and Special Tests. Accessory movement is fairly limited in a normal SI joint. However, mobility testing can assist a determination of what motion(s) increase or decrease symptoms, and may identify the presence of ligamentous instability or joint locking. The therapist may evaluate accessory movement using the same techniques described for special tests in the following paragraph.

The therapist performs special tests to further localize the site of pathology. Some suggest the Fabere, Gaenslen (19), and Lasègue (42) tests for evaluation of SID. However, these tests in isolation yield ambiguous clinical results because they move more than one joint, i.e., hip, lumbar spine, and the SI joint. Consequently, the reliability of many SI tests is poor (43). In order to reduce ambiguity, the special tests included in this examination form focus primarily on the SI joint (Fig. 3.70). In order for a test to be positive, symptoms should be reproduced in rhythm with the therapist oscillating movement.

Anterior distraction, or a "pelvic rock" test, assesses anterior ligamentous pathology. The patient lies supine for this test, as the therapist applies pressure with his arms crossed and palms over the ASIS (Fig. 3.72). He monitors mobility as well as any change in symptoms. He can also stress the anterior ligaments in the prone position by applying downward pressure over the sacrum (Fig. 3.73). In order to differentiate origin of symptoms from L5-S1, he should apply pressure centrally as well as laterally over the SI joint proper (Fig. 3.74).

Pelvic compression in side-lying position stresses the posterior ligaments. The therapist applies downward pressure with palmar contacts placed on the lateral aspect of the innominate bone (Fig. 3.75). A change in the symptoms may indicate posterior SI dysfunction. Caudal glide may also elicit symptoms of SI dysfunction (Fig. 3.69).

Neurologic Evaluation. Alterations in key muscles or the Achilles' tendon reflex may give clues to nerve root compression or irritation at the low lumbar or high sacral level (Fig. 3.76).

SACROILIAC JOINT MOBILIZATION

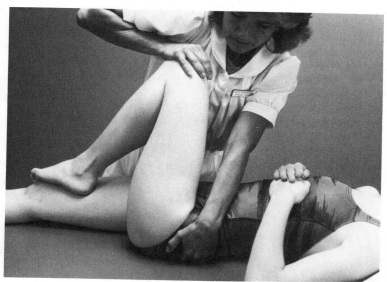

Figure 3.77. SI gapping; posterior innominate rotation (supine).
Patient position: Supine with hip flexed 100° and abducted knee flexed.
Therapist position: Standing on opposite side; S hand around ilium with fingers at PSIS; M hand grasps patient's knee with body resting over hand.
Technique: Use body weight through femur in direction of umbilicus to rotate innominate posteriorly. Oscillate to palpate SI gapping and accessory movement.
Comments: Effective for correcting anterior SID, or for assessing SI movement.

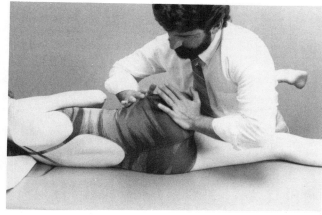

Figure 3.78. Posterior innominate rotation (side lying).
Patient position: Side lying with pillow supporting head.
Therapist position: Standing facing patient, between patient's legs in order to use uppermost leg to facilitate innominate rotation; hands grasp pelvis with palmar contacts over anterior iliac crest and ischial tuberosity.
Technique: Apply posterior rotary force through palms with forearms parallel to direction of force.
Comments: Effective for correcting anterior SID.

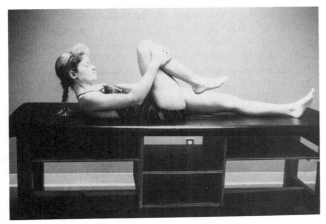

Figure 3.79.   Posterior innominate rotation (supine self-mobilization).

Patient position: Lying supine, pulling involved knee to chest.

Therapist position: Not applicable.

Technique: Patient pulls knee to chest bringing upper back off mat; sustains stretch for several seconds and then slowly releases.

Comments: Patient can oscillate unilateral SI joint during leg pull to ease any pain/symptoms associated with restoring innominate position/mobility. Effective for correcting anterior SID.

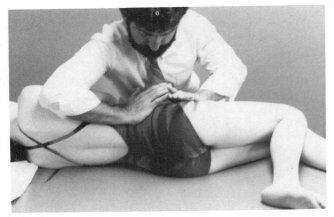

Figure 3.81.   Anterior innominate rotation. ⬆

Patient position: Side lying with pillow supporting head.

Therapist position: Standing facing patient; hands grasp pelvis with palmar contacts over posterior iliac crest and groin.

Technique: Apply anterior rotary force through palms with forearms parallel to direction of force.

Comments: Effective for correcting posterior SID.

Figure 3.82.   Anterior innominate rotation, through hip extension with patient prone. ➤

Patient position: Prone with opposite leg fixed on table.

Therapist position: Standing facing patient; S hand over opposite iliac crest; M hand grasps distal femur while forearm cradles patient's flexed knee.

Technique: Press ilium anteriorly with S hand while extending hip with M hand to rotate ilium anteriorly.

Comments: Effective for correcting posterior SID.

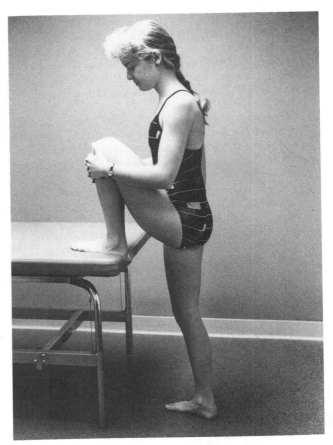

Figure 3.80.   Posterior innominate rotation (standing self-mobilization).

Patient position: Standing with foot flat on table. Hip and knee are fully flexed.

Therapist position: Not applicable.

Technique: Patient shifts weight forward onto flexed leg and uses arms to pull knee to chest; sustains stretch for several seconds and then slowly releases.

Comments: Patient can oscillate unilateral SI joint during weight shift and leg pull to ease any pain/symptoms associated with restoring innominate position/mobility. Effective correction of anterior SID.

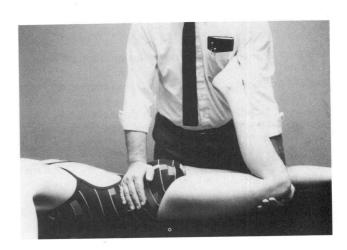

Recommendation of Other Tests. Other tests, such as x-rays, are helpful to verify osteoarthritis, spondylitis, or spondylolisthesis, but may not be adequate for detecting subtle changes in sacral angulation.

References

1. Moore KL: *Before We Are Born,* ed 2. Philadelphia, WB Saunders, 1983.
2. Fitzgerald MJT: *Human Embryology.* New York, Harper & Row, 1978.
3. Warwick R, Williams PL: *Gray's Anatomy,* British 35 ed. Philadelphia, WB Saunders, 1973.
4. Harrison RG: *Clinical Embryology.* New York, Academic Press, 1978.
5. Finneson BE: *Low Back Pain,* ed 2. Philadelphia, JB Lippincott, 1980.
6. Kapandji IA: *The Physiology of the Joints.* Edinburgh, Churchill Livingstone, 1974, vol 3.
7. Ramamurti CP: *Orthopaedics in Primary Care.* Tinker V (ed). Baltimore, Williams & Wilkins, 1979.
8. Bogduk N: The innervation of the lumbar spine. *Spine* 8:286–293, 1983.
9. Fisk JW: *The Painful Neck and Back.* Springfield, IL, Charles C Thomas, 1977.
10. Grieve GP: *Common Vertebral Joint Problems.* New York, Churchill Livingstone, 1981.
11. Cailliet R: *Low Back Pain Syndrome,* ed 2. Philadelphia, FA Davis, 1968.
12. Lockart RD, Hamilton GF, Fyfe FW: *Anatomy of the Human Body.* Philadelphia, JB Lippincott, 1965.
13. Kessler RM: Acute symptomatic disc prolapse. *Phys Ther* 59(8):978–984, 1979.
14. Farfan HF, Gracovetsky S: The nature of instability. *Spine* 9:714–719, 1984.
15. McKenzie RA: *The Lumbar Spine: Mechanical Diagnosis and Therapy.* Wellington, NZ, Spinal Publications, 1981.
16. White AA, Panjabi MM: *Clinical Biomechanics of the Spine.* Philadelphia, JB Lippincott, 1978.
17. Cyriax JH: *Textbook of Orthopaedic Medicine.* East Sussex, England, Baillière-Tindall, 1982.
18. Macnab I: *Backache.* Baltimore, Williams & Wilkins, 1977.
19. Hoppenfeld S: *Physical Examination of the Spine and Extremities.* East Norwalk, CT, Appleton-Century-Crofts, 1976.
20. Farfan HF: Scientific basis of manipulative procedures. *Clinics in Rheumatic Disease* 6:159–177, 1980.
21. Dillane JB, Fry J, Kalton G: Acute back syndrome: A study from general practice. *Brit Med J* 2:82–84, 1966.
22. Kelsey JL, White AA: Epidemiology and impact of low back pain. *Spine* 5:133–142, 1980.
23. Porter RW, Miller CG: Back pain and trunk list. *Spine* 11:596–600, 1986.
24. Raskin MM, Martinez-Lopez M, Sheldon JJ: Lumbar thermography in discogenic disease. *Radiology* 119:149–152, 1976.
25. Maitland GD: *Vertebral Manipulation,* ed 2. Kent, England, Butterworth, 1977.
26. Saunders HD: *Evaluation, Treatment, and Prevention of Musculoskeletal Disorders.* Minneapolis, MN, Viking Press, 1985, pp 257–284.
27. Bellamy N, Paru W, Rodney PJ: What do we know about the sacroiliac joint? *Semin Arthritis Rheum* 12:282–313, 1983.
28. Grieve EFM: Mechanical dysfunction of the sacro-iliac joint. *Int Rehabil Med* 5:46–52, 1983.
29. Stoddard A: Conditions of the sacroiliac joints and their treatment. *Physiotherapy* 44:97–101, 1958.
30. Hagen R: Pelvic girdle relaxation from an orthopedic point of view. *Acta Orthop Scand* 45:550–563, 1974.
31. Butler JM: Short leg backache. *Lancet* 66:10–11, 1946.
32. Brown LT: The mechanics of the lumbosacral and sacro-iliac joints. *J Bone Jt Surg* 19A:770–775, 1937.
33. Bird HA, Calcuneri M, Wright V: Changes in joint laxity occurring during pregnancy. *Ann Rheum Dis* 40:209–212, 1981.
34. Golightly R: Pelvic arthropathy in pregnancy and the puerperium. *Physiotherapy* 68:216–220, 1982.
35. Calin A: Ankylosing spondylitis. *Clin Rheum Dis* 11:41–60, 1985.
36. Smith-Petersen NM: Clinical diagnosis of common sacro-iliac conditions. *Am J Rotengenol* 12:546, 1924.
37. Mennell JM: *Back Pain: Diagnosis and Treatment Using Manipulative Techniques.* Boston, Little, Brown & Co, 1960.
38. Walker JM: Age-related differences in the human sacroiliac joint: A histological study; implications for therapy. *J Orthop Sports Phys Ther* 7:325–334, 1986.
39. Porterfield JA: A new innovation in sacroiliac management. *Bull Orthop Section APTA* 3:17–18, 1978.
40. Don Tigny RL: Dysfunction of the sacroiliac joint and its treatment. *J Orthop Sports Phys Ther* 1:23–35, 1979.
41. Fraser DM: Postpartum backache: A preventable condition? *Bull Orthop Section APTA* 3:14–16, 1978.
42. Don Tigny RL: Function and pathomechanics of the sacroiliac joint. *Phys Ther* 65(1):35–44, 1985.
43. Patter NA, Rothstein JM: Intertester reliability for selected clinical tests of the sacroiliac joint. *Phys Ther* 65:1671–1675, 1985.

Suggested Readings

Course Notes, Graduate Diploma in Manipulative Therapy, Western Australian Institute of Technology, Perth, Western Australia, 1982.
Edwards BC: Combined movements in the cervical spine (C2–7), their value in examination and technique choice. *Australian Journal of Physiotherapy* 26:165–171, 1980.
Elvey RL: Brachial plexus tension tests and the pathoanatomical origin of arm pain. In Glasgow EF, Twomey LT, Scull ER, et al. (eds): *Aspects of Manipulative Therapy,* ed 2. New York, Churchill Livingstone, 1985, pp 116–122.
Maitland GD: Palpation examination of the posterior cervical spine: The ideal, average and abnormal. *Australian Journal of Physiotherapy* 28:3–12, 1982.
Maitland GD: *Vertebral Manipulation,* ed 5. Stoneham, MA, Butterworth, 1986.

CHAPTER 4

THE SHOULDER

CLINICAL ANATOMY AND MECHANICS OF THE SHOULDER GIRDLE

Three bones, four joints, associated ligaments, and muscles comprise the shoulder girdle, a unit that links the upper limb to the trunk while permitting innumerable positions of the limb. The shoulder's major role is to place the hand in a functional position. Freedom of motion and synergy of muscle action facilitate accomplishing this task.

Osteology

Clavicle. The clavicle, serving as a strut, maintains the lateral projection of the shoulder, allowing the arm to swing clear of the chest wall (Fig. 4.1). Absence of the clavicle doesn't cause the shoulder to actually "collapse," but does permit exaggerated approximation toward the opposite side (1). The clavicle provides a continuous base for insertion of trunk musculature and for origin of arm musculature. It also furnishes protection for major nerves and blood vessels.

The clavicle is S-shaped: its medial two-thirds is convex anteriorly, and its lateral one-third is concave anteriorly. This configuration resembles a crankshaft, allowing greater range of motion on the outer end during long axis rotation that is essential to arm elevation described later. The additional motion occurring at the outer end, however, may account for the fact that a greater incidence of degenerative changes occurs at the acromioclavicular joint than at the sternoclavicular joint (1). The medial curve creates a space for the internal jugular vein, the subclavian artery and vein, and the brachial plexus. The clavicular curves confer elasticity and absorb shock from a direct fall upon the shoulder or an indirect force transmitted through the humerus. The junction between the curves is the weakest part of the bone and the most common site of fractures in the body (2, 3).

The clavicle runs obliquely in a posterolateral direction, forming a 30° angle with the frontal plane, and a 60° angle with the scapula (Fig. 4.1). Its upper surface is smooth and palpable throughout its length, whereas its lower surface is roughened in areas of ligamentous and muscular attachments.

Scapula. The scapula, a flat triangular bone, occupies the posterolateral chest wall between the 2nd and 7th ribs. Muscles attach it to the chest wall in what is termed the "scapulothoracic articulation." Its lateral border does not rest on the ribs, but projects outward to form the axilla.

The subscapular fossa occupies the anterior surface of the scapula. The scapular spine divides the posterior surface into the supraspinatus and infraspinatus fossae. The spine provides excellent leverage for the trapezius muscle, which inserts along its upper border, and the deltoid muscle, which originates along its lower border. The scapular spine's lateral projection, the acromion, forms the tip of the shoulder and articulates with the clavicle in a synovial joint (Fig. 4.1). The coracoid process projects anteriorly from the upper border of the scapula. This process is the site of origin for the short head of the biceps brachii and coracobrachialis muscles, of insertion for the pectoralis minor muscle, and the point of attachment for ligaments, to be described later. The projections of the acromion and the coracoid process protect the glenohumeral joint and prevent upward displacement of the humeral head.

The glenoid fossa, a pear-shaped cavity that is wider inferiorly, lies on the lateral side of the scapula, inferior to the acromion. The plane of the glenoid fossa is 30° anterior to the scapula and is directed slightly inferior when the arm rests at the side. This fossa provides a shallow base for articulation with the humerus. During abduction, the humeral head moves inferiorly into the wider area, preventing impingement by the overhanging coracoacromial arch.

Humerus. The humerus typifies a long bone, being comprised of a shaft and expanded, specialized ends. Its proximal head resembles about ⅓ of an irregular sphere, and is covered with articular cartilage. The surface area of the head is two to three times greater than the glenoid fossa with which it articulates. The humeral head is retroverted 20° and inclined 130–150° relative to the shaft; a therapist should take this anatomical feature into account when designing an exercise program (1, 4).

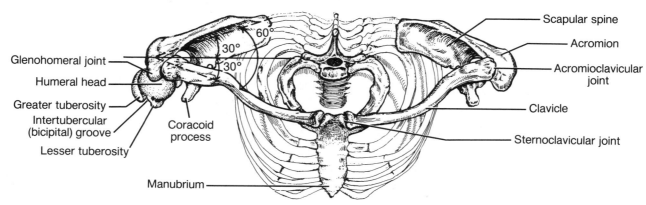

Figure 4.1. Bones of the shoulder girdle.

The anatomical neck of the humerus is a slight constriction located just distal to the head. It designates the margin between the head and the greater and lesser tuberosities. The greater tuberosity, located laterally on the upper humerus, produces the rounded surface contour of the shoulder; the lesser tuberosity occupies the anterior surface of the upper humerus (Fig. 4.1). Between the tuberosities lies the intertubercular sulcus (bicipital groove), which contains the long head of the biceps (LHB) tendon. The humeral shaft narrows just distal to the tuberosities, an area referred to as the surgical neck because of its high incidence of fractures.

Arthrology

Glenohumeral (GH) Joint. The GH joint is a ball-and-socket joint with three degrees of freedom. Normal passive ROM for the GH joint is listed in Table 4.1.

Circumduction occurs when these motions are combined. This joint acquires mobility at the expense of stability, however, giving it the dubious distinction of being the most frequently dislocated joint in the body (3). The relative sizes of the humeral head and the glenoid fossa dictate that only ⅓ of the humerus contacts the glenoid fossa at one time; the fossa therefore represents a base, rather than a receptacle, against which the convex head can be stabilized (3). The shallowness of the glenoid fossa and the ligamentous laxity of this joint allow for a wide range of accessory movements in addition to the physiologic movements noted previously. In the loose-packed position of 45–65° abduction and 45° flexion, the articular surfaces can be separated about 3 cm (3, 5). In contrast, full abduction and external rotation of the humerus pro-

duce the close-packed position in which there is minimal accessory movement (4, 6).

The GH joint depends primarily on nonosseous structures (i.e., capsule, ligaments, and muscles) for its limited stability. The joint capsule arises from the circumference of the glenoid fossa just proximal to the labrum, and inserts into the anatomical neck of the humerus (Fig. 4.2). Anteriorly, the capsule is prolonged into a sheath for the LHB tendon, rendering the tendon intracapsular but extrasynovial (7). The capsule is continuous with the subscapularis bursa anteriorly. The inferior aspect of the capsule is very loose and redundant when the arm is adducted, but stretches significantly to accommodate abduction. This large pouch of redundant tissue is termed the inferior joint recess, and is commonly obliterated in frozen shoulder (8).

Three thickenings, the superior, middle, and inferior glenohumeral ligaments, reinforce the capsule anteriorly. They arise from the superior-medial margin of the glenoid fossa, and run laterally and inferiorly to attach to the anterior humerus (Fig. 4.2). Between these bands lie two points of weakness—the foramen of Weitbrecht, opening into the subscapularis bursa between the superior and middle GH ligaments (7, 9); and the foramen of Rouviere through which the synovial cavity can communicate with the subcoracoid bursa (9). Lateral rotation tenses up all three ligaments; abduction tenses only the middle and inferior.

The coracohumeral ligament, the rotator cuff, and the LHB tendon contribute the most to GH joint stability (2). The coracohumeral ligament originates on the coracoid process and inserts into the greater tuberosity and capsule (Fig. 4.2). Its location between the supraspinatus and subscapularis tendons provides anterior superior reinforcement to the joint and contributes to vertical stability of the humeral head. Four short muscles arising from the scapula and inserting on the humerus by broad flat tendons which fuse with the fibrous capsule of the GH joint comprise the rotator cuff (1, 10). They serve as "active ligaments," reinforcing the anterior, superior, and posterior aspects of the joint capsule. The LHB tendon arises from the supraglenoid tubercle, where it is continuous with the

Table 4.1.
Passive ROM at the GH Joint[a]

Flexion	120°	Adduction	45°
Extension	55°	Medial rotation	90°
Abduction	120°	Lateral rotation	90°

[a]Does not include scapular nor clavicular movement, which add to the total range of shoulder motion.

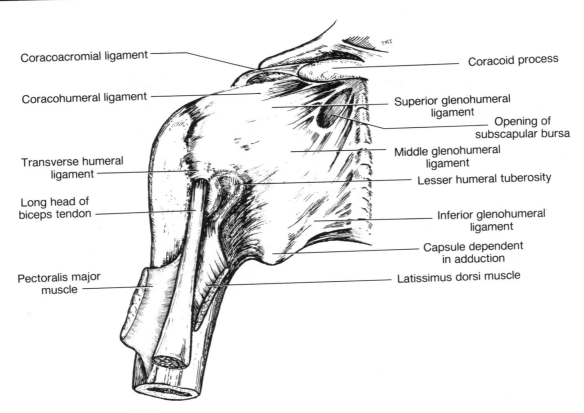

Coracoacromial ligament

Coracohumeral ligament

Transverse humeral ligament

Long head of biceps tendon

Pectoralis major muscle

Coracoid process

Superior glenohumeral ligament

Opening of subscapular bursa

Middle glenohumeral ligament

Lesser humeral tuberosity

Inferior glenohumeral ligament

Capsule dependent in adduction

Latissimus dorsi muscle

Figure 4.2.   The glenohumeral joint.

labrum, and runs within the capsule until it emerges to lie in the intertubercular groove, ensheathed in synovium (Fig. 4.2). Biceps brachii muscle contraction or shoulder movement does not displace this tendon; rather the humerus moves on the fixed tendon. When the LHB tendon is taut, it acts to prevent upward displacement of the humeral head (1). The transverse humeral ligament runs between the tuberosities and serves as a retinaculum for the LHB tendon (Figs. 4.2 and 4.3).

A ring of fibrocartilage attached to the margin of the glenoid fossa forms the glenoid labrum. It deepens the fossa, enhances GH joint stability, and improves the congruency of the articular surfaces (3, 9). When traumatic shoulder dislocations tear the labrum, subsequent instability often results (11).

The subacromial bursa (which includes the subdeltoid bursa) lies between the coracoacromial arch and the supraspinatus tendon (Fig. 4.3). It cushions the supraspinatus tendon and the greater tuberosity of the humerus inferiorly from pressure against the arch superiorly when the arm is elevated. If this bursa becomes irritated and inflamed, the resulting pain and thickening may block abduction. Normally, the bursa does not communicate with the joint cavity, but attrition or rupture of the rotator cuff and capsule will join the two spaces.

Other bursae in the shoulder region include: the subscapularis bursa, separating the scapula from the subscapularis tendon; the subcoracoid bursa, separating the subscapularis tendon from the coracoid pro-

cess; the infraspinatus bursa, separating the joint capsule from the infraspinatus tendon; and the superficial acromial bursa, separating the acromion from the skin.

Acromioclavicular (AC) Joint.   The AC joint, between the lateral end of the clavicle and the acromium, is a plane joint. It permits movement of the scapula in three planes: about a vertical axis to allow the vertebral border to separate from the chest wall (winging); about an A-P axis to allow protraction and retraction; and about a frontal axis to allow the inferior angle of the scapula to tilt away from the chest wall in shoulder shrugging (5, 11). Perhaps the most important function of the AC joint is to allow scapular movement to be enhanced by movement of the SC joint: the 30° of axial rotation occurring at the AC joint combines with approximately 30° of elevation at the SC joint to allow the scapula to effectively rotate through 60°. Maximal AC joint motion occurs after 90° of abduction, so noting the range at which the onset of pain occurs is helpful in identifying AC joint lesions.

The concave acromial facet faces anteriorly, medially, and superiorly, whereas the convex clavicular surface faces posteriorly, laterally, and inferiorly. This orientation explains the fact that the clavicle usually overrides the acromium in dislocations of this joint. A disc is often found in the AC joint, but varies in extent among individuals and undergoes thinning with age (11).

A weak joint capsule surrounds the AC joint. The acromioclavicular ligament reinforces the joint capsule (Fig. 4.3). The main suspensory ligament of the upper

Acromioclavicular ligament (covers acromioclavicular joint)

Coracoacromial ligament

Trapezoid ligament

Conoid ligament } Coracoclavicular ligament

Subacromial (subdeltoid) bursa

Synovial capsule of glenohumeral joint

Transverse humeral ligament

Long head of biceps tendon

Coracoid process

Subscapularis bursa

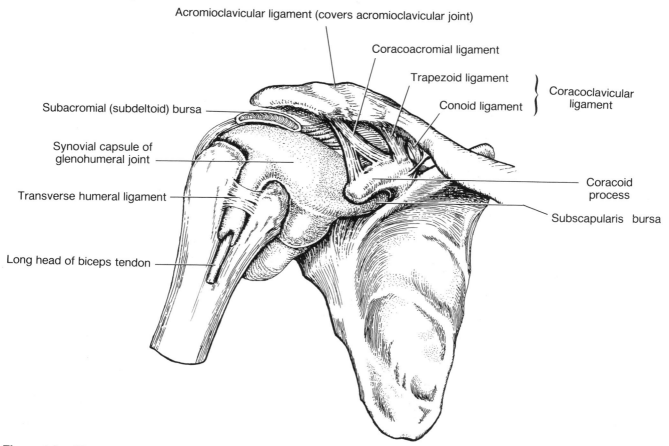

Figure 4.3. The acromioclavicular joint and coracoacromial arch.

extremity, the coracoclavicular ligament, enhances lateral stability of the clavicle (1). This ligament is divided into two portions: the trapezoid ligament anterolaterally and the conoid ligament posteromedially (Fig. 4.3). A fall on the tip of the shoulder which forces the scapula inferiorly and dislocates the AC joint may rupture these ligaments. A fall on the outstretched arm in which the force from the ground is transmitted up through the humerus, displacing the acromion superiorly relative to the clavicle may also dislocate the AC joint; in this case the coracoclavicular ligament is compressed rather than stretched, and is not disrupted.

Clinically, the most significant structure in this area is the coracoacromial arch. Comprised of the coracoacromial ligament attached between the acromion and the coracoid process, it forms a roof over the supraspinatus muscle and the humeral head (Fig. 4.3). It prevents upward dislocation of the humerus, but is actually not essential to stability if the other ligaments are intact (2). The coracoacromial arch is often associated with an impingement syndrome, in which the superior GH joint capsule, subacromial bursa, LHB tendon, or supraspinatus tendon may be compressed within the unyielding space between the arch and the humeral head. The potential for impingement occurs between 80–120° of elevation, when the greater tub-

erosity must pass beneath the arch. Impingement occurs if the space beneath the arch is restricted or component movements (caudal glide of the humeral head, lateral humeral rotation during abduction, medial humeral rotation during adduction) are prevented. Irritation from impingement can cause inflammation, attrition, degeneration, calcific deposits, and rupture, with major implications for shoulder function.

Sternoclavicular (SC) Joint. The articulation of the clavicle with the manubrium and first costal cartilage defines the SC joint, the only direct attachment of the upper extremity to the axial skeleton (Fig. 4.4). The sternocostal joint surface is saddle-shaped, and the clavicle is reciprocally shaped, but flatter (9). A disc improves the congruency of the joint surfaces and acts as a shock absorber.

Although technically saddle joints allow movement in two planes, the SC joint resembles a ball-and-socket joint with movement in three planes (12). Elevation (45°) and depression (5°) occur in the frontal plane, in which the convex clavicle moves upon the concave sternum (5). Protraction (15°) and retraction (15°) occur in the horizontal plane in which the concave clavicle moves on the convex sternum (5). Axial rotation (50°) occurs in a sagittal plane (5, 13).

Approximately 30° of angulation of the SC joint occurs during elevation of the arm to 90°; for every 10°

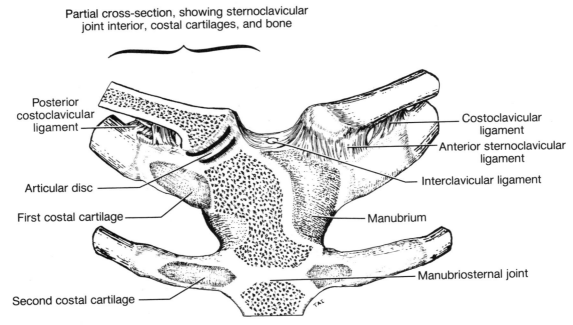

Partial cross-section, showing sternoclavicular
joint interior, costal cartilages, and bone

Posterior
costoclavicular
ligament

Articular disc

First costal cartilage

Second costal cartilage

Costoclavicular
ligament

Anterior sternoclavicular
ligament

Interclavicular ligament

Manubrium

Manubriosternal joint

Figure 4.4.   The sternoclavicular joint.

of arm elevation there is a 4° of SC elevation (5, 13). After 90° of elevation, clavicular angulation is negligible (13). The crank-like action produced by rotation of the S-shaped clavicle provides an additional 30° elevation, as the clavicle accompanies the scapula through 60° of movement. Limited rotation of the clavicle on its long axis hinders arm elevation.

The anterior and posterior sternoclavicular ligaments reinforce the loose fibrous capsule of the SC joint (Fig. 4.4). The interclavicular ligament connects the clavicles to one another (Fig. 4.4). The costoclavicular ligament joins the clavicle and the 1st costal cartilage (Fig. 4.4). Its strength imparts stability to the clavicle while acting as a fulcrum for all motions of the shoulder girdle. It limits excessive protraction and elevation.

Scapulothoracic (ST) Joint.   The ST articulation is described as a physiologic joint, as it allows movement but is not bounded by a fibrous capsule and synovial membrane. The scapula glides on the rib cage, from which it is separated by muscles and bursae. The range of scapular elevation and depression is 10–20 cm, protraction and retraction is 15 cm, and rotation is 60°.

Mechanics

Of the numerous muscles in the shoulder region, some connect the girdle with the trunk, some connect the girdle with the humerus, and others connect the humerus with the trunk. They are all ultimately involved in the stability and mobility of the humerus. A thorough review of their origins, insertions, and actions is recommended, but due to comprehensive coverage elsewhere (3), it is not included in this text.

The following paragraphs describe selected kinesiologic concepts relating to shoulder function and impairment.

Scapulohumeral Rhythm.   E.A. Codman coined the term "scapulohumeral rhythm" to describe the integrated movement of all joints in the shoulder girdle during elevation of the arm. The classic work of Inman et al. reports that during the first 60° of flexion or 30° of abduction the scapula seeks a stable position on the thorax; thereafter, a ratio of 2° of GH movement for every one degree of ST movement occurs (14). Thus, each 15° of arm abduction results from 10° of GH joint abduction and 5° of ST rotation; at 180° arm abduction, there is 120° GH abduction and 60° scapula rotation (Fig. 4.5) (14). Rotation of the scapula during abduction lends mechanical stability to the shoulder by bringing the glenoid fossa directly under the humeral head, and it increases the efficiency of the deltoid muscle by placing it on stretch (13). Arm abduction also requires clavicular motion. For every 10° of arm abduction, the clavicle elevates 4°, up to 90° of arm abduction; thereafter, the crank-shaped clavicle rotates, to accompany the scapula through its full 60° of motion (Fig. 4.5) (7).

The total range of scapular rotation is 60°, so theoretically this would be the extent of abduction if GH joint motion were blocked. Likewise, the total range of GH abduction is 120°, which would be the extent of **passive** abduction in the absence of scapular movement. Scapular restriction limits **active** abduction to 90° by preventing stretch and subsequent increased efficiency of the deltoid (5, 12, 13). The humerus must rotate laterally during abduction in order to permit the greater tuberosity to pass under the acromium and the coracoacromial ligament. To permit clearance during flexion, the humerus must rotate medially (14).

Forces Affecting the Shoulder Girdle. Inmann et al. state that three forces are required to establish equilibrium at the GH joint in any position of the arm (14). The first is the weight of the extremity, acting at the center of gravity of the limb; the second is the abducting musculature (primarily deltoid); the third is the result of the former two, acting in a direction opposite the deltoid. This last force is the resultant of pressure and friction of the humeral head, plus the inferior pull of the rotator cuff muscles. The actions of the deltoid and the rotator cuff muscles combine to produce a force couple, i.e., two equal forces acting in opposite directions to rotate a part about its axis. The superior, lateral force of the deltoid muscle balances the inferior, medial force of the rotator cuff muscles during abduction of the arm (Fig. 4.5). Both

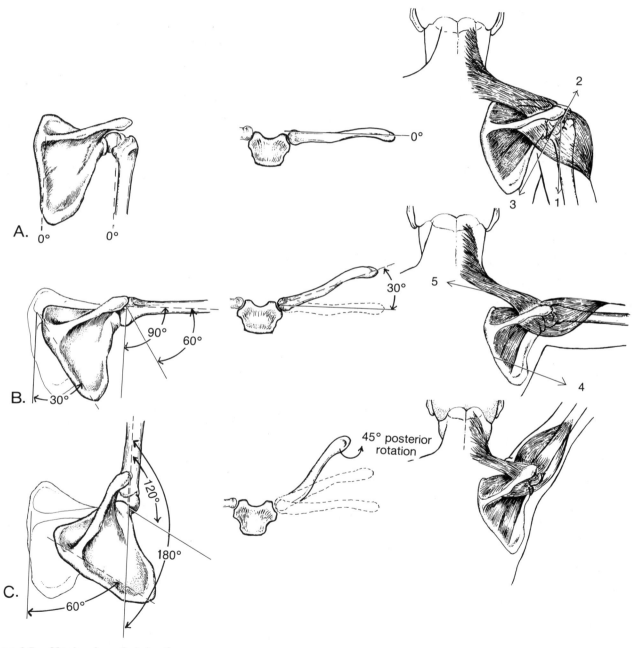

Figure 4.5. Mechanics of abduction.
A, Shoulder at 0° abduction, with scapula, humerus, and clavicle in neutral positions; the weight of the extremity (1) is balanced by a force couple comprised of the deltoid muscle (2) and rotator cuff muscles plus the pressure and friction of the humeral head (3). *B,* Shoulder at 90° abduction, with 30° scapular rotation and 60° humeral abduction; clavicle elevates 30°; serratus anterior muscle (4) and upper trapezius muscle (5) force couples balance and rotate scapula. *C,* Shoulder at 180° abduction, with 60° scapular rotation, and 120° humeral abduction; clavicle rotates 45° to reach an additional 30° elevation.

the deltoid and supraspinatus muscles act together throughout the entire ROM (14).

Acting alone, the deltoid muscle elevates the humerous against the coracoacromial arch; alone, the rotator cuff muscles depress the humeral head. Either alone can produce weak abduction, but such a disturbance in function may subject the joint to trauma and degenerative changes (10). At the beginning of abduction, the supraspinatus muscle is on stretch and maintains the humeral head against the glenoid, resisting the superior dislocating force of the deltoid. The downward (short rotator) force is maximal at 60° abduction (13, 14). As the arm is elevated, the deltoid muscle becomes more efficient, because its line of force changes from a position parallel to the humerus to near perpendicular. Deltoid muscle force becomes maximal at 90°, and as elevation continues, all forces progressively decline (5, 13, 14).

Inman et al. also state that three forces participate in scapular rotation (14). The first acts in a superior direction to counteract the weight of the shoulder girdle; the second acts on the inferior angles of the scapula in an anterolateral direction; the third acts on the acromion in a medial direction. The active components of the second and third forces are represented by the serratus anterior and upper trapezius muscles, which function as a force couple to rotate the scapula (Fig. 4.5). The upper trapezius muscle also acts to support the weight of the extremity. The forces rotating the scapula reach their maximum at 90° abduction (14).

The biceps mechanism is another means, although weaker, of abducting the arm. The LHB tendon crosses the humeral head at a right angle; rotating the arm 90° laterally brings the tendon into alignment with the muscle belly. Here it acts as a pulley by producing a horizontal force on the arm, while preventing upward displacement of the humeral head.

Neurology

Brachial Plexus. The anterior rami of C5,6,7,8,T1 pass between the scalenus anticus and scalenus medius muscles, and form the brachial plexus. They cross over the 1st rib, and behind the middle ⅓ of the clavicle, to enter the axilla and supply the upper limb. One can palpate the brachial plexus against the humeral head when the arm is abducted.

Motor innervation of the muscles of the shoulder girdle and sensory innervation of the shoulder girdle are listed in Table 4.2.

Structures of the shoulder, with the exception of the AC joint, are developmentally related to the 5th cervical segment; therefore, shoulder pathology may refer pain and sensory changes through the C5 dermatome. The AC joint develops with the 4th cervical segment; pathology of this joint produces localized pain.

Angiology

The axillary artery traverses the axilla, surrounded by the brachial plexus nerves and veins. The branches of this artery anastomose with each other and with

scapular arteries from the subclavian artery. The axillary artery becomes the brachial artery when it reaches the humerus.

Its four branches which supply the shoulder include: the thoracoacromial, which supplies the anterior region; the lateral thoracic, which supplies the medial chest wall; the subscapular, which supplies the posterior region; the anterior and posterior humeral circumflex, which supply the deltoid, shoulder joint, and humeral head.

Axillary Vein. The axillary vein is a continuation of the basilic vein, which becomes deep at the lower border of teres major; it ends at the outer border of the 1st rib, where it becomes the subclavian vein. It is joined by the cephalic vein just below the lateral clavicle.

SHOULDER GIRDLE EXAMINATION

History

The examiner initiates the history of a patient with suspected shoulder girdle dysfunction by obtaining identifying data (Fig. 4.6). He then requests a thorough description of symptoms, which may be depicted on a body chart and scales which indicate location, severity, impairment, and nature (Fig. 4.6).

A patient may occasionally be able to pinpoint his symptoms precisely, such as those arising from the AC or SC joints, which are characteristically localized. Often, however, shoulder lesions produce a vague reference of pain throughout the C5 dermatome. In other instances, a patient may experience pain proxi-

Table 4.2.
Motor innervation of the muscles of the shoulder girdle and sensory innervation of the shoulder and arm

Motor
  serratus anterior muscle—long thoracic nerve (C5,6,7)
  rhomboid muscle—dorsal scapular nerve (C5)
  levator scapula muscle—dorsal scapular nerve (C5)
  supraspinatus muscle—suprascapular nerve (C5,6)
  infraspinatus muscle—suprascapular nerve (C5,6)
  subclavicus muscle—nerve to the subclavicus (C5,6)
  pectoralis major muscle—medial and lateral pectoral nerve (C5,6,7,8,T1)
  pectoralis minor muscle—medial pectoral nerve (C8,T1)
  subscapularis muscle—subscapular nerve (C5,6)
  teres major muscle—subscapular nerve (C5,6)
  latissimus dorsi muscle—thoracodorsal nerve (C6,7,8)
  coracobrachialis muscle—musculocutaneous nerve (C5,6,7)
  biceps muscle—musculocutaneous nerve (C5,6,7)
  brachialis muscle—musculocutaneous nerve (C5,6,7)
  teres minor muscle—axillary nerve (C5,6)
  deltoid muscle—axillary nerve (C5,6)
  triceps muscle—radial nerve (C5,6,7,8,T1)

Sensory
  A-C joint—suprascapular nerve (C5,6)
  S-C joint—medial supraclavicular nerve (C3,4)
  G-H joint—suprascapular nerve (C5,6)
  G-H joint capsule—axillary nerve (C5,6)
  medial arm—medial cutaneous nerve of arm and forearm (C8,T1)
  lateral arm—upper lateral cutaneous nerve of arm and forearm (C5,6)
  posterior arm—posterior cutaneous nerve of arm and forearm (C5,6,7,8)

A. HISTORY

1. Identifying Data

Name _____ Age _____ Gender _____ Date _____

Provisional diagnosis _____ Precautions _____

Chief complaint _____

Dominant side R _____   L _____   Prior condition of involved part _____

2. Present Episode or Illness

a. Description of symptoms

1) location: //// = pain
             ==== = paresthesia
             ∘∘∘∘ = numbness
             xxxx = other _____

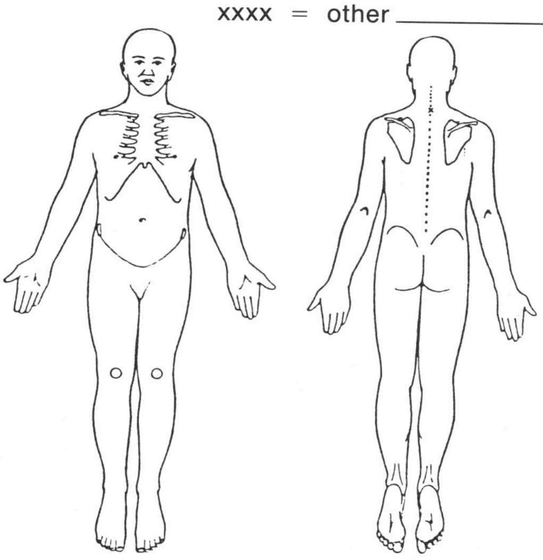

2) severity:

_____
none   worst

3) impairment:

_____
annoying   completely disabling

4) nature:

cramping _____ aching _____

shooting _____ burning _____

throbbing _____ tingling _____

stabbing _____ sore _____

other _____

5) behavior:

constant _____ intermittent _____ duration _____

occurs when _____ elicited by _____

aggravated by _____ relieved by _____

24-hour pattern _____

highly irritable _____ mildly irritable _____ not irritable _____

6) joint characteristics: catches _____ , locks _____ , swells _____ , gives way _____ , dislocates _____ ,

other _____

Figure 4.6. Examination form part 1: History.

mal to the shoulder, stemming from either cervical or shoulder structures. If the pain is accompanied by paresthesias or vascular disturbances, it is unlikely to be derived from the joints of the shoulder (1), but rather would be related to thoracic outlet or cervical pathology. The severity of pain may vary from mild (e.g., lesion which hurts only after activity) to moderate (e.g., lesion which hurts both during and after activity) to severe (e.g., lesion which hurts constantly) (15). The behavior of the symptoms, and factors related to their relief, assist a therapist in determining the irritability of the lesion and in planning the rest of the examination as well as treatment. Description of certain joint characteristics may also help to explain the lesion. For example, audible sounds in the GH joint may signify a loose body, labral defect, or other cartilage lesions (15).

The examiner asks for specifics regarding onset of the present illness or condition for which a patient seeks help. He notes treatment received, and the present status of the condition (Fig. 4.7). If an injury occurred, a patient should describe the date, nature,

b. Background and associated findings

Date of present injury _____ or onset _____ insidious _____

Dates of hospitalization _____ and/or other health care _____

Treatments; dates; results _____

_____

Status of condition: acute _____ or chronic _____

constant _____ or intermittent _____

better _____ or worse _____

Nature and mechanism of injury or events precipitating present episode _____

_____

Results of injury (if applicable): deformity (describe) _____

corrected _____ disability (type and cause) _____

loss of motion (specify) _____ when occurred _____

loss of strength (specify) _____ when occurred _____

swelling (specify) _____ when occurred _____

bleeding (specify) _____ when occurred _____

3. Relevant Past History and Family History

History of similar condition: dates _____ nature _____

_____

Treatment _____

Other relevant illnesses or disorders _____

General health status _____

Health problems of immediate family _____

4. Life-style

Occupation _____ ADL _____

Regular (3 times/week minimum) physical activities requiring: strength _____ agility _____ endurance _____

flexibility _____ other _____

What patient does to promote wellness _____

Patient's concept of cause of condition _____

Patient's concept of functional and/or cosmetic deficit(s) _____

Anticipated goals _____

5. Other

Current medications _____

Recent radiographs _____

6. Therapist's Interpretation and Plans for Objective Exam _____

_____

Figure 4.7.   Examination form part 2: History, continued.

and mechanism, including the position of the shoulder when it was struck or moved beyond its limit of motion. One should consider the force of a blow or fall because a force strong enough to produce a humeral fracture is likely to also traumatize one or more of the shoulder girdle joints, producing secondary complications (16).

A patient reports any deformity caused by the injury, and if and how it was corrected. Also, a patient portrays the extent and possible cause of the disability as he perceives it. For example, following AC joint subluxation, a patient may find movement across the midline difficult because the joint is unstable. The examiner requests a chronologic account of any loss of motion, loss of strength, swelling, or bleeding from the time of injury.

Many shoulder disorders have an insidious onset. Thus, the patient must attempt to recall when the condition began and if there were any precipitating factors. Overuse syndromes and degenerative changes are common at the shoulder, so one must be alert to minor repetitive stresses or environmental influences as etiologic factors.

The patient discusses his relevant past history, family history, lifestyle, and current medications with the examiner and provides recent radiographs (Fig 4.7). A review of the patient's general health status may identify a distant lesion which is referring symptoms to the shoulder. For example, diaphragmatic irritation secondary to gallbladder or hepatic disorders stimulates the phrenic nerve and may refer pain to the shoulder (17). A description of activities associated with occupation, or training habits relative to athletic participation, may reveal sources of repetitive trauma. For example, abduction, full flexion, and medial rotation of the shoulder during the crawl stroke commonly produces an impingement syndrome in swimmers (18). The examiner should also note what activities the patient has had to eliminate, secondary to the chief complaint (15, 17). After incorporating all of this information into the history, a therapist assesses the pertinent data and plans the physical examination.

Physical Examination

Inspection. The physical examination commences with inspection, which the superficial bony landmarks about the shoulder facilitate (Fig. 4.8). The therapist notes alignment of the axial skeleton, and the effects which deviations of the head, scoliosis, or kyphosis have on the shoulder girdle. He records the level of the shoulders and scapular alignment. Unilateral scapular elevation characterizes Sprengel's deformity. Severe drooping of the shoulder girdle is an etiologic factor in thoracic outlet syndrome (19, 20). Other alterations in alignment often indicate muscle imbalance, such as the winging associated with paralysis of the serratus anterior muscle. The therapist should carefully depict the general form and relations of the upper limb, girdle, and spine. Malalignment of clavicular or humeral fractures is one malady which can produce postural imbalance.

The examiner next describes changes in shape. Alterations in joint contour may occur following dislocation; anterior GH joint dislocation results in lateral prominence of the acromion, rendering a sharp angular outline to the shoulder; AC joint dislocation produces a step-off appearance between the clavicle and acromion. In addition to gross deformity accompanying some dislocations, localized swelling also characterizes AC and SC joint dislocation (1).

The location of swelling, masses, or atrophy often assists diagnosis. Subacromial bursitis produces a swelling laterally under the acromion. GH joint effusion is prominent anteriorly. Bulging of the biceps brachii muscle occurs after rupture of the LHB tendon. Atrophy of the spinati muscles, which is commonly associated with rotator cuff lesions, manifests as excessive prominence of the scapular spine. Deltoid muscle atrophy gives the shoulder a square appearance when viewed from the front.

The character and rhythm of movement during shoulder use often alert the examiner to a particular dysfunction. A patient with rotator cuff weakness or impingement initiates abduction by scapular elevation rather than humeral head depression, a reversal of scapulohumeral rhythm (Fig. 4.9) (1). Patients who lack GH joint motion, such as those with frozen shoulder or GH joint arthrodesis, also use shoulder hunching as a substitute mechanism. In contrast, patients who lack AC, SC, or ST joint motion demonstrate very little scapular rotation; abduction, which is weakened, is achieved only at the GH joint.

Inflammation, radiation treatment, surgery, etc., may produce visible skin changes. The examiner assesses a particular lesion in relation to the effect it may have on shoulder function. Lastly, he describes the characteristics and purpose of any slings, aids, etc., worn or used for the shoulder.

Palpation. The therapist first palpates the skin and subcutaneous tissues (Fig. 4.8). The superficial location of many structures around the shoulder girdle facilitates detection of signs of inflammation and adhesions. Next, he palpates the musculotendinous units, which are relatively easy to feel. He locates the supraspinatus muscle insertion over the greater tuberosity by having the patient medially rotate the arm to move the insertion anterior to the acromion. He palpates the infraspinatus muscle with the patient positioned prone on elbows with his forearm straight ahead; the therapist presses deeply behind the posterior border of the deltoid, below the acromion, to locate its insertion onto the greater tuberosity. He palpates the subscapularis muscle insertion on the lesser tuberosity with the arm laterally rotated. He may detect soft tissue crepitus in the above structures as a result of rotator cuff degeneration. He palpates the LHB tendon in the intertubercular sulcus; tenosynovitis may produce crepitus in this area. He palpates the subacromial bursa anterior to the acromion when the arm is extended; pain and swelling are indicative of bursitis.

Palpation of bone and joint structures may reproduce a patient's symptoms or reveal localized abnor-

B. PHYSICAL EXAMINATION

1. Inspection

   a. Posture

      neck and head alignment _____

      scoliosis _____ kyphosis _____

      shoulder level R _____ L _____ scapular alignment R _____ L _____

      general form & relations of upper limb—girdle & spine _____

      _____

   b. Shape

      GH joints R _____ L _____ SC joints R _____ L _____ AC joints R _____ L _____

      deformity (describe) _____ asymmetry _____

      swelling or masses _____ atrophy _____

   c. Use

      shoulder protected/use restricted _____

      handles clothing: independently _____ minimum assistance _____

                          maximum assistance _____

      movement: jerky _____ stiff _____ uncoordinated _____ limited by pain _____

   d. Skin

      color _____ condition _____ lesions _____ scars _____

   e. Aids

      sling _____ splint _____ orthosis _____ other _____

      purpose _____

2. Palpation (note location and nature of abnormality)

   a. Skin and subcutaneous tissue: tenderness _____ temperature _____ swelling _____ decreased mobility _____

      trigger points _____ other _____

   b. Muscles and tendons: tenderness _____ temperature _____ spasm _____ loss of continuity _____

      decreased mobility _____ other _____

   c. Tendon sheaths and bursae: tenderness _____ temperature _____ swelling _____ crepitus _____ other _____

   d. Bones and joints: tenderness _____ temperature _____ swelling _____ bony prominences _____ other _____

   e. Arteries and nerves: axillary artery _____ suprascapular nerve _____ brachial N-V bundle _____

Figure 4.8.   Examination form part 3: Inspection and palpation.

malities, such as bony crepitus from osteoarthritis. Palpation may also reveal the presence of synovial swelling. The examiner palpates the GH joint at the point of the shoulder. He palpates the SC joint just lateral to the sternoclavicular notch. The AC joint forms the superior frontal landmark; while the patient sits with the arm hanging dependently, the therapist may press up on the elbow to shift the acromion cranially and feel movement at this joint (Fig. 4.10) (10). The neurovascular structures accessible to palpation include the axillary arterial pulse, felt medially in the upper arm; the suprascapular nerve, palpated with the arm adducted by pressing over the supraspinatus muscle before it passes under the acromion; and the brachial neurovascular bundle, palpated anterior to the GH joint in the axilla.

Movement Assessment.   Assessment of functional active movement provides a quick indication of the amount of motion available in the shoulder. Using a given key (Fig. 4.11), the therapist records the ease with which the patient can achieve common positions. Also, if a painful arc is present, he indicates both of

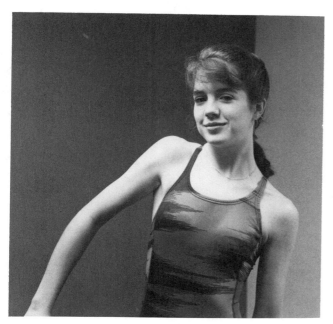

Figure 4.9. Shoulder haunching maneuver: if a patient attempts to substitute scapular elevation for arm abduction, the test is positive, implicating glenohumeral joint restriction.

its limits in degrees. The subacromial painful arc, associated with bursitis, occurs between 60–120° of abduction as the greater tuberosity passes beneath the coracoacromial ligament. AC joint lesions produce a painful arc during the last 30° of elevation when scapular rotation is maximal (1).

The therapist evaluates active, passive, and resistive physiologic movement at the GH joint, recording measurements in degrees, as well as the various qualities of movement, in the appropriate column on the form (Fig. 4.11). Selectively applying tension to the inert and contractile structures as described in Chapter 2 assists in identifying the site of the lesion, i.e., tendinous lesions usually do not limit passive movement, but may be weak and painful upon resisted movement (16). When testing a shoulder, one should be cautious to discern pain produced by impingement from pain produced truly by active or passive movement; passive abduction may impinge the rotator cuff tendons beneath the coracoacromial arch and elicit pain, an exception to the rule that passive movement of contractile structures in the direction of their action is painless.

It is not customary to measure the degrees of physiologic AC, SC, and ST joint movement, but a therapist can record the symptoms and quality of active movement, such as whether it is performed with ease or great effort. He records the symptoms related to passive movement and the strength and symptoms of resisted movement. Clavicular rotation is tested only actively during arm elevation. Scapular rotation is tested only passively.

A scale of 0–6 indicates accessory movement for the three true synovial joints (Fig. 4.12). A therapist also records the symptoms produced by accessory move-

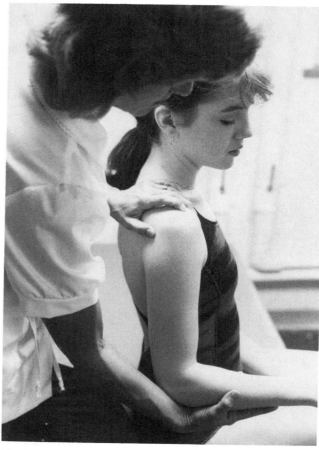

Figure 4.10. Acromioclavicular joint palpation: the examiner places his finger on the joint, while moving the acromion cranially by a long axis force through the humerus, to assess motion at the AC joint.

ment. Lack of certain accessory movements has direct functional implication, i.e., limited GH joint caudal glide increases the possibility of impingement of structures between the humeral head and the coracoacromial arch during abduction of the arm. Laxity in dorsal and ventral glide of the AC joint is the best way to identify subluxation or dislocation in the joint (10).

The examiner performs special tests to incriminate lesions in structures which behave in a characteristic manner (Fig. 4.12). A "drop arm test" may reveal a supraspinatus tendon or rotator cuff tear. The examiner instructs the seated patient to abduct his arm 90° against gravity, then to actively lower it or hold against resistance. This test is positive when the patient is unable to do either (Fig. 4.13). The examiner tests for an impingement syndrome (see page 92) by forcefully compressing the humerus against the acromion by passively flexing the arm while stabilizing the scapula; it is positive when this maneuver reproduces the pain or prevents full flexion (Fig. 4.14) (21). The examiner may also reproduce impingement symptoms by preventing lateral humeral rotation when the patient attempts to abduct the arm, or medial humeral rotation when he attempts to flex the arm; both techniques force the greater humeral tuberosity against the cor-

3. Movement assessment
   a. Functional active moment
      arms elevated _____
      arms crossed in front to touch opposite shoulders _____
      arms crossed behind neck to touch opposite superior angles of
         scapulae _____
      arms crossed behind back to touch opposite inferior angles of
         scapulae _____
      painful arc (in degrees) _____°

key: C = completes task
     D = completes task with
         difficulty or discomfort
     N = not able to complete
         task

b/c/d. Physiologic movement

GH joint	ACTIVE			PASSIVE			RESISTIVE	
	ROM	Symptoms	Quality	ROM	Symptoms	End-feel	Strength	Symptoms
flexion								
extension								
medial rot.								
lateral rot.								
abduction								
adduction								
horiz. abd.								
horiz. add.								

Shoulder girdle	Symptoms (indicate AC, SC, ST)	Symptoms (indicate AC, SC, ST)	Strength	Symptoms
elevation				
depression				
protraction				
retraction				
clavicular rotation (with arm elevation)				
scapular rotation upward				
downward				

Figure 4.11. Examination form part 4: Movement assessment.

acoacromial ligament or acromion. Horizontal adduction stresses the AC joint and may pinpoint the lesion by producing localized pain. The examiner performs an "apprehension test" by slowly moving the patient's arm into a position of abduction and lateral rotation; if positive, the patient will attempt to avoid this position because he fears it will reproduce a chronic GH joint subluxation. The examiner performs a Yergason test by resisting elbow flexion and shoulder medial rotation from a position of 90° elbow flexion and 90° forearm supination; a positive test occurs when the LHB tendon slips from the intertubercular groove, snaps, or when pain occurs (Fig. 4.15) (22). Winging of the scapula when a patient supports his weight on arms that are flexed to 90° indicates serratus anterior muscle paralysis.

e. Accessory movement

	Mobility	Symptoms
GH joint caudal humeral glide		
ventral humeral glide		
dorsal humeral glide		
lateral traction		
SC joint craniodorsal glide		
caudoventral glide		
AC joint dorsal glide		
ventral glide		

f. Special tests

	+	−	Comments
Drop arm test			
Impingement syndrome test			
Horiz. add. (stress AC joint)			
Apprehension test			
Yergason test			
Serratus anterior muscle paralysis			
Adson test			
Costoclavicular maneuver			
Hyperabduction maneuver			
Elevated arm stress test			

Figure 4.12. **Examination form part 5:** Accessory movement and special tests.

For a suspected thoracic outlet syndrome, the examiner performs an Adson test, to check for compression of the brachial plexus and subclavian artery by the scalenus anticus muscle. He first checks the patient's radial pulse with his arm dependent; then he instructs the patient to take a deep breath, hold it, and extend and rotate his head (to either side) while he again checks the pulse, but with the arm extended and laterally rotated (Fig. 4.16). Diminution of the pulse or reproduction of symptoms indicates a positive test.

Another test for thoracic outlet syndrome is the costoclavicular maneuver, which compresses the neurovascular structures between the clavicle and first rib in attempt to reproduce the symptoms. The therapist checks the patient's radial pulse with his arm in a dependent position, then after the patient assumes an exaggerated military position of shoulder retraction and depression, he repeats the pulse check. Diminution of the pulse or reproduction of symptoms indicates a positive test. Thoracic outlet syndrome may also occur when hyperabduction stretches the neurovascular bundle beneath the insertion of the pectoralis minor muscle and around the coracoid process. The examiner positions the patient's arm in full lateral rotation and 90° abduction. Diminution of the radial pulse or reproduction of symptoms in this position indicates a positive hyperabduction test. According to Roos (20), subclavian artery compression is responsible for symptoms in only 1% of thoracic outlet syndrome cases, so the pulse would be normal in 99% of these cases. Moreover, positional compression of the

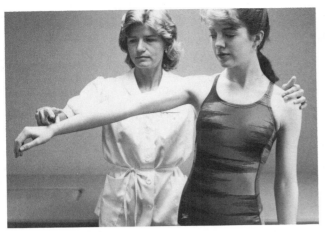

Figure 4.13. Drop arm test: if a patient can't sustain abduction against minimal resistance or lower his arm smoothly, the test is positive, implicating a supraspinatus tendon or rotator cuff tear.

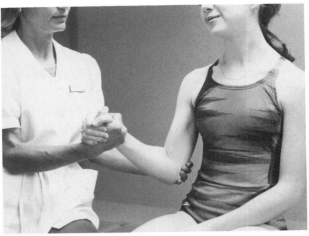

Figure 4.15. Yergason test: if resisted elbow flexion and shoulder medial rotation reproduce pain or snapping in the anterior upper arm, the test is positive, implicating instability of the long head of the biceps tendon in the bicipital groove.

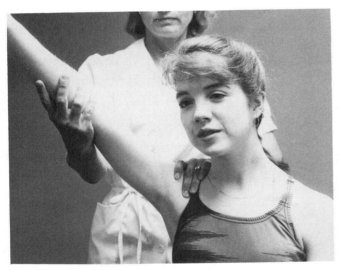

Figure 4.14. Impingement syndrome test: if passive compression of the greater tuberosity against the cora-coacromial ligament or acromion reproduces the patient's pain, the test is positive, implicating bicipital or supraspinatus tendon, or subacromial bursa pathology.

subclavian artery occurs in many people without thoracic outlet syndrome, and thus may produce a false-positive test. Neurologic symptoms such as pain, fatigue, numbness, and paresthesia are a better indication of compression within the thoracic outlet. For this reason, the most reliable test for thoracic outlet syndrome is an elevated arm stress test; a patient laterally rotates the shoulder and abducts to 90° with the elbow flexed 90°, then opens and closes his fist for 3 minutes (Fig. 4.17) (20). Reproduction of symptoms indicates a positive test.

Neurologic Evaluation. The deltoid muscle, representing the C5 neurological level (although the deltoid is also supplied by C6), is the only key muscle the examiner assesses in the shoulder region (Fig.

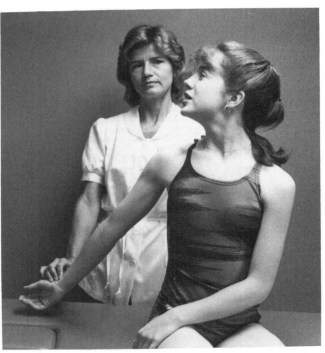

Figure 4.16. Adson test: if a combination of deep inhalation, cervical extension and rotation, and arm extension and lateral rotation reproduce medial arm pain or paresthesia and radial pulse diminution, the test is positive, implicating compression of neurovascular structures within the scalene triangle.

4.18). The examiner completes sensory testing as described in Chapter 2. Since the most common cause of referred shoulder pain is disorders of the cervical spine and the emerging nerve roots, identifying the pattern of sensory changes is essential (1). If certain neck movements reproduce the shoulder symptoms, cervical referral may be implicated. Bending the head

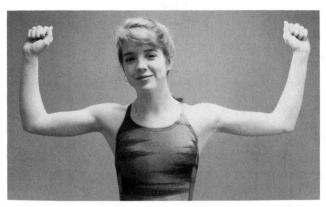

Figure 4.17. Elevated arm stress test: if exercising the forearm muscles by opening and closing the fingers for 3 minutes, with the shoulders abducted and laterally rotated, reproduces arm fatigue and pain, the test is positive, implicating neurologic impingement within the thoracic outlet.

and neck toward the side of pain increases the irritation of cervical nerve roots from extruded discs; head and neck motion away from the painful side aggravates scalene disorders (10). Another source of sensory change is a traction injury to the brachial plexus; this condition is commonly referred to as a stinger, and may produce hyperesthesia in the limb. The examiner performs motor function and coordination testing, as described in Chapter 2.

Recommendation of Other Tests. When a therapist has collected and interpreted all the data from the shoulder examination, he may desire additional diagnostic tests. Roentgenographic examination may reveal calcium deposits in the rotator cuff. A high-riding humeral head may suggest a rotator cuff defect (15). A Hill-Sachs lesion, demonstrated radiographically as a notch or crease defect on the posterior lateral surface of the humeral head when the arm is medially rotated in an A-P view, is indicative of recurrent shoulder

4. Neurological evaluation

   a. Key muscle (strength grade 0–5): C5 = deltoid muscle _____

   b. Key reflexes—none at shoulder

   c. Sensibility

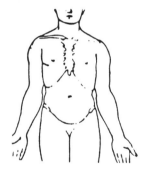 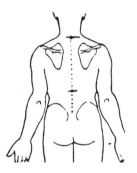

Key: lacking A = light touch sensation
                 B = sharp/dull discrimination
                 C = temperature discrimination
                 D = proprioception

   d. Motor control: spastic _____ flaccid _____ rigid _____ clonic _____

   e. Coordination

   Reciprocal arm swing _____

   Reciprocal shoulder shrug _____

   Shoulder circumduction _____

Key: C = completes task
       D = completes task with difficulty or discomfort
       N = not able to complete task

5. Recommendation of other tests

   a. Radiography _____

   b. Laboratory _____

   c. Electrodiagnostic _____

   d. Arthroscopy _____

   e. Arthrography _____

   f. Other _____

Figure 4.18. Examination form part 6: Neurologic evaluation and recommendation of other tests.

dislocation. Arthrography is necessary to make the definitive diagnosis of frozen shoulder by confirming a reduced joint volume. Arthrography is also useful in identifying a rupture of the rotator cuff by noting escape into the subacromial bursa of radiopaque dye injected into the GH joint. Arthroscopy may reveal tears of the glenoid labrum or lesions of the capsule-

and tendons. There are a variety of other tests which help confirm different shoulder lesions. When in doubt about a diagnosis, it is always wise to consult with other members of the health team. Table 4.3 includes a summary of the differential diagnosis and treatment of common shoulder disorders.

Table 4.3.
Summary of Differential Diagnosis and Treatment of Common Shoulder Disorders

Disorder	Chief Complaint	Onset	Symptom Characteristics	Static Physical Changes	Dynamic Physical Changes	Special Tests	Treatment[a]
AC Joint a. Acute syndrome b. Sprain c. Subluxation and/or dislocation	a. Pain b. and c. Instability	a. secondary to overhead activity b. and c. Trauma—fall on tip of shoulder or outstretched arm	a,b,c.—Local pain experienced when elevation >90° or horizontal adduction	a,b,c. Local swelling c. Step off appearance with dependent arm holding weight	a,b,c. Painful arc in last 30° elevation; ↑ joint play	a,b,c. Horizontal adduction or passive press humerus up through elbow and clavicle down	a. Avoid aggravating activities; heat or ice; ADL b. Active ROM, but avoid abduction for 3 wks and avoid lifting for 6 wks c. conservative: sling protection, avoid abd. 4 wks, avoid lifting 2 mos; surgical—ORIF
Bicipital tendinitis	Local snapping sensation over bicipital groove; pain	Following rigorous activity or repetitive training; common 45–65 y/o female	Local anterior tenderness; chronic pain over proximal arm; symptoms worse with abd. and lat. rotation	Arm held close to side	Resisted elbow flexion and supination increase pain	Yergason	Local rest with sling; heat; NSAIDS; injection along LHB tendon sheath but not into tendon; with repeated occurrences, surgical reattachment of tendon more distally onto humeral head, muscle reeducation
Calcific supraspinatus tendinitis	Severe, disabling pain	Acute, fulminating attack	Intense pain in deltoid region; rapidly increasing severity; not ↓ by rest	Swelling; arm held protected in adduction	Painful arc from 60°–120°	Impingement; radiographic: calcific deposits, sclerosis, and cystic changes	Self-limiting, but often too painful to wait; ice (don't use heat), analgesics, sedatives; multiple needle punctures with aspiration; progress to full PROM bid and resume function
Degenerative supraspinatus tendinitis	Low-grade ache	Chronic	Local, lateral pain and tenderness, ↑ by abduction; aching at night	Crepitus over supraspinatus insertion	↓ ROM	Impingement	Temporary rest in sling; modalities; anti-inflammatory drugs; ROM; functional activities
Frozen shoulder	Painfully restricted shoulder motion	Insidious or secondary to precipitating factors	Initial pain during both activity and rest in deltoid region; progressive to stiffness	Patient protective of arm and motion guarded	Motion limited in capsular pattern; ↓ joint play; girdle hunching	Arthrography reveals reduced joint volume	Modalities and medication for pain relief; exercise program including joint mobilization, active and resistive exercises; infiltration debrisement; manipulation under anesthesia
GH joint dislocation/ subluxation	Sensation of catching or lose control with subluxation; complete disability with dislocation	Forced abduction and lateral rotation; fall on extended arm	Severe pain and disability following acute dislocation	Square appearance	Motion difficult unless reduced; laxity; ↑ ventral glide joint mobility in chronic cases	Apprehension test Hill-Sachs lesion in radiographs if recurrent	Reduce by relaxing while lying prone with weighted arm hanging at 90° shoulder flexion; or caudal glide manipulation to reduce then 3 wks immobilization in adduction and medial rotation; surgical repair; rehab emphasizing strengthening subscapularis
Rotator Cuff Lesions	Catching sensation at 90°	Traumatic violent rupture; mild trauma if tendon degenerated	Pain with rotation or abduction; can't sleep on involved side	Atrophy; palpable cleft with rupture	Unable to resist abduction	Drop arm test; leakage of dye into bursa with arthrography	Young (complete tear)—surgical repair and partial anterior acromionectomy followed by 3–4 wks immobilization in abd. (incomplete tear)—conservative—8 wks immobil., then strengthening. Elderly—maintain ROM and strength
Subacromial bursitis	Painful to abduct	Acute, within 2–3 days of strenuous activity or immobilization for any reason	Severe, local tenderness; hard to distinguish from supraspinatus tendinitis	Lateral swelling	Painful arc 60°–120° (initially can't abduct this far)	Impingement; no pain if arm rotated at side	Rest and support 2 days; start active and PROM in 2–6 days; oral anti-inflammatory drugs; corticosteroid injections
Thoracic outlet syndrome	Paresthesias and hypethesias down medial arm; pain; swelling, cyanosis, cold limb	Chronic (scalene sapsm, hypertrophy, or clavicular drooping); congenital anomalies	Pain and sensory changes related to position and/or activity	Rounded, sagging shoulder posture	Weakness in C_8 T_1 musculature	Adson; costoclavicular; hyperabd.; elevated arm stress test; ↓ sensation in C_8 T_1 distribution	Strengthen upper trapezius and rhomboids; postural exercises to promote retracted, level shoulders and cervical alignment; surgical decompression

[a]AC, acromioclavicular; ROM, range of motion; GH, glensbumeral; ORIF, open reduction internal fixation; NSAID, nonsteroidal inflammatory drug; PROM, passive range of motion.

SHOULDER MOBILIZATION

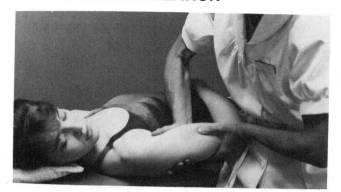

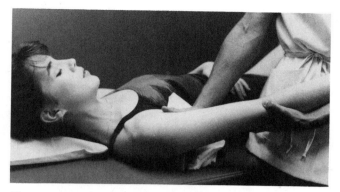

Figure 4.19.   Lateral Glenohumeral Joint Traction.

Patient Positon: Supine with arm at side; hand resting on abdomen

Therapist Position: Standing at P's side; web space of S hand grasps distal lateral humerus; web space of M hand grasps proximal medial humerus.

Technique: With forearms parallel to direction of force (perpendicular to humerus), hold distal humerus stationary with S hand, and apply lateral pressure to proximal humerus with M hand.

Comments: Effective for any painful limitation or hypomobility

Figure 4.20.   Caudal Humeral Glide.

Patient Position: Supine with scapula stabilized by T's hand or strap; arm supported against T's body.

Therapist Position: Standing at P's side with back toward P, but upper body rotated to face P; dorsum of S hand rests against P's thorax with web space in axilla; M hand grasps distal humerus.

Technique: Apply firm pressure with S hand to fixate scapula; rotate body away from P with M hand holding humerus to produce caudal glide of humerus.

Comments: Especially effective for increasing abduction.

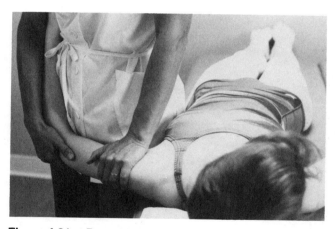

Figure 4.21.   Dorsal Humeral Glide.

Patient Position: Supine with scapula on firm table or sandbag, and humerus free of table; forearm supported against T's body.

Therapist Position: Standing at P's side; S hand cradles P's elbow; M hand rests on proximal anterior humerus.

Technique: With M arm parallel to force, press down upon P's arm using heel of hand to impart dorsal force to humeral head.

Comments: Especially effective for increasing flexion and medial rotation; may be used with varying amounts of shoulder abduction.

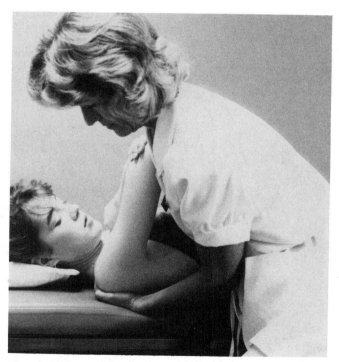

Figure 4.22.   Dorsal Humeral Glide (when flexion surpasses 70°).

Patient Position: Supine with shoulder and elbow maximally flexed; scapula stabilized by T's hand.

Therapist Position: Standing at P's side; S hand fixates scapula; M hand cups elbow.

Technique: Use chest contact upon M hand to apply dorsal force through the long axis of humerus.

Comments: Use as an alternate technique to achieve more flexion and medial rotation when flexion surpasses 70°.

SHOULDER MOBILIZATION

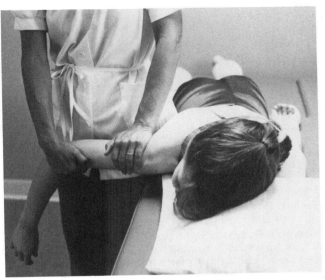

Figure 4.23.   Ventral Humeral Glide.

Patient Position: Prone with coracoid process of scapula on firm table or sandbag, and humerus free of table.

Therapist Position: Standing at P's side, S hand supports distal humerus; M hand rests on proximal posterior humerus.

Technique: With M arm parallel to force, press down upon P's arm using heel of hand to impart ventral force to humeral head.

Comments: Especially effective for increasing extension and lateral rotation. Therapist should carefully monitor endfeel and P's response, to avoid excessive force when anterior stabilizing structures are compromised.

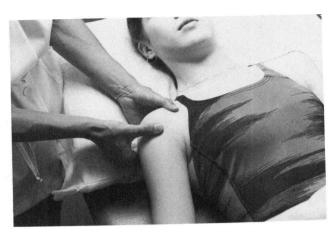

Figure 4.24.   Dorsal-Ventral Humeral Oscillation.

Patient Position: Supine with arm resting on abdomen.

Therapist Position: Standing; thumbs and fingers hold anterior and posterior humerus respectively.

Technique: Oscillate humeral head in dorsal and ventral directions while scapula remains relatively fixed by P's body weight.

Comments: Use to relieve pain and initiate motion in acute conditions.

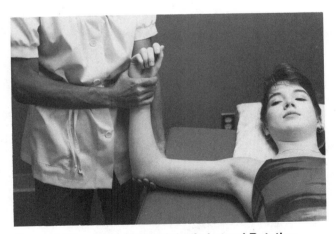

Figure 4.25.   Graded Physiologic Lateral Rotation.

Patient Position: Supine with shoulder abducted and in neutral rotation.

Therapist Position: Standing, facing P's feet; S hand cradles P's elbow; M hand grasps P's wrist.

Technique: Oscillate arm in designated range of lateral rotation, while providing a block to further motion with S arm contact against P's forearm.

Comments: T may use his leg or body instead of arm to block motion and enhance P's confidence in variations of this technique.

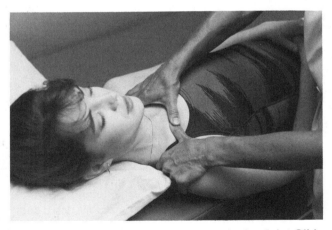

Figure 4.26.   Craniodorsal Sternoclavicular Joint Glide.

Patient Postion: Supine with arm resting on abdomen; trunk stabilized by friction against table.

Therapist Position: Standing at P's side; S thumb reinforces M thumb on medical inferior clavicle.

Technique: Move clavicle in a craniodorsal direction to accommodate obliquity of joint axis.

Comments: Adjust thumb pressure for comfort, avoiding pressure on supraclavicular nerve.

SHOULDER MOBILIZATION

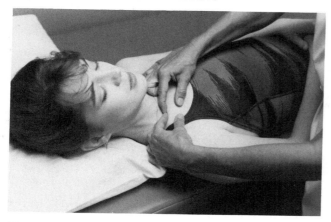

Figure 4.27.   Caudoventral Sternoclavicular Joint Glide.
Patient Position: Supine with arm resting on abdomen; trunk stabilized by friction against table.
Therapist Position: Standing at P's side; S and M fingers rest behind medical clavicle.
Technique: Move clavicle in a caudoventral direction to accommodate obliquity of joint axis.
Comments: Keeping fingers parallel to clavicle may alleviate uncomfortable pressure.

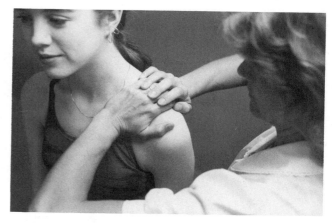

Figure 4.28.   Dorsal Acromioclavicular Joint Glide.
Patient Position: Seated with arm resting at side.
Therapist Position: Standing facing P; S hand rests on scapular spine; M hand rests on lateral clavicle.
Technique: With arms parallel to force, secure scapula with S hand and move clavicle posteriorly upon fixed acromion with M hand.

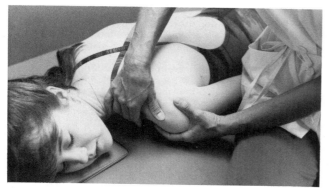

Figure 4.29.   Ventral Acromioclavicular Joint Glide.
Patient Position: Prone with arm resting at side.
Therapist Position: Sitting on table facing P's head; S hand grasps shoulder and fixates scapula by pressure against coracoid process; M thumb rests on dorsal lateral clavicle.
Technique: Anchor scapula with S hand and move clavicle ventrally upon fixed acromion with thumb pressure of M hand.

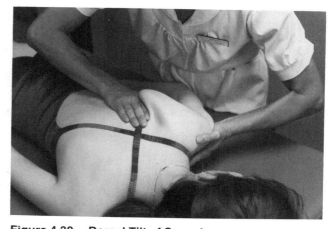

Figure 4.30.   Dorsal Tilt of Scapula.
Patient Position: Prone with arm resting at side.
Therapist Position: Standing facing P; S hand cups inferior angle of scapula; M hand grasps shoulder.
Technique: Apply parallel forces in opposite directions through forearms to lift scapula away from thorax.
Comments: P must completely relax to allow this scapular mobilization.

SHOULDER MOBILIZATION

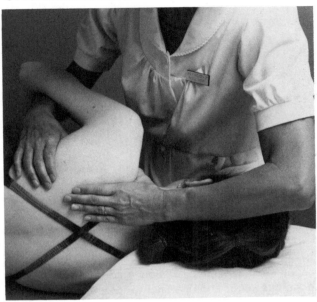

Figure 4.31. General Scapulothoracic Mobilization.

Patient Position: Side lying facing T, with arm resting on T's forearm.

Therapist Position: Standing facing P, supporting P's arm; web spaces of hands cup medial and lateral scapular borders.

Technique: Glide scapula in various directions as indicated: elevation and depression; abduction and adduction; and rotation.

Comments: Use to enhance relaxation and mobility of all shoulder girdle joints.

References

1. Kessel L: *Clinical Disorders of the Shoulder.* Churchill Livingstone, New York, 1982.
2. Carmichael SW, Hart DL: Anatomy of the shoulder joint. *J Orthop Sports Phys Ther* 6:225–228, 1985.
3. Williams PL, Warwick R (eds): *Gray's Anatomy,* 36th British Edition, WB Saunders, 1980.
4. Sarrafian SK: *Gross and functional anatomy of the shoulder. Clin Orthop* 173:11–19, 1983.
5. Peat M: The shoulder complex: a review of some aspects of functional anatomy. *Physiotherapy Canada* 29:241–246, 1977.
6. Hart DL, Carmichael SW: Biomechanics of the shoulder. *J Orthop Sports Phys Ther* 6:229–234, 1985.
7. Cailliet R: *Shoulder Pain,* ed 2, Philadelphia, FA Davis, 1981.
8. Rizk TE, Pinals RS: Frozen shoulder. *Semin Arthritis Rheum* 11, 1982.
9. Kapandji IA: *The Physiology of the Joints,* Edinburgh, Churchill Livingstone, 1974, vol 1.
10. Bateman JE: *The Shoulder and Neck,* Philadelphia, WB Saunders, 1978.
11. Halbach JW, Tank RT: The shoulder. In Gould GA, Davies GJ (eds): *Orthopaedic and Sports Physical Therapy,* St. Louis, CV Mosby Co., 1985.
12. Kent BE: Functional anatomy of the shoulder complex. *Phys Ther* 51:867–887, 1971.
13. Lucas DB: Biomechanics of the shoulder joint. *Arch Surg* 107:425–432, 1973.
14. Inman VT, Saunders JBdeCM, Abbott LC: Observations on the function of the shoulder joint. *J Bone Jt Surg* 26:1–30, 1944.
15. Jobe FW, Jobe CM: Painful atheletic injuries of the shoulder. *Clinical Orthop* 173:117–124, 1983.
16. Cyriax J: *Textbook of Orthopaedic Medicine,* ed 6 Baltimore, Williams & Wilkins, 1975, vol 2.
17. Yocum LA: Assessing the shoulder. In Jobe FW (ed): *Clinics in Sports Medicine,* Philadelphia, WB Saunders Co., 1983, vol. 2.
18. Simkin PA: Tendinitis and bursitis of the shoulder. *Postgrad Med* 73:177–190, 1983.
19. Britt LP: Nonoperative treatment of the thoracic outlet syndrome symptoms. *Clinical Orthop* 51:45–48, 1967.
20. Roos DB: Congenital anomalies associated with thoracic outlet syndrome. *Am J Surg* 132:771–778, 1976.
21. Neer CS: Impingement lesions. *Clin Orthop* 173:70–77, 1983.
22. Simon WH: Soft tissue disorders of the shoulder. *Orthop Clin North Am* 6:521–539, 1975.

THE ELBOW

CLINICAL ANATOMY AND MECHANICS OF THE ELBOW

Clinicians may erroneously depict the elbow as a simple joint, when actually it is a complex mechanism depending upon the integrated action of three bones within three distinct articulations. These closely related joints must operate congruously; otherwise, mechanical alterations in one or more of the structures can impose severe restrictions on the overall function of the elbow and interfere with the use of the hand.

Osteology

Humerus. The humerus transforms from a cylindrical shape at midshaft to become flattened anteroposteriorly and broadened laterally at its distal end. Its sharp lateral and medial supracondylar ridges terminate in jutting epicondyles that are easily visible and palpable. Adjacent to the epicondyles, the distalmost condyles bear two convex articular surfaces that distinctly differ from one another. The lateral condyle, the capitulum, presents a dome-shaped surface (which does not extend posteriorly) for articulation with the radius. The medial condyle, the trochlea, embodies a pulley-shaped surface for articulation with the hooked olecranon (Fig. 5.1).

Three nonarticulating fossae also occupy the distal humerus. They serve to increase the range of elbow flexion and extension by delaying the impact of the respective bony prominences upon the humeral shaft (1). The olecranon fossa is a deep hollow on the posterior surface that contains the tip of olecranon when the elbow is extended. The coronoid fossa is a smaller hollow anteromedially that accommodates the coronoid process of the ulna during elbow flexion. The radial fossa is a depression above the capitulum anterolaterally that receives the margin of the radial head on full flexion.

The transverse axis of the trochlea dips medially, directing the forearm into abduction. The forearm thus forms an angle with the arm that normally ranges from 5–15° and is referred to as the carrying angle. Because there is a single axis for elbow flexion and extension,

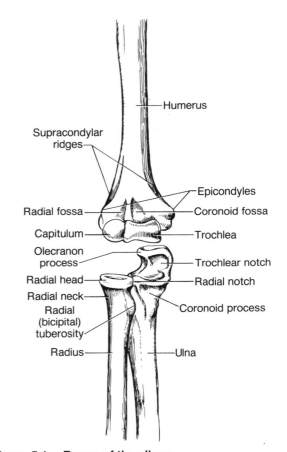

Figure 5.1. Bones of the elbow.

Labels: Humerus; Supracondylar ridges; Epicondyles; Radial fossa; Coronoid fossa; Capitulum; Trochlea; Olecranon process; Trochlear notch; Radial head; Radial notch; Radial neck; Coronoid process; Radial (bicipital) tuberosity; Radius; Ulna

the carrying angle remains constant throughout the full range of elbow motion (2). Cubitus valgus deformity increases the carrying angle and is clinically significant because it may stretch the ulnar nerve and produce an ulnar nerve palsy (3). Cubitus varus (gunstock) deformity decreases the carrying angle; it commonly results from improperly reduced supracondylar fractures or epicondylar epiphyseal injuries (4). Cubitus varus does not appear to cause functional disability, but rather becomes a cosmetic problem (5).

Another feature of the distal humerus is the 45°

angle that the anterior projection of its articular surface makes with the frontal plane (6). Since the ulnar trochlea also joins its shaft at a 45° angle, this arrangement provides space for the interposing soft tissue, while theoretically allowing 180° elbow flexion (1). This anatomical relationship becomes clinically significant because displaced fractures and joint trauma can alter the bony configuration and thus impede function.

Ulna. Anatomists sometimes refer to the ulna as an extension of the humerus. The trochlear notch occupies its thick, hook-like proximal end. A lengthwise groove marks the notch that articulates with the pulley-shaped trochlea. An anterior projection, the coronoid process, and a large posterior projection, the olecranon process, deepen the concave articular notch and increase bony elbow stability (Fig. 5.1). Its subcutaneous position makes the olecranon particularly vulnerable to direct trauma. Most olecranon fractures are intraarticular and, therefore, can compromise the stability of the elbow joint (7). A lateral indentation on the ulna, the radial notch, provides a surface for articulation with the radial head and an area to which the annular ligament attaches.

The olecranon tip and the humeral epicondyles lie in a transverse line when viewed from behind with the elbow extended to 0° (see Fig. 5.8A)(6). These landmarks define an isosceles triangle when viewed from behind with the elbow flexed 90° (see Fig. 5.8B). Elbow dislocation or olecranon or intercondylar fractures may disrupt these relationships, providing diagnostic evidence of such pathology. However, a displaced supracondylar fracture would not alter the relationship between the three landmarks but would change their relationship with the shaft of the humerus.

The distal ulna projects medially as the ulnar styloid process (Fig. 5.2). Adjacent to the styloid process is the small rounded head of the ulna, which forms the convex partner of the distal radioulnar joint (Fig. 5.2). A triangular fibrocartilage disc attaches between the ulnar styloid process and the base of the radius; it anchors the radius to the ulna and provides a dual articular surface at the radioulnar and radiocarpal joints.

Radius. The radius participates with the humerus and ulna in the elbow joint. A disc-shaped head occupies its proximal end, providing a shallow concave surface for articulation with the capitulum (Fig. 5.1). The articular circumference of the head is smooth and widest medially where it articulates with the radial notch of the ulna (8). The proximal surface of the radial head and its articular circumference are covered with hyaline cartilage. Just distal to the head the radius constricts into a neck. Below the neck a small area known as the radial (bicipital) tuberosity protrudes anteromedially; this is the site of insertion of the biceps brachii tendon.

The radial head, lateral humeral epicondyle, and tip of the olecranon form a triangle when the elbow is viewed from the side. Within this triangle lies the posterolateral capsule of the elbow. Following an

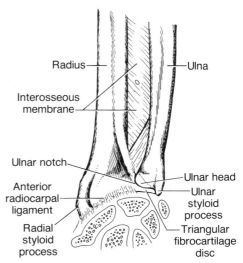

Figure 5.2.   The inferior radioulnar joint.

intraarticular fracture of the elbow, an examiner often can palpate swelling secondary to hemarthrosis in this triangle (3).

The shaft of the radius is slightly convex laterally, allowing it to clear the ulna during pronation. The radius is widest distally, where the radial styloid process and two articulating surfaces are found (Fig. 5.2). The medial articular surface is a small ulnar notch that forms the convex partner in the inferior radioulnar joint. A large inferior articulating surface forms the concave portion of the radiocarpal joint.

When the long axis of the radius is projected proximally, it should always pass through the capitulum, regardless of the degree of elbow flexion and extension or forearm rotation. This anatomical essential provides a relevant landmark for assessing elbow joint integrity radiographically (3).

The overall shapes of the radius and ulna serve to provide a compatible relationship within an area where there is little room for error. It is quite conceivable how such postfracture situations as malunion and extensive callus formation can restrict their movement (8, 9). The midregion of the forearm seems to be most critical in this respect; Tarr et al. found that deformities in the middle third of the bones produced statistically significantly greater supination losses than deformities in the distal third (10).

Arthrology

Three joints, which work together as a unit to produce elbow flexion and extension and forearm rotation, form the cubital complex. Within a single joint cavity lie the hinged (ginglymus) humeroulnar articulation, the gliding (plane) humeroradial articulation, and the pivotal (trochoid) superior radioulnar articulation (Fig. 5.3).

Humeroulnar and Humeroradial Joints. The combined articulations between the humerus and the forearm bones form a joint that is uniaxial, permitting 145° active (160° passive) flexion to full extension. Flex-

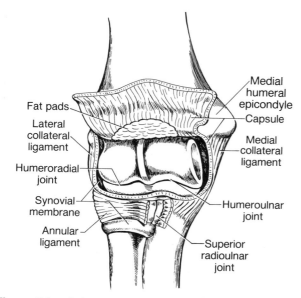

Fat pads

Lateral
collateral
ligament

Humeroradial
joint

Synovial
membrane

Annular
ligament

Medial
humeral
epicondyle

Capsule

Medial
collateral
ligament

Humeroulnar
joint

Superior
radioulnar
joint

Figure 5.3.   Joint structures of the elbow.

ion and extension occur about an axis that passes through the centers of arcs described by the trochlear sulcus and the capitulum (2).

The trochlea articulates with the corresponding trochlear notch and radial head, which are not perfectly congruent and, therefore, produce the following accessory movements: a slight screw action (the ulna is slightly supinated during flexion and pronated during extension); abduction and adduction; and gliding of the radial head on both the humerus and ulna. Extension is the close-packed position of the humeroulnar joint.

The capitulum and radial head are reciprocally curved; the close-packed position of the humeroradial joint is midflexion and midpronation (11).

Elbow flexion and extension depend upon the harmonious function of both the humeroulnar and humeroradial joints. It becomes obvious that reduction of a fracture involving both joints is especially critical; otherwise the joint function may resemble that of a door with its hinges improperly aligned (3).

An articular capsule encloses the humeroulnar, humeroradial, and superior radioulnar joints and extends from somewhat proximal to the radial and coronoid fossae, distally to the annular ligament and adjacent coronoid process and olecranon. The capsule is continuous laterally with the ulnar and radial collateral ligaments, where it is strongest. The anterior and posterior parts of the capsule are broad and thin. Forty-five degrees of flexion permits maximum volume of the joint, which is the position a patient assumes to accommodate diffuse swelling secondary to joint trauma or supracondylar fracture (4). A synovial membrane lines the capsule and reflects into the coronoid, radial, and olecranon fossae, over parts of the trochlea, and beneath the annular ligament (Fig. 5.3). It also projects as a fringe between the radial head and both the capitulum and ulna, an area where

it may be nipped and become one of the numerous etiologies of the tennis elbow syndrome (9). Fat pads exist between the fibrous capsule and the synovial membrane over the fossae; thus, they are intracapsular but extrasynovial. The classic radiographic "fat pad sign," used to detect joint effusion usually associated with the presence of a fracture, is positive when a translucent area appears between the soft tissue and the bone in the area of the fat pads.

An ulnar collateral (medial) ligament is a triangular structure formed by anterior and posterior bands and thin uniting fibers. Its apex is on the medial epicondyle, from which it fans anteriorly to the coronoid process and posteriorly to the olecranon process. The ulnar collateral ligament is the primary stabilizer of the elbow, increasingly resisting valgus stress and anterior distraction as flexion progresses to 90° (12). Its anterior band may also contribute to limiting full extension in cases of restricted range (13).

A radial collateral (lateral) ligament runs from the lateral epicondyle to the annular ligament, with some fibers inserting into the ulna. It provides lateral stability against varus stress. Some fibers of both collateral ligaments remain taut through the range of flexion and extension and serve to restrain excessive lateral movement. The strength of the ulnar collateral ligament is much greater, however, than that of the radial collateral ligament, an anatomical feature that corresponds to the nature of the stresses most frequently experienced. A person seldom encounters varus-producing forces, whereas the elbow is subjected to valgus stress in a variety of activities, such as throwing, golfing, the use of a hammer, and falling on the outstretched hand. The mass of the wrist and finger flexor muscles reinforces the medial ligament against valgus stress, but it is the ligament rather than the muscle that is usually ruptured in violent injuries (14). The humeroradial articulation also affords some lateral compression support against valgus elbow stress; following excision of either the radial head or capitulum, an elbow may exhibit varying degrees of instability. Damage of both the ulnar collateral ligament and the humeroradial articulation requires that a prosthesis be inserted after radial head excision.

The annular (orbicular) ligament is a strong band that encircles the peripheral margin of the radial head and retains it in contact with the ulna. The quadrate ligament is a small strip of fibrous tissue between the radial notch and radius that checks extremes of supination and pronation and reinforces the inferior aspect of the joint capsule. The oblique cord is a small anterior band running from the lateral aspect of the ulnar tuberosity to a point just distal to the radial tuberosity, its fibers being perpendicular to those of the interosseous membrane. Distal-medial fibers between the interosseous borders of the radius and ulna comprise the interosseous membrane (Fig. 5.2). It is taut midway between pronation and supination and serves the questionable function of transferring forces from the hand and radius to the ulna and humerus.

An olecranon bursa lies just deep to the skin over

the olecranon process. Friction or pressure from desk or armchair activities may cause olecranon bursitis. A bicipito-radial bursa exists in the angle between the biceps brachii muscle tendon and radius, just proximal to the insertion of the tendon into the tuberosity. Repetitive supination and flexion may irritate this bursa.

Superior Radioulnar Joint. The articular surfaces of the superior radioulnar joint include the cylindrical rim of the radial head and a fibro-osseous ring, comprised by the radial notch of the ulna and the annular ligament (Fig. 5.3). The palmar and dorsal parts of the annular ligament, which are subjected to tension, are made of firm connective tissue. Near the radial notch where the annular ligament is subjected to compression, cartilage cells are embedded in the ligament (11). Flexibility within this fibro-osseous ring accommodates the slightly oval configuration of the radial head.

Movement of the radius upon the ulna reaches about 85° of both pronation and supination. Accessory movements include rotation and gliding of the radial head relative to the capitulum, lateral displacement of the radial axis during pronation due to a larger anteroposterior head diameter (allowing room for the radial tuberosity), and distal-lateral tilt of the plane of the proximal surface of the radial head during pronation (1). The close-packed position is midway between supination and pronation (11).

The mechanical axis for forearm pronation and supination is a line passing between the head of the radius and head of the ulna (15). In supination, the long axes of the radius and ulna are parallel, whereas in pronation the radius sweeps over the ulna (the posterior concavity of the radius facilitates spacing between the bones), and the axis of the forearm then becomes parallel to the arm and the carrying angle becomes negligible (1).

Inferior Radioulnar Joint. The inferior radioulnar joint is also a critical component in forearm rotation (Fig. 5.2). It anchors the distal radius and ulna, and along with the superior radioulnar joint, provides a pivot for radial movement. This joint is discussed further in Chapter 6.

Mechanics and Soft Tissue Relationships

The skin and subcutaneous tissue overlying the elbow region move freely over the brachial and forearm fascia. The deep fascia, on the other hand, consists of a tough inelastic membrane that surrounds each muscle group and anchors it to bone. The fascia may constrain extravasated blood sufficiently to compromise circulation and produce ischemia, which, in severe instances, results in Volkmann's ischemic contracture.

The muscles that power the elbow are few in number and are easily identified as flexors or extensors. Their chief action is at the elbow, but the biceps brachii and triceps muscles also contribute to shoulder movement. In addition to the prime movers of the elbow, other muscles cross the elbow joint, whose primary function is wrist and finger motion. Due to extensive

coverage elsewhere (8, 9), muscle origins, insertions, and actions are not included here. Instead, selected functional concepts are presented in the following paragraphs.

The brachialis muscle has an extensive origin along the anterior humeral shaft and the lateral and medial intermuscular septa. This large area of bony contact may contribute to the relatively high incidence of myositis ossificans encountered in this muscle.

In general, the power of the elbow flexors is greater with the forearm pronated. Also, the position of the shoulder influences elbow strength somewhat, e.g., an overhead position facilitates elbow flexion and an anatomical position facilitates elbow extension (positions that can be said to facilitate climbing postures) (1). The pronators are less powerful than the supinators; the industrial design of nuts, bolts, and screws, which are tightened by a supinative movement in right-handed individuals, reflects this feature.

During investigation of a representative sample of functional activities, Morrey et al. found the functional arc of elbow flexion was 30–130°; the functional arc of forearm rotation was 55° supination to 50° pronation (16). Others investigators have studied the structures that normally constrain elbow motion. Active flexion is checked by (in order of descending importance) opposition of flexor muscles, bony contact, and the posterior capsule (1). Checks to passive flexion, in contrast, are bony contact, posterior capsule, passive triceps muscle tension, and soft tissue bulk (1). According to Kapandji, extension, both active and passive, is checked by bony contact, anterior capsule, and passive biceps brachii and brachialis muscle tension (1). However, Cummings found that elbow extension is first limited by muscles in the normal, relaxed subject (17). These studies have ramifications for goals involving mobility and strength when planning treatment.

Neurology

The median nerve (C5–8, T1) crosses the elbow anteromedially in relation to the humerus and medial to the brachial artery (Fig. 5.4). It gives off articular branches to the elbow and superior radioulnar joint and travels distally to give off branches to the pronator teres muscle, pronator quadratus muscle, and many of the wrist and finger flexor muscles (see Chapter 6). The median nerve is susceptible to compression by a vestigial ligament (of Struthers) between the heads of the pronator teres muscle.

The ulnar nerve (C7–8, T1) crosses the elbow in a groove on the dorsum of the medial epicondyle where one may palpate and roll it against the bone. It is susceptible to compression within the cubital tunnel behind the medial epicondyle (Fig. 5.4). It gives off a few small articular branches to the elbow, then muscular branches to the flexor carpi ulnaris muscle, the medial half of the flexor digitorum profundus muscle, and many of the hand intrinsic muscles (see Chapter 6).

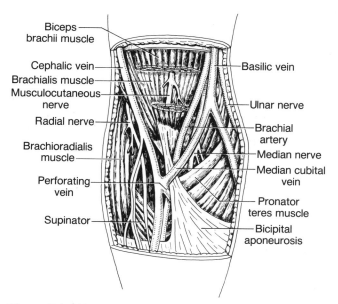

Figure 5.4. **Nerves and vessels crossing the elbow joint.**

The radial nerve (C5–8, T1) spirals around the posterior lateral humerus where it is frequently injured by a humeral fracture. It then crosses the elbow anterior to the lateral epicondyle, after which it divides into its terminal rami, the superficial and deep branches (Fig. 5.4). The deep branch, also known as the posterior interosseous nerve, may be entrapped either proximal or distal to the point where it enters the supinator muscle, producing the "posterior interosseous syndrome." Its muscular branches supply the triceps, anconeus, supinator, brachioradialis, extensor carpi radialis longus and brevis, abductor pollicis longus, and extensor muscles of the thumb and fingers. It also sends articular branches to the elbow joint.

The posterior and medial cutaneous nerves of the arm and forearm, the lower lateral cutaneous nerves of the arm, and the lateral cutaneous nerve of the forearm provide sensory innervation for the elbow. The musculocutaneous nerve supplies the anterior capsule, the radial nerve supplies the lateral and posterior capsule, the ulnar nerve supplies the posteromedial capsule, and the median nerve supplies the anteromedial capsule (9). An examiner may elicit the biceps brachii and triceps muscle reflexes at the elbow and the brachioradialis muscle reflex at the distal forearm.

The elbow is derived from the C6–7 neurologic segments, an important fact to consider when seeking the source of referred pain.

Angiology

The brachial artery serves as the main arterial supply to the arm. It is a continuation of the axillary artery, running from a position medial to the humerus to a midline position more distally (Fig. 5.4). It is superficial and palpable along much of its course.

The brachial artery gives off numerous branches proximal to the elbow. The three major branches are the profunda brachii artery, which accompanies the radial nerve, the superior ulnar collateral artery, which runs with the ulnar nerve, and the inferior ulnar collateral artery. These branches anastomose with the recurrent branches of the radial and ulnar arteries, proving collateral circulation around the elbow that is functionally and surgically important in instances of brachial artery occlusion.

In the cubital fossa the brachial artery lies between the biceps brachii muscle tendon laterally and the median nerve medially and is protected by the bicipital aponeurosis, which bridges over it (Fig. 5.4). At the level of the radial neck, the brachial artery divides into its terminal branches, the radial and ulnar arteries.

Two sets of veins, the superficial and the deep, drain blood from the upper extremity. The superficial include the cephalic vein laterally, the basilic vein medially, and the median antebrachial vein (Fig. 5.4). Just distal to the front of the elbow the cephalic vein gives off the median cubital vein, which connects with the deep venous system and also joins the basilic vein; the median cubital vein is quite superficial over the cubital region and is commonly used for venopuncture.

The deep veins accompany the arteries (vena comitantes), after which they are named, and are usually found in pairs. They anastomose freely with the superficial veins.

ELBOW EXAMINATION

History

The examiner first requests the specified identifying data from the patient (Fig. 5.5). Age often contributes to problem identification because certain elbow pathologies are unique to various age groups. Children rarely sustain elbow sprains, but frequently incur epiphyseal trauma, supracondylar fractures, and elbow dislocation (3, 18). Sprains occur more often in teenagers and young adults. In adults the dicondylar and olecranon types of fractures are most common (3).

The examiner asks the patient for a description of current symptoms, which are recorded on the given body chart with the accompanying key (Fig. 5.6). Some examples of pathologies that would produce symptoms with specific locations include compression of the sensory portion of the musculocutaneous nerve between the biceps brachii tendon and brachialis fascia causing vague, aching pain in the anterior region of the elbow (19); epiphyseal trauma producing linear tenderness that is maximal along the epiphyseal plate; tennis elbow evoking pain over the area of the lateral humeral epicondyle and radial neck (20, 21). The examiner also rates the severity and nature of the patient's symptoms and the impairment they impose by the given scales. Factors that affect the behavior, onset, and intensity of symptoms lend valuable information for subsequent diagnosis and treatment. For example, the symptoms of many sports-related dis-

A. HISTORY

  1. Identifying Data

      Name _____ Age ____ Gender ____ Date _____

      Provisional diagnosis _____ Precautions _____

      Chief complaint _____

      Dominant side R _____ L _____ Prior condition of involved part _____

  2. Present Episode or Illness

     a. Description of symptoms

        1) location: //// = pain
                 ==== = paresthesia
                 oooo = numbness
                 xxxx = other _____

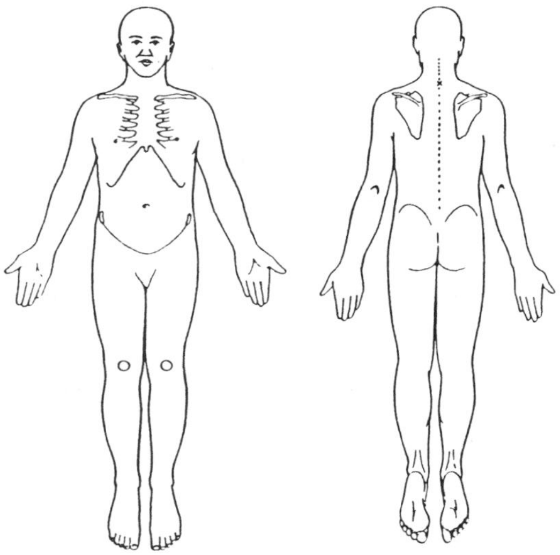

        2) severity:

              _____
              none   worst

        3) impairment:

              _____
              annoying   completely disabling

        4) nature:

            cramping _____ aching _____

            shooting _____ burning _____

            throbbing _____ tingling _____

            stabbing _____ sore _____

            other _____

      5) behavior:

        constant _____ intermittent _____ duration _____

        occurs when _____ elicited by _____

        aggravated by _____ relieved by _____

        24-hour pattern _____

        highly irritable _____ mildly irritable _____ not irritable _____

      6) joint characteristics: catches _____ , locks _____ , swells _____ , gives way _____ , dislocates _____ ,

        other _____

Figure 5.5. Examination form part 1: History.

orders correlate directly with the aggravating activity. The examiner also asks the patient to identify any abnormal characteristics of involved joints.

The patient descibes the present episode or illness, including pertinent dates, treatments, and status of the condition (Fig. 5.6). He recounts the nature or mechanism of injury or onset. Direct trauma, such as

a fall, "side swipe," or crush injury, often fractures the elbow. A fall right onto the elbow typically wedges the ulna up between the humeral condyles, splitting the bone with a resultant dicondylar "T" fracture. A fall onto the hand with the elbow extended is the mechanism that produces a supracondylar fracture.

Indirect trauma, i.e., lateral or distractive forces,

b. Background and associated findings

Date of present injury _____ or onset _____ insidious _____

Dates of hospitalization _____ and/or other health care

Treatments; dates; results _____

_____

Status of condition: acute _____ or chronic _____

constant _____ or intermittent _____

better _____ or worse _____

Nature and mechanism of injury or events precipitating present episode _____

_____

Results of injury (if applicable): deformity (describe) _____

corrected _____ disability (type and cause) _____

loss of motion (specify) _____ when occurred _____

loss of strength (specify) _____ when occurred _____

swelling (specify) _____ when occurred _____

bleeding (specify) _____ when occurred _____

3. Relevant Past History and Family History

History of similar condition: dates _____ nature _____

_____

Treatment _____

Other relevant illnesses or disorders _____

General health status _____

Health problems of immediate family _____

4. Life-style

Occupation _____ ADL _____

Regular (3 times/week minimum) physical activities requiring: strength _____ agility _____ endurance _____

flexibility _____ other _____

What patient does to promote wellness _____

Patient's concept of cause of condition _____

Patient's concept of functional and/or cosmetic deficit(s) _____

Anticipated goals _____

5. Other

Current medications _____

Recent radiographs _____

6. Therapist's Interpretation and Plans for Objective Exam _____

_____

Figure 5.6.   Examination form part 2: History, continued.

usually produces sprains, avulsions, or dislocations. Elbow dislocations are quite common: the elbow is the most frequently dislocated joint in children and ranks second to shoulder dislocations in adults (6, 18). A sudden traction force at the wrist may cause distal dislocation of the radial head (nurse-maid's elbow) in children under the age of 8 in whom the incompletely ossified radial head does not yet overhang the annular ligament. Due to the proximity of the forearm bones, certain types of elbow dislocations are inherently associated with a fracture, such as a Monteggia fracture of the ulnar shaft and accompanying radial head dislocation. Also, because of this proximity, a dislocation of the superior radioulnar joint often implicates a dislocation of the inferior radioulnar joint as well (15). Usually the patient has no difficulty describing the deformity and disability associated with fractures or dislocations.

The patient next reports the chronological onset of loss of motion, loss of strength, swelling, or bleeding. Loss of either motion or strength, or both, may occur 24 hours after a supracondylar fracture from swelling that compromises neurovascular structures at the elbow. A supracondylar fracture, or its treatment, may also cause brachial artery spasm, rupture, or contusion. The first signs of this severe complication are pain, pallor, pulselessness, and paresis; if not resolved, Volkmann's ischemic contracture and paralysis result. Another example of an injury which produces delayed loss of motion is a radial head fracture. Its accompanying hemarthrosis limits joint motion within two to three hours after injury.

Relevant past and family history are taken (Fig. 5.6). A patient describes any similar disorders experienced previously. Also a life-style summary, including occupation, sports, and hobbies, may help to explain the nature of the pathology. For example, sports requiring overhand throwing or racquet motion place tension stress over the medial (leading) side of the elbow, rendering it susceptible to ligament tears, tendon avulsions, or ulnar nerve injury; compression of the lateral side produces osteophytes, cartilage frag-

B. PHYSICAL EXAMINATION

1. Inspection

   a. Posture

      cubitus varus _____ cubitus valgus _____

      bony landmark relationships (olecranon and epicondyles)

	0°	90°
posterior view	_____	_____
lateral view	_____	_____

      general appearance of extremity _____

      attitude of hand _____

   b. Shape

      deformity (describe) _____ asymmetry _____

      swelling or masses _____ atrophy _____

   c. Use

      elbow protected/use restricted _____

      handles clothing: independently _____ minimum assistance _____

      maximum assistance _____

      movement: jerky _____ stiff _____ uncoordinated _____ limited by pain _____

   d. Skin

      color _____ condition _____ lesions _____ scars _____

   e. Aids

      sling _____ splint _____ orthosis _____ other _____

      purpose _____

Figure 5.7. Examination form part 3: Inspection.

ments, and loose bodies (22). It is particularly important, when examining radiographs of the elbow, to compare them with films of the uninvolved extremity, due to the large number of ossification centers in this area.

Finally, a review of current medications and recent radiographs completes the history. The therapist reviews all of the subjective data obtained in the history and proceeds with planning the physical portion of the examination.

Physical Examination

Inspection. The examiner inspects the arms for proper alignment (Fig. 5.7). He measures and records a cubitus varus or valgus deformity in degrees. The relationship of the three bony landmarks of the elbow, the olecranon and the humeral epicondyles, allows the examiner to assess the integrity of the joint. When viewed posteriorly, with the elbow extended, the landmarks should lie on a horizontal line (Fig. 5.8*A*);

with the elbow flexed 90°, they should form an inverted isoceles triangle (Fig. 5.8*B*) (4). Nonconformity to these rules may indicate posterior, anterior, or lateral dislocation or olecranon, epicondylar, or intercondylar fractures. When viewed laterally in extension, the epicondyles should lie slightly anterior to the olecranon process (Fig. 5.8*C*); at 90° flexion, the landmarks should lie on a vertical line (Fig. 5.8*D*). If the olecranon lies posterior to the epicondyles in flexion, then posterior dislocation is likely, whereas if the landmarks are properly related to one another but lie posterior to the humeral shaft, a supracondylar fracture is likely (18). The general appearance of the extremity, as well as the posture of the hand, may reveal evidence of nerve or vessel damage at the elbow.

Dislocations generally alter the shape of the elbow and often produce major soft tissue damage. A posterior elbow dislocation may tear the brachialis muscle extensively. Of the three peripheral nerves crossing the elbow, the ulnar nerve is the most commonly injured by elbow dislocation (3). Soft tissue swelling

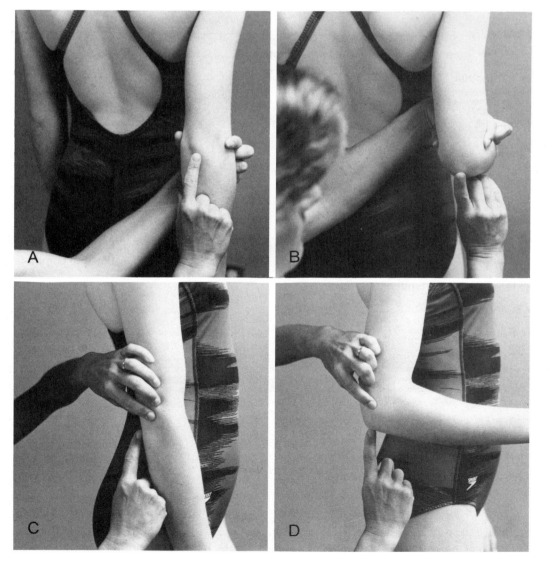

Figure 5.8. Elbow inspection. *A,* Posterior view. When the elbow is extended, the medial and lateral humeral epicondyles and the olecranon process should lie in a straight line. *B,* Posterior view. When the elbow is flexed, the medial and lateral humeral epicondyles and the olecranon process should form an isoceles triangle. *C,* Lateral view. When the elbow is extended, the medial and lateral humeral epicondyles should lie slightly anterior to the olecranon process. *D,* Lateral view. When the elbow is flexed, the medial and lateral epicondyles and olecranon process should lie in a straight line.

secondary to a fracture also alters shape, as does a hemarthrosis secondary to intraarticular fracture, which produces a bulging, tense joint capsule. The manner in which a patient uses the elbow for functional activities may indicate the severity or irritability of the condition. The examiner notes any skin lesions or color changes and the type and purpose of aids worn by the patient (Fig. 5.7).

Palpation.   The examiner palpates the elbow area to identify structural abnormalities, painful lesions, etc. (Fig. 5.9). Palpating the skin and subcutaneous tissue may reveal tissue tension resulting from swelling and inflammation. Rupture of the long head of the biceps tendon produces bulging of the biceps brachii muscle. Myositis ossificans of the brachialis muscle manifests as a firm lump or mass, in the antecubital region, that may be tender. Bursitis may enlarge the olecranon bursa that is superficial and accessible to palpation. Bony landmarks and joints, described pre-

viously, are superficial and easy to palpate in this area. The examiner may discover a fracture by indirect maneuvers, i.e., pushing proximally on the humeral shaft or percussing at some distance from the fracture site, which produces tenderness at the fracture (3). To locate the pulse of the brachial artery, the examiner palpates just medial to the insertion of the biceps brachii tendon (4). To elicit Tinel's sign from the ulnar nerve as it superficially crosses the elbow joint, one taps where it crosses posterior to the medial humeral epicondyle; localized tingling indicates nerve regeneration to that point.

Movement Assessment.   Assessment of functional active movement demonstrates a patient's capability to perform certain gross elbow movements (Fig. 5.9). Mechanical problems that limit movement, i.e., radial head irregularity, loose bone fragments, joint adhesions, and swelling, commonly follow elbow injury and immobilization. Ankylosis, with or without

2. Palpation (note location and nature of abnormality)

   a. Skin and subcutaneous tissue: tenderness _____ temperature _____ swelling _____ decreased mobility _____

       trigger points _____ other _____

   b. Muscles and tendons: tenderness _____ temperature _____ spasm _____ loss of continuity _____

       decreased mobility _____ other _____

   c. Tendon sheaths and bursae: tenderness _____ temperature _____ swelling _____ crepitus _____ other _____

   d. Bones and joints: tenderness _____ temperature _____ swelling _____ bony prominences _____ other _____

   e. Arteries and nerves: brachial artery _____ Tinel's sign (ulnar nerve) _____

3. Movement assessment

   a. Functional active moment

       flex elbow until extended thumb touches shoulder _____

       extend elbow to reach in front of body _____

       pronate and supinate with elbow flexed 90° _____

       pronate and supinate with elbow extended to 0° _____

       painful arc (in degrees) _____°

key: C = completes task
D = completes task with difficulty/discomfort
N = not able to complete task

   b/c.d. Physiological movement

	ACTIVE			PASSIVE			RESISTIVE	
	ROM	Symptoms	Quality	ROM	Symptoms	End-feel	Strength	Symptoms
Elbow flexion								
extension								
Forearm supination								
pronation								

Figure 5.9.   Examination form part 4: Palpation and movement assessment. ROM, range of motion.

myositis ossificans, is the most frequent complication after elbow injury (7). Also fibrosis and shortening of the collateral ligaments following trauma are primary causes of elbow stiffness (7). If a painful arc occurs, the examiner records its beginning and end ranges.

The therapist should examine physiological movements more specifically in the active, passive, and resistive categories (Fig. 5.9). He or she measures active movements that involve both inert and contractile structures, in degrees; in addition, associated symptoms and quality of movement are reported. Passive movement that generally involves inert structures (but may stretch antagonist contractile structures) is assessed for degree, symptoms, and end feel. The examiner grades muscle strength and assesses symptoms while the patient performs isometric resisted tests.

The examiner next tests accessory movement, which is graded on a scale of 0–6. Symptoms associated with accessory movement are also recorded (Fig. 5.10).

Special tests also aid the examiner in clarifying a disorder. To test the collateral ligaments (Fig. 5.11), the examiner stresses the elbow in both directions. This test may reveal laxity in the collateral ligaments

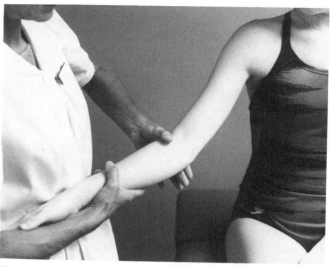

Figure 5.11.   Collateral ligamentous stability. If passive varus or valgus (shown here) force on an elbow in a few degrees of flexion reproduces pain or excessive motion, the test is positive, implicating laxity or rupture of the lateral or medial collateral ligaments, respectively.

e. Accessory movement

	Mobility	Symptoms
Humeroulnar joint traction		
medial glide		
lateral glide		
Humeroradial joint traction		
approximation		
Superior radioulnar joint dorsal (ventral) glide		
Inferior radioulnar joint ventral (dorsal) glide		

f. Special tests

	+	−	Comments
Collateral ligamentous stability: lateral			
medial			
Tennis elbow: resisted wrist extension			
passive wrist flexion			

Figure 5.10.   Examination form part 5: Accessory movement and special tests.

or reproduce any symptoms experienced by the patient (4).

A tennis elbow test attempts to reproduce the patient's symptoms by stressing the wrist extensor muscles. The therapist positions the patient's arm in elbow extension and forearm pronation, then resists wrist extension (Fig. 5.12*A*), then passively flexes the wrist fully (Fig. 5.12*B*). Pain felt in the area between the radial neck and lateral humeral epicondyle with either maneuver indicates a positive test.

Neurological Evaluation.   An examiner begins neurologic evaluation with the key muscles (Fig. 5.13). The biceps brachii muscle represents the C5–6 neurological level, and the triceps muscle represents the C7 neurological level. Key reflexes include the biceps brachii muscle, representing C5–6; the brachioradialis muscle, representing C6; and the triceps muscle, representing C7. The examiner maps sensibility on a body chart (Fig. 5.13). The pattern of sensory involvement may distinguish peripheral nerve lesions from nerve root lesions. All three peripheral nerves are subject to contusion, laceration, or stretching at the elbow. Radial tunnel syndrome, for example, results when fibrous bands, recurrent vessels, or the supinator tunnel (arcade of Frohse) compresses the radial nerve, producing pain, paresthesias, and paresis in the forearm extensors (23).

Recommendation of Other Tests.   When the examination is complete, the examiner begins to integrate and interpret the data. If there is a need for other tests or consultation, the patient is referred to the appropriate source.

The outcome of the final interpretation of results should provide information contributing to the definitive diagnosis, the current status of the condition, the functional ability of the patient, and the treatment planning process. Table 5.1 is a summary of the differential diagnosis and treatment of common elbow disorders.

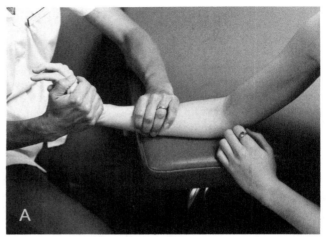

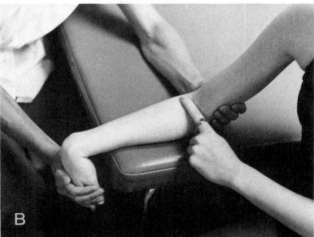

Figure 5.12.   Tennis elbow test. If resisted wrist extension *(A)* or passive wrist flexion *(B)* with the forearm pronated reproduces pain over the lateral humeral epicondyle, the test is positive, implicating pathology in the area of wrist extensor muscle origins.

4. Neurological evaluation

    a. Key muscles (strength grade 0–5):   C5–6 = biceps brachii muscle _____

                                              C7   = triceps muscle _____

    b. Key reflexes (graded +1 through +3);

        C5–6 = biceps brachii muscle _____   C6 = brachioradialis muscle _____

        C7 = triceps muscle _____

    c. Sensibility

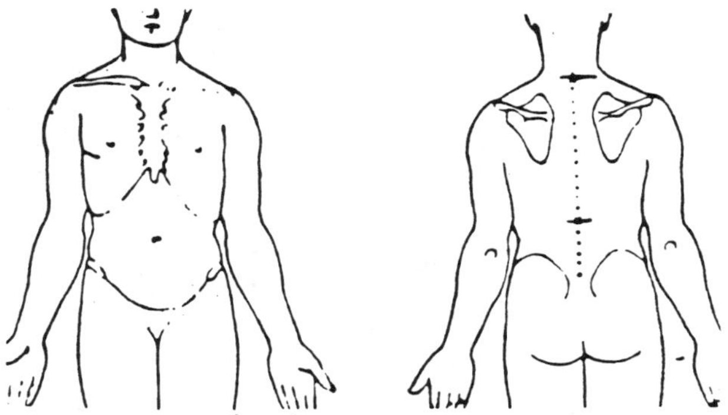

Key: lacking
    A = light touch sensation
    B = sharp/dull discrimination
    C = temperature discrimination
    D = proprioception

    d. Motor control: spastic _____ flaccid _____ rigid _____ clonic _____

    e. Coordination

        Index finger from distant moving object to nose _____

        Reciprocal pronation and supination _____

key: C   = completes task
       D   = completes task with
               difficulty/discomfort
       N   = not able to complete
               task

5. Recommendation of other tests

    a. Radiography _____

    b. Laboratory _____

    c. Electrodiagnostic _____

    d. Arthroscopy _____

    e. Arthrography _____

    f. Other _____

Figure 5.13.   Examination form part 6: Neurologic evaluation and recommendation of other tests.

Table 5.1.
Summary of Differential Diagnosis and Treatment of Common Elbow Disorders

Disorder	Complaint	Onset	Symptom Characteristics	Static Physical Changes	Dynamic Physical Changes	Special Tests	Treatment[a]
Bursitis non-inflammatory (olecranon)	Lump	Direct trauma or repetitive stress	Painless	Cystic swelling			Local measures to prevent injury such as resting splint and compression; aspiration; surgical excision
Dislocation (posterior)	Incapacitating pain and deformity	Fall on out-stretched hand and/or severe hyperextension	Pain, loss of function; associated soft tissue injury	Deformity and/or swelling	Loss of motion is a late complication	Olecranon palpated posteriorly	Prereduction neurovascular assessment; closed reduction (anesthesia if necessary); splint; week 1—start active flexion; 2—active assistive exercise; 3—ROM and strengthening exercise
Fractures a. Intraarticular (T or Y condylar)	Pain, swelling deformity for a, b, c, d	a. Blow to flexed elbow or longitudinal loading to extended elbow	Pain and dysfunction for a, b, c, d	Swelling a. Disruption of isosceles triangle	Loss of motion is a late complication of a, b, c, d	Radiography (for a, b, c)	Depending on alignment and comminution: a. Closed reduction and immobilization, traction, early motion, or ORIF
b. Olecranon		b. Direct trauma or triceps avulsion		b. Disruption of isosceles triangle			b. Immobilization with gentle ROM 3–7 days; ORIF; excision with triceps reconstruction and avoid full flexion for 4 weeks
c. Radial head		c. Axial load on pronated forearm or valgus compression		c. Lateral swelling from hemarthrosis, and disruption of lateral triangle			c. Aspiration of hemarthrosis and early motion; 2–3 weeks' immobilization; ORIF; operative excision, with or without implant
d. Supracondylar		d. Fall on out-stretched hand	Neurovascular compromise	d. Posterior displacement of distal fragment		Fat pad sign	d. Closed reduction; traction; ORIF; active ROM and strengthening
Lateral epicondylitis	Dull or sharp lateral pain	Insidious; overuse	Swelling, pain, weakness of wrist extension and grip	Lateral swelling		Decreased wrist extensor and grip strength	*Acute:* ice, prevent stress *Subacute:* heat, counter-force armband, passive stretch, friction massage, high-voltage galvanic stimulation *Chronic:* modify activity/equipment, steroid injection, excision of ECRB origin
Myositis ossificans	Painful swelling of brachialis muscle	Direct muscle trauma or secondary to fracture or dislocation	Rapidly enlarging painful mass	Mass in muscle or soft tissue	Limited motion	Well-circumscribed osseous mass	Prevent additional trauma; spontaneous regression may occur after 9–12 months; surgical excision only after maximal regression complete
Nurse-maid's (pulled) elbow	Pain localized to superior radioulnar joint	Longitudinal pull on forearm	Avoids use of arm	Arm held in pronation	Inability to supinate without pain	Palpate sulcus proximal to radial head	Closed reduction by flexion/supination maneuver; no immobilization necessary
Volkmann's contracture	Severe pain in forearm; sensation of pressure if compartment syndrome	Nerve and muscle ischemia, secondary to arterial compromise	Pain within 2 hours increased by passive finger extension; pallor; paresis; pulselessness	Wrist extension and finger flexion contractures	Paralysis and contractures are late complications		*Early:* remove restrictions; fasciotomy *Late:* functional activity, splinting, surgical reconstruction

[a]ROM, range of motion; ORIF, open reduction internal fixation; ECRB, extensor carpi radialis brevis.

ELBOW MOBILIZATION

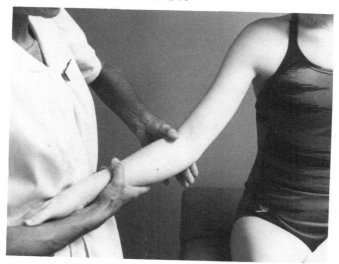

Figure 5.14.   Medial-Lateral Ulnar Oscillation.

Patient Position: Seated at edge of table with shoulder flexed and elbow slightly flexed.

Therapist Position: Standing at edge of table facing P; S hand supports wrist and hand against body; M hand contacts proximal forearm with web space.

Technique: Apply medial force with M hand web space against radius and ulna, perpendicular to arm; passive tension in joint structures produces a rebound lateral movement.

Comments: Indicated for painfully restricted elbow flexion and extension.

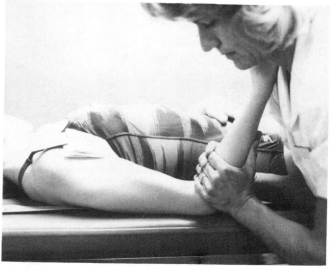

Figure 5.15.   Humeroulnar Joint Traction.

Patient Position: Supine with stabilizing strap in axilla and humerus stabilized against table; wrist rests on T's shoulder.

Therapist Position: Standing facing P's head; hands grasp around proximal forearm.

Technique: Use body movement to impart force through hypothenar contacts on ulna parallel to long axis of humerus.

Comments: General technique for treatment of elbow pain and hypomobility; using dorsal pressure during technique moves the olecranon away from the olecranon fossa, providing for greater mobility.

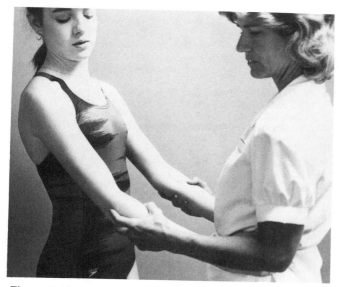

Figure 5.16.   Humeroradial Joint Test.

Patient Position: Standing with forearms supported by T.

Therapist Position: Standing, facing P; hands grasp P's elbows, forearms fixate P's hands; palpate humeroradial joints with index fingers.

Technique: Flex and extend P's elbows by leaning body toward or away from P; supinate and pronate P's forearms by rotating elbows.

Comments: Compare involved and uninvolved sides by palpating joint spaces and radial head mobility.

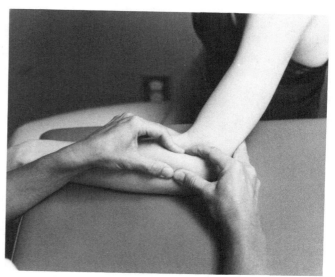

Figure 5.17.   Dorsal-Ventral Radial Glide, Superior Radioulnar Joint.

Patient Position: Seated with forearm resting on table and stabilized by friction against table.

Therapist Position: Seated facing lateral aspect of P's arm; thumbs and index fingers grasp radial head.

Technique: Move radius dorsally and ventrally with pressure through fingers and thumbs respectively upon fixed ulna.

Comments: Effective for increasing pronation, supination, and radial head mobility.

MANUAL THERAPY TECHNIQUES

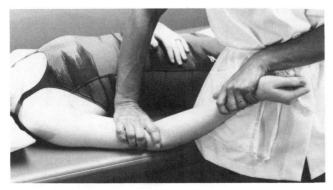

Figure 5.18. Humeroradial Joint Traction (Radioulnar Joints Caudal Glide).

Patient Position: Supine with arm stabilized against table.

Therapist Position: Standing with back toward P, but upper body rotated to face P; S hand fixates distal humerus on table; M hand grasps distal radius only (avoid holding ulna too).

Technique: Rotate body away from P with M hand restraining radius to produce traction on radius parallel to long axis of radius.

Comments: Effective for increasing joint space and improving elbow and forearm mobility.

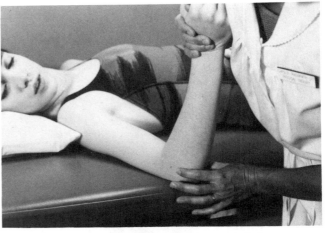

Figure 5.19. Humeroradial Joint Approximation (Radioulnar Joints Cranial Glide).

Patient Position: Supine with shoulder abducted, elbow flexed to 90°, and olecranon stabilized against table.

Therapist Position: Standing facing P's head; S hand holds elbow and palpates proximal humeroradial joint; M hand clasps P's hand with thenar to thenar contact.

Technique: Use chest contact over thenar contact only (avoid contact over entire palm) to apply dorsal force through long axis of radius.

Comments: Effective for reducing joint space and improving elbow and forearm mobility.

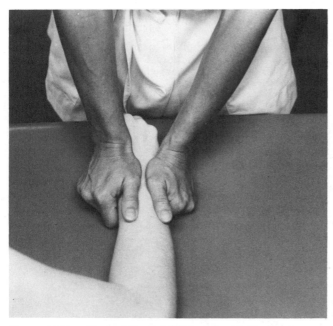

Figure 5.20. Ventral Radial Glide, Inferior Radioulnar Joint.

Patient Position: Seated with forearm resting on table.

Therapist Position: Standing facing P; S hand fixates distal ulna on table; M hand grasps distal radius.

Technique: Apply ventral force to radius through M hand thenar contact with arm parallel to force.

Comments: Use this technique to increase pronation. To increase supination, reverse hands so that M hand becomes S hand that fixates ulna, then impart a dorsal glide to the radius with the other hand.

References

1. Kapandji IA: *The Physiology of the Joints.* Edinburgh, Churchill Livingstone, 1974, vol. 1.
2. London JT: Kinematics of the elbow. *J Bone Joint Surg* 63A:529–535, 1981.
3. Smith FM: *Surgery of the Elbow.* Philadelphia, WB Saunders, 1972.
4. Hoppenfeld S: *Physical Examination of the Spine and Extremities.* New York, Appleton-Century-Crofts, 1976.
5. Dowd GSE, Hopcroft PW: Varus deformity secondary to supracondylar fractures in children. *Injury* 10:297–303, 1979.
6. Wadsworth TG: *The Elbow.* New York, Churchill Livingstone, 1982.
7. Morrey BF: *The Elbow and Its Disorders.* Philadelphia, WB Saunders, 1985.
8. Warwick R, Williams PC (eds): *Gray's Anatomy,* 35th British Edition. Philadelphia, WB Saunders, 1973.
9. Lockart RD, Hamilton GF, Fyfe FW: *Anatomy of the Human Body.* Philadelphia, JB Lippincott, 1965.
10. Tarr RR, Garfinkel AI, Sarmiento A: The effects of angular and rotational deformities of both bones of the forearm. *J Bone Joint Surg* 66A:65–70, 1984.
11. Bartz B, Tillman B, Schleicher A: Stress in the human elbow joint II. Proximal radio-ulnar joint. *Anat Embryol* 169:309–318, 1984.
12. Morrey BF, An K-N: Articular and ligamentous contributions to the stability of the elbow joint. *Am J Sports Med* 11:315–319, 1983.
13. Johnson C, Glasheen-Wray MB: Effect of forearm abduction on the ulnar collateral ligament. *Phys Ther* 63:660–663, 1983.
14. Schwab GH, Bennett JB, Woods GW, Tullos HS: Biomechanics of elbow instability: the role of the medial collateral ligament. *Clin Orthop* 146:42–51, 1980.
15. Vesely DG: The disto radio-ulnar joint. *Clin Orthop* 51:75–91, 1967.
16. Morrey BF, Askew LJ, An KN, Chao EY: A biomechanical study of normal functional elbow motion. *J Bone Joint Surg* 63A:872–877, 1981.

17. Cummings G: Comparison of muscle to other soft tissue in limiting elbow extension. *J Orthop Sports Phys Ther* 5:170–174, 1984.
18. Conwell HE: Injuries to the elbow. *Clin Symp* 21:35–62, 1969.
19. Bassett FH, Nunley JA: Compression of the musculocutaneous nerve at the elbow. *J Bone Joint Surg* 64A:1050–1052, 1982.
20. Bernhang AM: The many causes of tennis elbow. *NY State Med J* 79:1363–1366, 1979.
21. Priest JD, Braden V, Gerberich SG: The elbow and tennis, part 2: a study of players with pain. *Physician & Sports Med* 8:77–85, 1980.
22. Priest JD: Elbow injuries in sports. *Minn Med* 65:543–545, 1982.
23. Moss S, Switzer H: Radial tunnel syndrome: a spectrum of clinical presentations. *J Hand Surg* 8:414–420, 1983.

CHAPTER 6

THE WRIST AND HAND

CLINICAL ANATOMY AND MECHANICS OF THE WRIST AND HAND

Numerous structures interact in the wrist and hand to produce the remarkable dexterity and precision that characterize this unit. The following section describes the respective bones, joints, soft tissues, and nerves, detailing both their individual and collective functions.

Osteology

Radius and Ulna. The distal radius and ulna, in conjunction with the 27 bones of the hand proper (excluding sesamoids), comprise the wrist and hand skeleton (Fig. 6.1). The radius widens near the wrist, providing a large articular surface. Shallow depressions mark the concave radial articular surface where it contacts the scaphoid and lunate. A radial styloid process projects distally from the lateral side of the radius. A cartilage-covered ulnar notch occupies the distal medial side of the radius. Posteriorly, a dorsal (Lister's) tubercle arises near the center of the radius.

The distal end of the ulna expands slightly into a rounded head laterally and an ulnar styloid process medially. The convex articular surface of the ulnar head contacts both the ulnar notch of the radius laterally and the triangular fibrocartilaginous disc distally. The ulnar styloid process is one-half inch shorter than the radial styloid process, allowing ulnar deviation to exceed radial deviation.

Carpal Bones. Most anatomists divide the bones of the hand into units: the carpals, i.e., bones of the wrist; the metacarpals, i.e., bones of the palm; and the phalanges, i.e., bones of the fingers (Fig. 6.1). The carpal bones lie in two transverse rows. The proximal row contains (lateral to medial) the scaphoid (navicular), lunate, triquetrum, and pisiform. The distal row holds the trapezium (greater multangular), trapezoid (lesser multangular), capitate, and hamate. Collectively, the proximal carpal row presents a convex surface that articulates with the radius and triangular fibrocartilage disc. The between-row configuration of the conjoined carpals is S-shaped; the prox-imal row is convex laterally and concave medially, while the distal row is reciprocally shaped. The following paragraphs describe characteristics of individual carpal bones (Fig. 6.1).

The scaphoid resembles a boat, the basis for its name (1). Its proximal convex surface articulates with the radius; its distal lateral convex surface articulates with the trapezium and trapezoid; its distal medial concave surface articulates with the capitate and lunate. A prominent tubercle arises palmarly, to which the flexor retinaculum attaches. Because it transmits forces from the hand to the radius, and it lies across the midcarpal joint's plane of motion, the scaphoid commonly is fractured at its midsection, the waist (1,2). Arteries from the distal pole that cross the waist furnish the sole blood supply to the proximal pole in one-third of the population; therefore it is not uncommon for a fracture to produce loss of blood supply to the proximal pole.

The lunate, the keystone of the proximal carpal row, derives its name from its semilunar shape. This configuration results from its curving around a lateral facet that articulates with the scaphoid. The lunate is the most frequently dislocated carpal bone and may potentially compress the overlying median nerve when dislocated volarly. The triquetrum is a three-cornered bone, characterized by an oval facet for pisiform articulation. The small pea-shaped pisiform, other than a smooth dorsal articular facet, presents a generally roughened surface for attachment of the flexor and extensor retinacula, the pisometacarpal and pisohamate ligaments, and the tendons of the flexor carpi ulnaris and abductor digiti minimi muscles.

The trapezium, in the distal row, possesses a tubercle on its palmar surface to which the flexor retinaculum and origins of the thenar muscles attach. A groove on its palmar surface retains the flexor carpi radialis tendon. Its distal lateral surface is saddle-shaped for articulation with the reciprocally shaped first metacarpal bone. The trapezoid is small and irregular in shape, with four articular surfaces. The capitate is the largest and most central carpal bone, the focus of direction of many carpal ligaments. It articulates with seven other bones. The hamate occupies the medial end of the distal row. A hook-like hamulus projects from the palmar surface of the hamate. It protects the deep branchs of the ulnar nerve and artery, and provides attachment for the flexor retinaculum.

Metacarpal Bones. The five metacarpals resemble miniature long bones, with elongated shafts and expanded ends (Fig. 6.1). Their widened, proximal bases articulate with the carpals and with one another in plane joints. Their biconvex distal heads are broader anteriorly than posteriorly, a feature with mechanical significance to be discussed later. The first metacarpal is unique because its base is separate from the common joint formed by the others, and its head is pulley-shaped like the phalanges.

Phalanges. The fourteen phalanges are similar in configuration to the metacarpals, each comprised of a base, shaft, and head (Fig. 6.1). Two shallow depressions, which correspond to the pulley-shaped heads of the adjacent phalanges, mark the concave proximal bases. (The bases of proximal phalanges 2–5 are biconcave, however, to accommodate the metacarpal heads at that metacarpophalageal (MP) joints.) Two distinct condyles produce the pully-shaped configuration of the phalangeal heads, the convex members of the interphalangeal (IP) joints. The congruency of the IP joint surfaces contributes greatly to finger joint stability.

The bones of the hand form three separate arches that are all concave volarly. The arches enhance prehensile function, such as cupping an object in the palm. A longitudinal arch spans the hand lengthwise, with its keystone at the MP joints. A relatively mobile

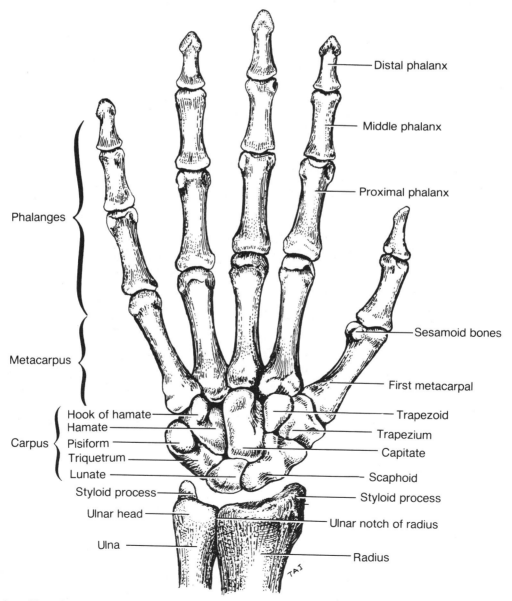

Figure 6.1. Wrist and hand skeleton.

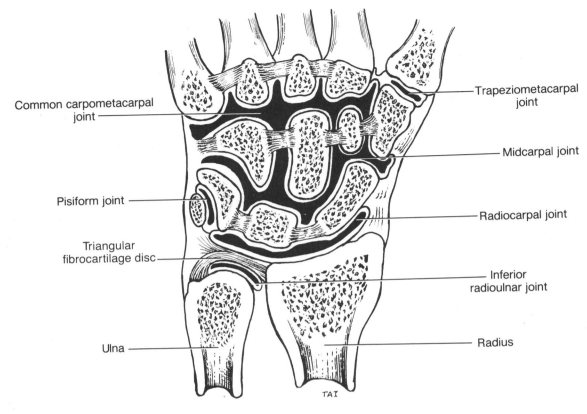

Figure 6.2. Wrist joints.

transverse arch occurs at the metacarpal heads. Another, immobile, transverse arch occurs within the palmar concavity of the carpal bones. This carpal arch is deepened by the volar projections of the scaphoid and trapezium laterally and the pisiform and hamate medially. The overlying flexor retinaculum transforms the carpal arch into the carpal tunnel through which the long flexor tendons and the median nerve pass.

The wrist contains another tunnel, the distal ulnar tunnel through which the ulnar artery and nerve pass. The space between the hamulus and pisiform marks its location. The palmar (volar) carpal ligament, palmaris brevis muscle, and the palmar aponeurosis form its roof, and the flexor retinaculum (transverse carpal ligament), pisohamate ligament, and pisometacarpal ligament form its floor (3–6) (Fig. 6.3).

Arthrology

Inferior Radioulnar Joint. The inferior radioulnar joint plays an important role in wrist and forearm function (Fig. 6.2). It is a double pivot, uniting the distal radius and ulna, as well as the ulna and articular disc. During forearm rotation, the concave ulnar notch of the radius sweeps around the peripheral surface of the convex ulnar head. Thus, in pronation, the radius crosses the ulna so that its distal end lies medially while its proximal end remains lateral. When the forearm supinates, the radius lies parallel to the ulna on its lateral side. Although the radius produces most of the supination-pronation motion, the ulna also moves

slightly in the opposite direction (e.g., during pronation the ulna moves in a posterior-lateral direction) (1,7,8). This uniaxial pivot joint, along with the superior radioulnar joint, provides up to 170° of forearm rotation, and allows the hand and radius to be positioned relative to the ulna. Accessory movements include anterior and posterior glide of both the radius and the ulna upon one another.

A triangular fibrocartilaginous disc assists in binding the distal radius and ulna. Its apex attaches to the ulnar styloid process and its base to the radius. The disc's anterior and posterior borders are thickened, and both its superior and inferior articular surfaces are smooth and concave. The disc also separates the distal radioulnar joint from the radiocarpal joint, as will be described later in this chapter. The articular capsule enclosing the inferior radioulnar joint is lax. It attaches to the articular margins of the radius and ulna and to the disc. Volar and dorsal radioulnar ligaments strengthen the capsule anteriorly and posteriorly. Supination tightens the anterior capsule while pronation tightens the posterior part; excessive forces may rupture these respective areas of the capsule. The capsule projects proximally between the bones in a pouch known as the recessus sacciformis.

Carpal Joints. The wrist forms a ''link joint'' between the forearm and hand. It contains several superimposed segments whose movements, when combined, create a total range of motion that is greater than that of its individual parts. However, the presence of intercalated bones inherent to this system creates the potential for instability. For instance, an unbalanced extrinsic tendon force may produce hand deformity when supporting ligaments are weakened by trauma or arthritis (9,10). The bones forming the wrist joint occupy and articulate with one another in a large synovial cavity. Joint capsules and interosseous ligaments divide this cavity into the separate joints described below (Fig. 6.2).

The radiocarpal joint marks the articulation of the concave radius and disc with the convex proximal row of carpals. In a neutral wrist position, the scaphoid contacts the radius, and the lunate contacts the radius and disc. Ulnar deviation brings the triquetrum into contact with the disc. The midcarpal joint lies between the two rows of carpals. It is a "compound" articulation because each row has both a concave and convex segment; the proximal row is convex laterally and concave medially, and the distal row is reciprocally arranged. Together, the radiocarpal and midcarpal joints produce the motion occurring at the biaxial wrist joint. The ranges are 70–80° of extension, 75–85° of flexion, 15–20° of radial deviation, and 30–40° of ulnar deviation. The wrist also allows relatively extensive traction and gliding accessory movement. Extension is the close-packed position of the wrist (8). During measurement of motion one must be aware that finger joint positions may affect wrist joint ranges (and vice versa) due to the constant length of the extrinsic tendons that cross multiple joints. For example, greater wrist flexion occurs with finger extension than with finger flexion because the extensor digitorum tendons aren't stretched maximally. The important clinical ramifications arising from this principle are as follows: a therapist should maintain all joints in a consistent position, except the one being measured; a therapist should identify wrist and finger joint position when measuring the strength of related muscles; a therapist may take advantage of tenodesis effects in certain disorders, such as a spinal cord-injured patient with no active finger flexion who can passively flex his fingers by extending his wrist.

Many of the wrist ligaments are not separate entities and remain unnamed. Numerous short intercarpal ligaments bind the carpal bones together on their dorsal and palmar surfaces. Deeper interosseous ligaments also attach the carpals to one another. Some of the major ligaments include the volar radiocarpal, volar ulnocarpal, dorsal radiocarpal, radial collateral, and ulnar collateral ligaments (Fig. 6.3).

The common carpometacarpal joint is an irregular combination of plane articulations between the distal row of carpals and the bases of the 2–5 metacarpals (Fig. 6.2). It allows the metacarpals, which progress in mobility toward the 5th, to glide slightly and cup the palm. The volar and dorsal carpometacarpal and intermetacarpal ligaments stabilize this joint.

The trapezium joins the first metacarpal in an isolated synovial joint. This trapeziometacarpal joint is a saddle-shaped articulation that theoretically possesses two degrees of freedom, but practically displays

a third also. Flexion and extension reach 50–60°, abduction and adduction 40–50°, and axial rotation 17°(11). Convention dictates that thumb flexion and extension occur in a plane (frontal) that is perpendicular to the plane (sagittal) of finger flexion and extension. Thumb abduction and adduction occur in a plane (sagittal) that is perpendicular to the plane (frontal) of finger abduction and adduction. During thumb flexion and extension, the concave first metacarpal articular surface moves on the convex trapezium. During thumb abduction and adduction, the convex metacarpal surface moves on the concave trapezium. Lateral, volar, and dorsal oblique ligaments span this joint.

The pisiform-triquetral joint is a small, plane joint with its own synovial cavity. The pisiform glides slightly on the triquetrum. The ulno-menisco-triquetral joint joins the ulna, disc, and triquetrum. It does not possess a separate capsule and synovial cavity, but is significant clinically because it allows gliding between the carpals, disc, and ulna during pronation and supination. Also, lack of direct ulnar-triquetral articulation permits a greater range of ulnar deviation (7).

Metacarpophalangeal Joints. The 2nd–5th metacarpals articulate with the respective proximal phalanges in biaxial joints (Fig. 6.3). Movement increases progressively from the 2nd–5th MP joints. The approximate range of motion for these joints is 90° of flexion, 25° of extension, and 20° of abduction. Traction, gliding, and rotatory accessory movement occurs at all of the MP joints. Joint capsules, attached to the articular margins of the metacarpals and phalanges, surround the joints. The dorsal hood apparatus reinforces (or replaces) the dorsal joint capsules, and likewise, the volar plates reinforce the palmar aspects of the joints. The volar plates are fibrocartilaginous units, which attach firmly to the phalangeal bases but connect only loosely to the metacarpal heads by membraneous fibers (12). Their dorsal surface contributes to the joint area, and their palmar surface channels the finger flexor tendons (Fig. 6.3). Finger flexion causes the membranous portions of the volar plates to overlap, and prolonged immobilization in this position may lead to adhesion formation.

Collateral ligaments provide lateral support for the MP joints. They are strong cords that run obliquely from the dorsal aspect of the metacarpal head to the ventral aspect of the phalangeal base (Fig. 6.3). Due to their location and the eccentric axis of rotation of the metacarpal head, which is broader anteriorly, they tighten in flexion, thereby preventing MP joint abduction in this position. Contracture of these ligaments is a major cause of loss of MP flexion. To prevent contracture during immobilization of the hand, a therapist should splint a patient's fingers with the MP joints flexed 70–90°. Superficial and deep transverse metacarpal ligaments, connecting the metacarpal heads to one another, also provide indirect support for the MP joints.

The thumb MP joint is a hinge joint. Its bony configuration, which resembles the IP joints, provides it with some inherent stability. Its range of motion is 50°

of flexion to 0° of extension. Traction, gliding, and rotatory accessory movement are also present. Volar and collateral ligaments support this joint.

Interphalangeal Joints. The adjacent phalanges articulate in hinge joints that allow motion in only one plane. Flexion approximates 110° at the proximal interphalangeal (PIP) joints, 90° at the distal interphalangeal (DIP) joints, and 90° at the thumb interphalangeal (IP) joint. Extension reaches 0° at the PIP joints, and 25° at the DIP joints and thumb IP joint. Traction, gliding, and accessory movement also occur at the IP joints.

Joint capsules, attached to the articular margins of the phalanges, surround the IP joints. Volar and collateral ligaments, similar to those of the MP joints, are present but not as essential to stability (Fig. 6.3). The collateral ligaments are maximally taut at 25° of finger flexion, unlike the MP joint collateral ligaments, which are taut from 70–90° (12). For this reason a therapist

should initially splint the fingers in 25° of flexion to prevent IP joint contractures resulting in loss of IP joint extension; during rehabilitation this position changes as a patient resumes function.

Mechanics

Physical therapists frequently treat disorders of the hand related to soft tissue pathology. The following paragraphs discuss the interrelationships and common disorders of soft tissue structures.

The dorsal subcutaneous tissue differs structurally from the palmar tissue. The dorsal areolar tissue is thin and elastic to permit stretching when making a fist. Its loose attachment and preponderance of lymphatics and veins account for the fact that swelling manifests predominantly on the dorsum of the hand, although its source often lies elsewhere (13). The palmar subcutaneous tissue, in contrast, contains many

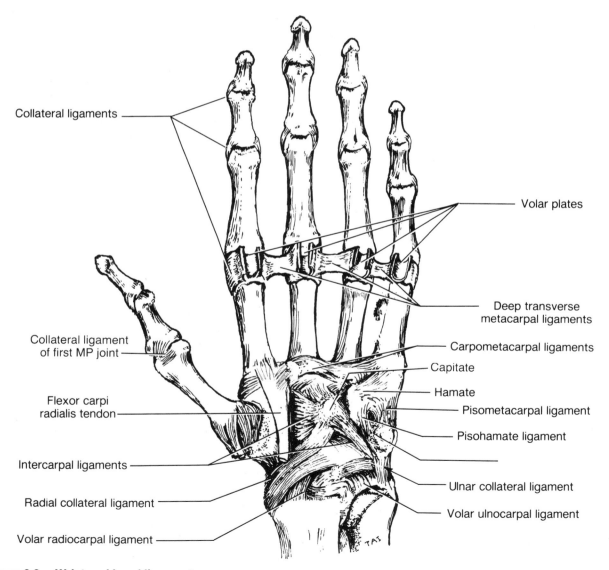

Figure 6.3. Wrist and hand ligaments.

Labels in figure:
- Collateral ligaments
- Volar plates
- Deep transverse metacarpal ligaments
- Collateral ligament of first MP joint
- Carpometacarpal ligaments
- Capitate
- Flexor carpi radialis tendon
- Hamate
- Pisometacarpal ligament
- Pisohamate ligament
- Intercarpal ligaments
- Radial collateral ligament
- Ulnar collateral ligament
- Volar ulnocarpal ligament
- Volar radiocarpal ligament

strong fibrous fasciculi that connect the skin tightly to the adjacent palmar aponeurosis, permitting relatively little sliding of the skin and enhancing secure grasp.

The palmar aponeurosis, just deep to the subcutaneous tissue, is a dense fibrous structure continuous with the palmaris longus tendon and fascia covering the thenar and hypothenar muscles (Fig. 6.4). It continues distally to attach to the transverse metacarpal ligaments and flexor tendon sheaths. It offers some protection for the ulnar artery and nerve, and digital vessels and nerves. Nodule formation or scarring in this structure produces a clinical entity known as Dupuytren's contracture, which may ultimately cause finger flexion contractures.

The flexor retinaculum (transverse carpal ligament), deep to the palmar aponeurosis, spans the area between the pisiform, hamate, scaphoid, and trapezium. It converts the carpal arch to a tunnel through which pass the median nerve and some of the tendons of the hand (Fig. 6.4). This retinaculum offers attachment for the thenar and hypothenar muscles, helps maintain the transverse carpal arch, prevents bowstringing of the extrinsic flexor tendons, and protects the

median nerve. In a condition known as carpal tunnel syndrome, the median nerve is compressed in this relatively unyielding space.

Extrinsic muscles whose bellies lie proximal to the wrist join with intrinsic muscles located entirely within the hand to produce the intricate precision and power maneuvers that characterize hand function. This design provides for a large number of muscles to activate the hand without inordinate bulkiness. Table 6.1 lists both the extrinsic and intrinsic muscles that move the hand. A thorough review of muscle origins, insertions, and actions is recommended, but due to comprehensive coverage elsewhere (1,8,14), it is not included in this text. The extrinsic tendons enhance wrist stability through a balance of flexor and extensor forces, as well as their resultant force in a proximal direction that compresses the carpals (2). As stated earlier, this purported stabilizing force can become a deforming force in the presence of ligamentous laxity.

The extrinsic finger flexor tendons pass into the hand deep to the flexor retinaculum. The flexor digitorum superficialis muscles, whose main function is to flex the PIP joints and whose secondary function is

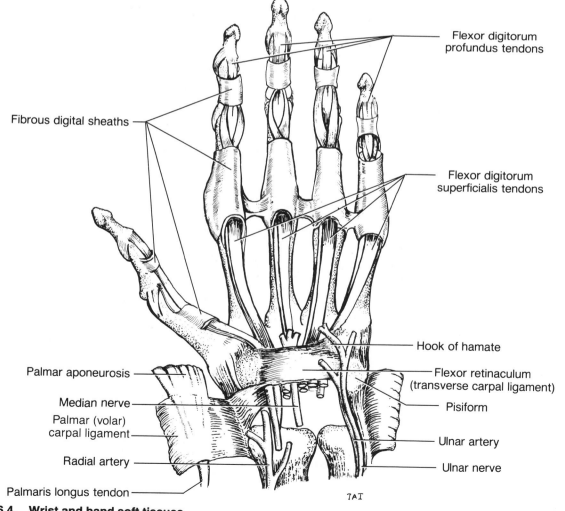

Figure 6.4.   Wrist and hand soft tissues.

Table 6.1.
Extrinsic and Intrinsic Muscles of the Wrist and Hand

Extrinsic Muscles	Intrinsic Muscles
Extensor carpi radialis longus and brevis	Lumbricals
Extensor carpi ulnaris	Dorsal and palmar interossei
Flexor carpi radialis	Adductor pollicis
Flexor carpi ulnaris	Flexor pollicis brevis
Palmaris longus	Abductor pollicis brevis
Extensor pollicis longus and brevis	Opponens pollicis
Abductor pollicis longus	Flexor digiti minimi
Extensor indicis	Abductor digiti minimi
Extensor digiti minimi	Opponens digiti minimi
Extensor digitorum	Palmaris brevis
Flexor digitorum superficialis	
Flexor digitorum profundus	
Flexor pollicis longus	

to assist MP joint flexion, possess tendons that are capable of relatively independent action at each finger. The flexor digitorum profundus muscles, which, alone, flex the DIP joints, and assist in flexion of the PIP and

MP joints, also supply tendons for each finger. Unlike the superficialis tendons these tendons cannot operate independently. To isolate the PIP joint flexor function of these two muscles, a therapist holds the adjoining finger(s) in extension while the patient attempts to flex the finger being tested. This anchors the profundus muscle of the finger being tested distally, and allows the superficialis muscle to act alone at the PIP joint (15).

Fibrous sheaths between the distal palmar crease and the PIP joints tether the flexor tendons to the fingers. Some surgeons refer to the area where the sheaths contain two tendons as "no man's land." Severed tendons within a common sheath demonstrate a tendency to adhere to surrounding tissues following primary repair (Fig. 6.4).

The extensor retinaculum retains the extensor tendons on the dorsum of the wrist. Proximal to the metacarpal heads, juncturae tendinea connect the four tendons of the extensor digitorum muscles (ED), limiting their independent motion (Fig. 6.5). Flexion of

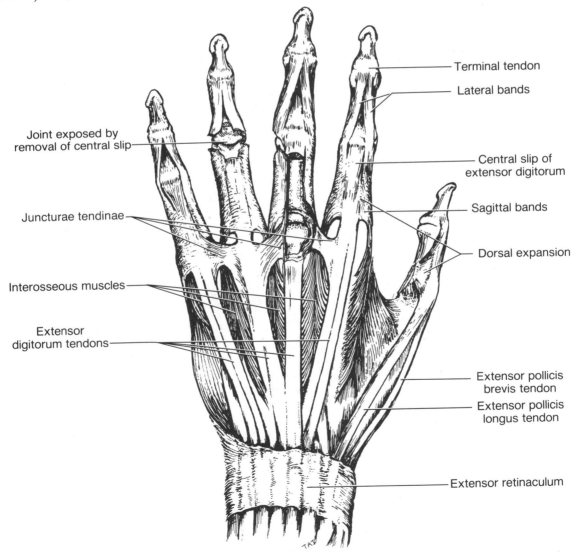

Figure 6.5. Dorsal hood, extensor tendons, and finger ligaments.

the middle and little fingers thus restricts extension of the ring finger MP joint because the juncturae tendinae pull the ring finger extensor tendon distally, rendering it lax. Conversely, extension of the ring finger exerts an extensor force upon its neighbors, such that they can be actively extended even if the middle and little extensor tendons are severed proximal to the juncturae (16).

As the ED tendons cross the region of the MP joints, their primary connection to the proximal phalanx is through the sagittal bands, which pass palmarward to attach to the volar plate (Fig. 6.5). The main function of the sagittal bands is to transmit the extension force of the ED to the proximal phalanges, thus extending the MP joints, but they also prevent bowstringing of the extensor tendon dorsally (16–18). Active extension of the MP joint transmits all of the force of the ED to the proximal phalanx; excursion of the tendon is blocked so that any extension of the IP joints which is to occur must be performed by the intrinsic muscles (8,16,18). Thus, to differentiate function of the extrinsic and intrinsic extensor muscles, a therapist should have a subject maintain full active MP joint extension, then attempt IP joint extension; only the intrinsic muscles can produce this latter action.

Between the MP and PIP joints the ED tendon divides into three parts, the central slip, which inserts into the proximal dorsal edge of the middle phalanx, and two lateral bands (Fig. 6.5). These lateral bands rejoin over the middle phalanx into a terminal tendon which inserts into the proximal dorsal edge of the distal phalanx. Rupture of the tendon insertion into the distal phalanx produces a mallet finger. Fibers from the lumbrical and interosseous muscles join the ED tendons over the proximal phalanx, contributing to the dorsal hood apparatus. The tendons of the intrinsic muscles pass volar to the MP joint axes, but dorsal to the PIP and DIP joint axes. Thus, the intrinsic muscles exert a flexion force on the MP joints and an extension force on the IP joints.

The lateral bands, comprised of fibers from both extrinsic and intrinsic tendons, are prevented from dislocating dorsally by the transverse retinacular ligaments which link them to the volar plates of the PIP

joints (Fig. 6.6). Stretching or laxity of these ligaments allows bowstringing of the lateral bands, which transmit excessive extension force to the PIP joint. This abnormal tension may contribute to a hyperextension deformity of the PIP joint. Volar plate rupture or joint laxity enhances this deforming force. In addition, such a hyperextended position of the PIP joint tightens the flexor digitorum profundus tendon, flexing the DIP joint and producing a classic "swan neck" deformity (Fig. 6.6).

The oblique retinacular ligament (Landsmeer's ligament) also contributes to interdependence of interphalangeal joint movement. It attaches between the PIP volar plate, where it is volar to the PIP joint axis, and the terminal tendon, where it is dorsal to the DIP joint axis (Fig. 6.7). When the PIP joint extends, the oblique retinacular ligament exerts a passive extensor force on the DIP joint, and when the PIP joint flexes, it allows the DIP joint to flex. In the normal hand, the oblique retinacular ligament has a minor influence on function. Following a burn or trauma injury, this ligament may shorten, producing a tenodesis effect, e.g., when the PIP joint is extended, the DIP joint will be brought into fixed extension by this ligament (18).

Proximal interphalangeal joint position also may influence DIP joint position through lateral band action. The lateral bands normally slip volarly upon PIP joint flexion, decreasing the excursion required for full DIP joint flexion. If scar tissue tethers the lateral bands so that they do not move volarly, then a person cannot fully flex both the PIP and DIP joints at the same time. Proximal interphalangeal joint flexion also affects DIP joint active extension. Full flexion of the PIP joint anchors the central slip and the ED distally; the lateral bands become completely lax, thus permitting only weak and limited distal joint extension (13,18). In contrast, when the central slip ruptures from its insertion and retracts proximally, the proximal tension in the ED renders the lateral bands taut. The PIP joint is pulled into flexion by the unopposed flexor digitorum superficialis muscle, and the lateral bands drop volar to the PIP joint axis and become flexors. The force of the ED and intrinsic muscles is transmitted through the lateral bands to the distal phalanx, extending it,

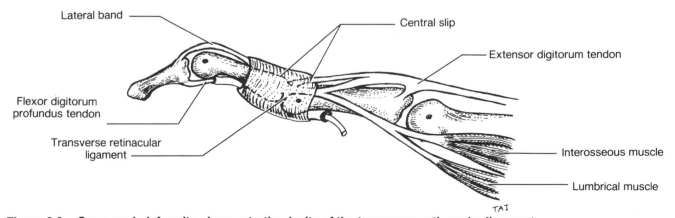

Figure 6.6.   Swan neck deformity, demonstrating laxity of the transverse retinacular ligament.

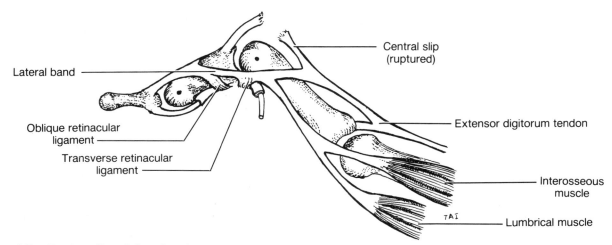

Figure 6.7.   Boutonnière deformity, demonstrating rupture of the central slip.

and producing a "boutonnière" deformity (16–19) (Fig. 6.7). A therapist should consider these interrelationships when evaluating the DIP joint in cases of PIP joint contracture.

The lumbrical muscles originate from the flexor digitorum profundus tendons and insert into the dorsal hood apparatus. During contraction, they pull the profundus tendons distally, thus prossessing the unique ability to relax their own antagonist. The lumbrical muscles serve as a primary organ of feedback in the hand. They are ideally located to provide feedback as to position and movement of the hand and finger joints (16).

In instances of lumbrical spasm or contracture, attempts to flex the fingers via the profundus result in transmission of force through the lumbricals into the extensor apparatus, producing extension rather than flexion. "Lumbrical plus" deformity occurs when there is excessive lumbrical force, or if there is imbalance of opposing forces. This produces exaggerated lumbrical action, i.e., MP joint flexion and IP joint extension.

Neurology

Motor Innervation.   The median nerve supplies the following muscles while coursing through the forearm: pronator teres, flexor carpi radialis, palmaris longus, and flexor digitorum superficialis. It gives off an anterior interosseous branch that supplies the flexor pollicis longus, pronator quadratus, and flexor digitorum profundus muscle to the index and middle fingers and sometimes the ring finger. It then passes under the flexor retinaculum and enters the palm, splitting into 4 sensory branches and a motor branch that supply the following muscles: abductor pollicis brevis, opponens pollicis, and superficial head of the flexor pollicis brevis. Other branches supply the first and second lumbricals. High median nerve paralysis results in loss of thumb opposition and IP flexion, and flexion of the first two fingers. A hand with a median nerve lesion may assume a resting "benediction" atti-

tude with the thumb adducted and the first two fingers extended. Loss of median nerve function severely hinders the ability to perform precision maneuvers due to loss of critical sensory and motor function in the thumb, index, and middle fingers (20).

The ulnar nerve supplies the following muscles in the forearm: flexor carpi ulnaris and flexor digitorum profundus muscle to the little and the ring fingers. In the hand it innervates the following muscles: flexor digiti minimi, abductor digiti minimi, opponens digiti minimi, adductor pollicis, palmaris brevis, 3rd and 4th lumbricals, deep head of the flexor pollicis brevis, and the interossei. A potential site of ulnar nerve compression in the hand is the distal ulnar tunnel. Paralysis of the ulnar nerve produces loss of thumb adduction (lateral pinch), weakness in power grip, and difficulties in finger spreading and coordinated activities, such as piano playing (20). A hand with an ulnar nerve lesion in which MP joint extension and IP joint flexion are unopposed, may assume a "claw hand" or "intrinsic minus" deformity. This deformity is more severe in lesions distal to innervation of the flexor digitorum profundus muscle, which leave it intact so that it adds to the flexion force upon the IP joints.

All motor branches of the radial nerve are located in the forearm, where it supplies the following muscles: extensor carpi radialis longus and brevis, extensor carpi ulnaris, supinator, extensor digitorum, abductor pollicis longus, extensor pollicis longus and brevis, extensor indicis, and extensor digiti minimi. Radial nerve paralysis results in loss of extension of the wrist and MP joints of the fingers, and thumb extension and abduction. Since the wrist extensor muscles are synergists and stabilizers for the finger flexor muscles, this loss can significantly hamper hand function.

Sensory Innervation.   The hand serves in many respects as a "sense organ." Twenty-five percent of all the pacinian (touch) corpuscles in the body are located in the hand. The motor system is totally dependent upon the constant feedback it receives from the sensory receptors. The three major peripheral nerves and their branches carry sensation from the hand in the following manner (Fig. 6.8A):

1. *Median*—lateral portion of palm and thenar surface; volar part of thumb, index, and middle fingers, and lateral half of ring finger, extending over the dorsum of the terminal phalanges; innervation is most constant at the tip of the index finger.

2. *Ulnar*—ulnar side of hand, medial half of ring finger, and little finger (both dorsal and palmar surfaces); innervation is most constant at the tip of the little finger.

3. *Radial*—dorsum of hand, lateral to 4th metacarpal, and dorsal surfaces of thumb and first 2 1/2 digits to DIP joints; innervation is most constant at the dorsal web space between thumb and index finger.

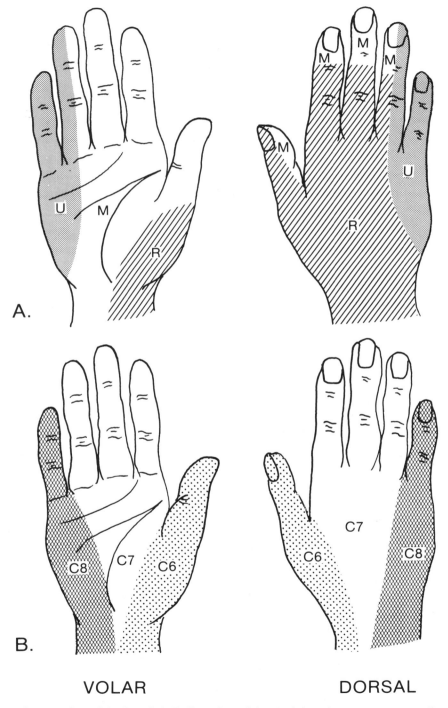

VOLAR   DORSAL

Figure 6.8.   Sensory innervation of the hand. *A,* Delineation of the peripheral cutaneous sensation supplied by the radial (R), median (M), and ulnar (U) nerves. *B,* Delineation of sensation derived from cervical root levels C6, C7, and C8. (Adapted from Calliet R: Hand Pain and Impairment, ed 2. Philadelphia, FA Davis, 1975.)

Cervical nerve root compression may produce sensory changes that one experiences in the distal-most areas of the dermatomes, thus involving the hand. Knowledge of dermatomal distribution assists the examiner in differentiating between nerve root and peripheral nerve lesions. Root level representation includes C6 to the thenar area and thumb, C7 to the midpalm and dorsal areas, and index, middle, and ring fingers, and C8 to the hypothenar area and little finger (21) (Fig. 6.8B). Because of the similar patterns of C8 and ulnar nerve sensory distribution, additional motor tests may be necessary for making a differential diagnosis.

Angiology

Arterial. The radial and ulnar arteries supply blood to the hand. The radial artery courses along the lateral side of the forearm to the wrist, where its pulse is palpable just lateral to the flexor carpi radialis tendon. After giving off the superficial palmar branch, it winds laterally around the dorsum of the wrist and enters the palm between the first and second metacarpals, where it forms the deep palmar arch by uniting with the deep branch of the ulnar artery. The radial artery gives off a superficial palmar branch proximal to the scaphoid which anastomoses with the corresponding ulnar branch, forming the superficial palmar arch. This arch is usually larger and more significant than the deep arch.

The ulnar artery crosses the wrist medially, deep to the volar carpal ligament, and superficial to the flexor retinaculum. It lies between the pisiform and the ulnar nerve, which it parallels. Just distal to the pisiform, it divides into a superficial branch, which continues across the palm as the superficial palmar arch, and a deep branch, which anastomoses with the radial artery, completing the deep arch. An ulnar artery thrombosis sometimes occurs where the superficial branch passes between the flexor retinaculum and volar fascia (4,22).

From the deep palmar arch arise the palmar metacarpal arteries, which join the palmar digital arteries from the superficial arch. They extend into the fingers as digital arteries.

Venous. A plexus of superficial and deep veins drains the hand. The superficial system is most significant. It is developed best over the dorsal surface of the hand and becomes increasingly prominent with age. At the level of the wrist, this system converges into the cephalic vein laterally and the basilic vein medially which ascend superficially up the forearm. The deep veins of the hand travel in pairs with the arteries (venae comitantes). They ascend from the digits to the palmar arches to the radial and ulnar arteries.

WRIST AND HAND EXAMINATION

When examining a wrist and hand, one must thoroughly understand the complex interaction of struc-

tures in this area. For example, any particular position or motion relies on the combined function of extrinsic and intrinsic motors, and passive and active restraints; in addition, rarely is one joint's position independent of others', because musculotendinous units may span up to four joints in the wrist and hand. Normal function also requires an intricate sensory feedback mechanism. This section explains many of these relationships, providing tests for evaluating various structures in isolation when applicable and a format for evaluating the structure and function of the wrist and hand as a unit.

History

The physical therapist begins by requesting identifying data, chief complaint, etc., from the patient (Fig. 6.9). Next, he asks for details of the present disorder beginning with a description of symptoms. A body chart is useful for detailing the location of particular types of symptoms. A lesion may lie within, or outside, the area of pain; the therapist may be misled if he is always expecting the former. For instance, ligamentous injury produces localized pain over the involved structure, whereas peripheral nerve compression may produce both local and radiating pain (23). The examiner also documents severity, impairment, and nature of the condition as described in Chapter 2. The behavior of the patient's symptoms may depict aggravating factors related to the pathology. The patient is often able to discern particular activities or postures which affect his symptoms. An unusual condition in which the severity of symptoms appears unrelated to other events is posttraumatic sympathetic dystrophy. It manifests as inappropriate, constant pain immediately after surgery or injury, to the degree that the patient avoids all contact with the hand (23). In addition to symptom behavior, peculiar characteristics of the joints, such as abnormal sensations during movement (e.g., catching or locking), swelling, and instability assist in problem identification (Fig. 6.9). Chronic popping or snapping is often indicative of a tendon problem; whereas popping or snapping at the original incident may suggest an intercarpal ligament tear or fracture.

The examiner next requests more background information on the precipitating event and associated findings (Fig. 6.10). He notes the date of injury or onset. Many hand conditions are insidious, in which the date of onset may be ambiguous. Examples of insidious conditions include a flareup of an overuse syndrome such as De Quervain's disease or a gradual increase in joint laxity from an old sprain.

If an injury occurred, its nature and mechanism assist the examiner in identifying the damaged structures. Owing to its vulnerable anatomic position and wide range of function, the hand sustains an inordinate amount of trauma (24). Table 6.2 lists some structures commonly traumatized, and the typical mechanisms of injury.

It is often necessary to ask the patient to be very specific when describing an injury. If he states "I fell

A. HISTORY

1. Identifying Data

Name _____ Age _____ Gender _____ Date _____

Provisional diagnosis _____ Precautions _____

Chief complaint _____

Dominant side R _____ L _____ Prior condition of involved part _____

2. Present Episode or Illness

a. Description of symptoms

1) location: //// = pain
              ==== = paresthesia
              °°°° = numbness
              xxxx = other _____

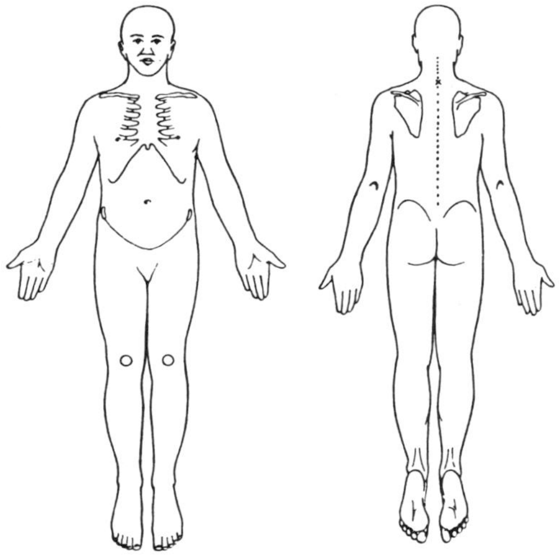

2) severity:

_____
none   worst

3) impairment:

_____
annoying   completely disabling

4) nature:

cramping _____ aching _____

shooting _____ burning _____

throbbing _____ tingling _____

stabbing _____ sore _____

other _____

5) behavior:

constant _____ intermittent _____ duration _____

occurs when _____ elicited by _____

aggravated by _____relieved by _____

24-hour pattern _____

highly irritable _____ mildly irritable _____ not irritable _____

6) joint characteristics: catches _____ , locks _____ , swells _____ , gives way _____ , dislocates _____ ,

other _____

Figure 6.9. Examination form part 1: History.

b. Background and associated findings

Date of present injury _____ or onset _____ insidious _____

Dates of hospitalization _____ and/or other health care

Treatments; dates; results _____

_____

Status of condition: acute _____ or chronic _____

constant _____ or intermittent _____

better _____ or worse _____

Nature and mechanism of injury or events precipitating present episode _____

_____

Results of injury (if applicable): deformity (describe) _____

corrected _____ disability (type and cause) _____

loss of motion (specify) _____ when occurred _____

loss of strength (specify) _____ when occurred _____

swelling (specify) _____ when occurred _____

bleeding (specify) _____ when occurred _____

3. Relevant Past History and Family History

History of similar condition: dates _____ nature _____

_____

Treatment _____

Other relevant illnesses or disorders _____

General health status _____

Health problems of immediate family _____

4. Life-style

Occupation _____ ADL _____

Regular (3 times/week minimum) physical activities requiring: strength _____ agility _____ endurance _____

flexibility _____ other _____

What patient does to promote wellness _____

Patient's concept of cause of condition _____

Patient's concept of functional and/or cosmetic deficit(s) _____

Anticipated goals _____

5. Other

Current medications _____

Recent radiographs _____

6. Therapist's Interpretation and Plans for Objective Exam _____

_____

Figure 6.10. Examination form part 2: History, continued.

on my wrist," the examiner should probe whether the wrist was flexed or extended, the forearm supinated or pronated, and what position the arm was in. Also, he should determine on which side of the wrist the impact occurred. The ulnar side is more vulnerable to sharp objects due to the location of all of the extrinsic finger flexor tendons as well as the median and ulnar nerves. In contrast, the radial side is at risk for a scaphoid fracture from a blunt impact. Following an industrial accident, it may be necessary to clarify technical jargon, and follow a question like "What happened to your hand?" with "What size space was your hand caught in?", "How large were the rollers, and what type of surface did they have?", "How quickly was your hand released?", etc. (23).

The results of injury on a hand also assist interpretation. The examiner should inquire about any deformity sustained, such as bone or joint malalignment or loss of tendon continuity. Disability is another parameter which he explores, determining both a description (e.g., "decreased pinch strength") and a reason (e.g., "thumb metacarpophalangeal (MP) joint instability" or "thumb MP joint pain"). The **sequence** of injury and development of disability may be relevant. For example, a patient who falls onto an extended wrist and dislocates his lunate may experience immediate pain, but may not notice symptoms of median nerve compression until later. Another instance is hyperextension of a finger which produces immediate loss of active movement when a musculotendinous unit is ruptured, but loss of passive movement only after 12–24 hours when capsular injury results in joint effusion.

The examiner next requests the patient's relevant past history and a history of family health problems. He also asks the patient to summarize his lifestyle with regard to occupation, habits, living conditions,

and physical activities. Repetitive occupational or recreational postures may increase the risk of developing certain conditions, such as thumb extension in assembly line work which predisposes one to tenosynovitis. Another example of activity-related pathology is ulnar nerve compression within the distal ulnar tunnel from bicycling, which may produce intrinsic paralysis and sensory changes. Finally, the patient's concept of the cause of his condition, along with the functional and cosmetic impact on his anticipated lifestyle, cue the examiner as to the overall severity of the case and the goals of rehabilitation. Occupational and recreational demands placed upon the hand, plus cosmetic and economic factors will all affect reconstructive or replantation considerations, postsurgical care, and rehabilitation.

Physical Examination

Inspection.   While taking the history, the examiner has observed the patient's relationship with his involved limb. A closer inspection of the appearance and posture of the hand should now ensue (Fig. 6.11). The attitude of a resting hand often portrays common deformities such as clawing, ulnar drift, and joint contractures and subluxations. The examiner may detect collapse of the normal longitudinal or transverse arch framework, resulting from skeletal malalignment, muscle imbalance, or joint instability. Early postural deviations may later become contractures. Photographs are a valuable asset to defining postural deformities.

A hand chart and key to typical changes allows the examiner to describe a hand's shape easily and accurately (28) (Fig. 6.11). He can document changes in contour, which may result from protuberances or nodules, such as ganglia or Heberden's nodes, loss of arches, absence of digits, narrowed web spaces,

Table 6.2.
Commonly Traumatized Wrist and Hand Structures and Associated Mechanisms of Injury

Mechanisms of Injury	Structures Commonly Damaged
1. Sudden forced (striking) flexion of distal phalanx	1. Mallet finger produced by: tear of extensor tendon, avulsion of lateral bands, volar fracture/subluxation DIP joint
2. Forceful flexion of middle phalanx or dorsal blow over PIP joint	2. Boutonniére deformity produced by ruptured insertion of central slip of extensor digitorum tendon
3. Sudden forced finger extension while FDP contracted	3. FDP avulsion
4. Sudden hyperextension of PIP joint	4. Volar plate rupture from middle phalanx
5. Longitudinal compression with some hyperextension of PIP joint	5. Dorsal fracture/dislocation of PIP joint
6. Sudden twisting of finger or blow over MP joint	6. Tear of dorsal hood with ulnar subluxation of extensor digitorum tendon
7. Sudden, forceful forearm pronation or supination	7. Dorsal or volar dislocation of ulnar head with damage to triangular fibrocartilage disc
8. Fall on hand with thumb abducted	8. Tear ulnar collateral ligament of thumb MP joint
9. Fall onto extended wrist	9. Scaphoid fracture
10. Fall onto flexed wrist with pronation	10. Rupture of dorsal radioulnar ligaments; Smith's fracture
11. Fall onto outstretched hand with hyperpronation or hypersupination	11. Dislocation of distal radioulnar joint

B. PHYSICAL EXAMINATION

1. Inspection

   a. Posture

   Position or attitude of resting hand _____

   Longitudinal arch _____ carpal arch _____ metacarpal arch _____

   General appearance of extremity _____

   b. Shape

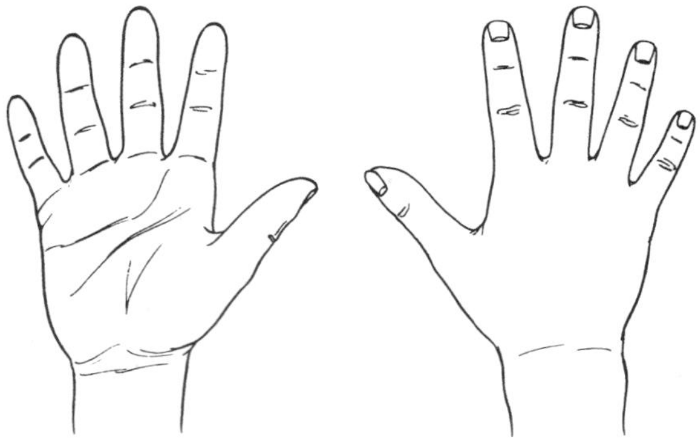

   Key: X = missing digit
          At = atrophy
          S = swelling
          D = deviation
          θ = lacks web
          An = ankylosis
          SN = swan neck
          B = boutonniere
          D/S = dislocation/subluxation
          M = mallet finger
          Z = collapse deformity
          N = nodule

   Circumferential measurements: arm _____ forearm _____ wrist _____ hand _____

   Volumetric measurement: involved hand _____ ml displaced

                            uninvolved hand _____ ml displaced

   c. Use

   Hand protected/use restricted _____

   Handles clothing: independently _____ minimum assistance _____   maximum assistance _____

   movement: jerky _____ stiff _____ uncoordinated _____ limited by pain _____

   d. Skin

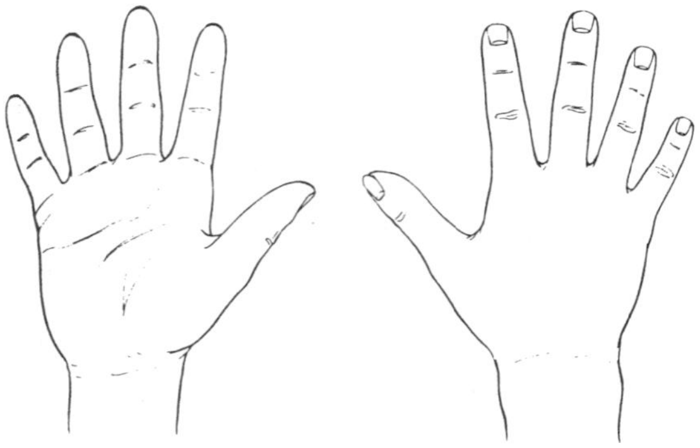

   Key: C = cyanotic
          R = redenned
          W = whitened
          S = scar
          L = lesion
          F = fixation
          Na = nail deformity
          T = texture changed
          Ne = necrosis
          H = abnormal hair pattern

   e. Aids

   sling _____ splint _____ orthosis _____ other _____

   Description _____

   Purpose _____

Figure 6.11.   Examination form part 3: Inspection.

deviations in length and alignment, etc. by this system. The examiner performs circumferential measurements of the upper limb at designated anatomic sites: 7 cm proximal to the elbow flexion crease (arm), 11 cm proximal to the distal wrist flexion crease (forearm), at the distal wrist flexion crease (wrist), and at the distal palmar flexion crease (hand) (29). Bilateral comparison portrays individual deviations. Often the site of shape deviation is pathognomonic. A small immobile swelling beneath the proximal digital crease is almost always a tendon sheath ganglion; whereas significant swelling around a bone or joint is evidence of underlying skeletal injury (23). Atrophy of only the thenar eminence follows median nerve compression in carpal tunnel syndrome. Hypothenar and interossei muscle atrophy follow an ulnar nerve lesion. Immobilization may produce generalized atrophy, although it is sometimes masked by edema following trauma or reflex sympathetic dystrophy. Volumertric water displacement is a useful test for detecting subtle differences.

The patient's functional use of his hand indicates much about its condition. The examiner notes unused parts as well when observing function. Persistent drooping of the distal phalanx during active movement of other joints typifies a mallet finger (25). Extensor lag at the middle phalanx may signify a boutonnière deformity, although it may be concealed by swelling following initial trauma (25).

The examiner inspects the skin for color, texture, hair pattern, and lesions (Fig. 6.11). He assesses scars and skin grafts for signs of contracture, adhesions, incomplete healing, and hypertrophy. Denervation produces skin changes such as smoothness (skin ridges less pronounced), absence of calluses, dryness (loss of sympathetic innervation), and lesions from loss of protective sensation.

Completing the inspection portion of the examination, the therapist reviews external aids worn or used by the patient. He should describe each device, its purpose, and how well it appears to be working. For example, is a ''reverse knuckle bender'' splint preventing a boutonnière deformity, or is it failing to maintain extension of the PIP joint?

Palpation. Palpation is the next procedure in the examination sequence (Fig. 6.12). Structural and physiological changes are relatively easy to detect in the hand because of its superficial nature. The examiner palpates the skin and subcutaneous tissues for tenderness, dryness, edema, alteration of temperature, and decreased mobility. The dorsal tissues are normally thin and loosely attached, allowing maximal mobility for hand flexion. The lack of fascial attachments in this area permits the collection of edematous fluid over the dorsum of the hand, which may be deceiving if the source of inflammation is located elsewhere. By contrast, the palmar tissue feels thick upon palpation, with relative lack of mobility. Excessive moisture over the plam may suggest vasomotor instability or neurosis; dryness occurs following sympathetic nerve loss.

Muscles and tendons may be tender to palpation in overuse syndromes. Some individual muscle bellies are distinguishable in the hand, and most of the extrinsic tendons can be felt beneath the skin when movement is resisted. The examiner can usually determine if a tendon is severed, adherent, or not gliding smoothly within its sheath. To assess continuity of the extrinsic finger flexors, the examiner exerts firm pressure about one-third of the way up the forearm on the ulnar side; normally this produces 1–2 cm of passive finger flexion and if it doesn't, one should suspect tendon adhesions or severance (23). Pain at a tendinous insertion may signify partial avulsion. Tendon sheaths and bursae may present as swollen or tender.

Palpation of bones and joints commonly reveals tenderness, swelling, instability, or deformity following injury or joint disease. The examiner should not stress a bone if he suspects a fracture, and should be cautious during examination of an injured joint. To systematically palpate the wrist and hand bones, the examiner begins with the wrist and proceeds distally. Pain or abnormal mobility of the ulnar head may signify distal radioulnar joint instability. Rupture of the extensor carpi ulnaris tendon retinaculum produces snapping over the distal ulna during attempted wrist extension or ulnar deviation. The ulnar styloid process lies at the level of the radiocarpal joint. Just distal to it is the triquetrum, which becomes prominent on the ulnar aspect of the hand with radial deviation. The pisiform, resting upon the triquetrum, is easily felt; its position coincides with the distal wrist skin crease. By placing his thumb IP joint over the pisiform, pointing the tip of the thumb toward the thenar web space, and pressing the thumb tip into the tissue beneath it, the examiner can palpate the hook of the hamate. Strangely, fracture of the hamulus may produce dorsal pain (26).

Just dorsal and distal to the radial styloid process lies the anatomic snuffbox, outlined by the extensor pollicis longus and brevis tendons. Tenderness in the snuffbox is a classic sign of scaphoid fracture. The scaphoid tubercle is prominent volarly at the distal wrist skin crease. The trapezium lies just distal to the scaphoid, where pain is present after a wrist radial collateral ligament injury (26). The trapezoid is located on the ulnar side of the trapezium. Ulnar to the trapezoid is the capitate. The capitate, along with the lunate, are most easily palpated dorsally. A line extending between the dorsal radial tubercle and the base of the 3rd metacarpal bisects both the capitate and lunate. When the wrist is in a neutral position, the distal aspect of the capitate is prominent, but the lunate lies in a depression; flexing the wrist brings the lunate up to fill out the depression. Palpation may reveal displacement of the lunate, which is the most frequently dislocated bone in the hand. Palpating the metacarpals and phalanges is a good method for detecting joint instability and related symptoms.

Palpation reveals certain qualities of arteries and nerves. The Allen test is a clinical method of assessing the patency of the palmar arch, and radial, ulnar, and

2. Palpation (note location and nature of abnormality)

a. Skin and subcutaneous tissue: tenderness _____ temperature _____ swelling _____ moisture _____

decreased mobility _____ other _____

b. Muscles and tendons: tenderness _____ temperature _____ spasm _____ loss of continuity _____

decreased mobility _____ other _____

c. Tendon sheaths and bursae: tenderness _____ temperature _____ swelling _____ crepitus _____ other _____

d. Bones and joints: tenderness _____ temperature _____ swelling _____ bony prominences _____

deformity _____

e. Arteries and nerves: radial artery pulse _____ ulnar artery pulse _____ Allen test _____ Tinel's sign _____

Phalen's test _____

3. Movement assessment

a. Functional active moment

		key: C = completes task
Power grip _____ (hammer)	Lateral pinch _____ (key)	D = completes task with
Precision grip _____ (writing)	Cylinder grasp _____ (2.5-cm cylinder)	difficulty/discomfort
Hook grip _____ (suitcase)	Spherical grasp _____ (5-cm ball)	N = not able to complete
		task

Gross range of motion

Distance (cm)	I	M	R	L
Fingertips to PP crease				
Fingertips to MP crease				
Fingertips to dorsal plane				

Grip and pinch strength

Grip (Jaymar dynamometer) _____ kg   handle position _____

Grip, alternative (sphygmomanometer) _____ mm Hg

Pinch (pinch meter)

Key (lateral) _____ g

Pulp   I _____ g   M _____ g   R _____ g   L _____ g

Special tests

	+	−	Comments
Finklestein			
Bunnell-Littler			
Oblique retinacular ligament			
Weightbearing on extended wrist			
Froment's sign			
Circle with index finger & thumb			

Figure 6.12.   Examination form part 4: Palpation and measurement assessment.

digital arteries. The examiner compresses the radial and ulnar arteries, then requests the patient to pump the blood from his hand by repeatedly clenching a fist. Then he instructs the patient to open his hand, releases pressure on one of the arteries, and observes the recovery of color in the palm. An occlusive lesion in the uncompressed artery delays recovery of palmar color, thus producing a positive test (30). To reduce the incidence of false-negative or -negative tests, the examiner should not stretch the skin forcibly around the wrist or hyperextend the wrist. Instead, he should confirm the arterial location, compress only enough to occlude flow, and have the patient clench powerfully enough to produce pallor (30).

Tinel's sign indicates palpation or percussion sensitivity of an injured nerve. The examiner gently taps the injured nerve, beginning at the site of injury, and moving distally. The level of regeneration correlates with production of tingling (31). Phalen's test may reproduce symptoms of median nerve compression within the carpal tunnel. A patient maximally flexes the wrist, and maintains this position with overpressure for 60 seconds (32). Paresthesias in a median nerve distribution distal to the carpal tunnel represent a positive test.

Movement Assessment. "Functional," "physiological," and "accessory" divisions of movement facilitate testing. Functional movement includes the ability to perform basic types of grasp and pinch; gross range of motion; and grip and pinch strength (Fig. 6.12). The basic types of grasp and pinch indicate indicate whether a hand can adopt positions required for common use, and reveal neuromuscular integrity. The median nerve innervates the radial side of a hand, which performs precision maneuvers. The ulnar nerve supplies the ulnar side, which produces power grip. The radial nerve innervates the dorsum of a hand and wrist extensors, agonists of the finger flexors. Loss of function in any one of these areas may assist in identification of a lesion of one of the peripheral nerves. The therapist may also elect to evaluate the patient's functional capacity, depending upon home and job requirements.

The therapist measures the range of gross finger flexion (of all three finger joints) by determining the distance from the plane of a nail to the proximal palmar crease (Fig. 6.13A). Gross flexion of just the PIP and DIP joints is measured as the distance between a nail plane and the MP crease. Gross finger extension is the distance from the plane of a nail to the projected dorsal surface of the hand (Fig. 6.13B). Table 6.3 lists common restrictions of finger flexion and extension.

A dynamometer provides objective grip strength data. Males normally can generate about 46 kg of force, and females about 23 kg (33, 34). Grip strength of only 4 kg is required to perform 90° of ADL activities. Patients normally generate their maximum force when the dynamometer handle is at the 2nd setting, followed by the 3rd, 4th, 5th and 1st settings; a graph of forces at these settings should approximate a bell curve. Malingering may be detected by a flat curve in all five dynamometer settings (35). With a rapid exchange of dynamometer grips between hands, strength normally decreases due to fatigue in normals, but may increase in malingerers, who are confused by the effort (23). If stiffness or pain prevent a patient from being able to grip a dynamometer, the examiner may use a rolled up sphygmomanometer cuff for test-

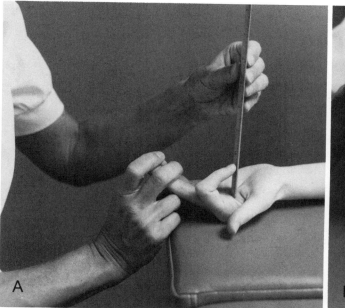

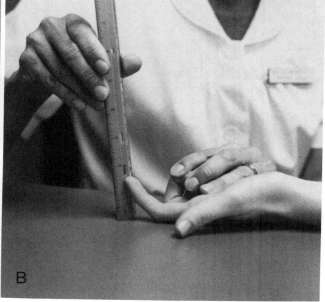

Figure 6.13. *A*, **Gross finger flexion measurement:** distance between the fingernail plane and proximal palmer crease provides a gross estimate of flexion in the finger joints. *B*, **Gross finger extension measurement:** distance between the fingernail plane and dorsal metacarpal plane provides a gross estimate of extension in the finger joints.

Table 6.3.
Factors Contributing to the Stiff Hand

	Dorsal structures shortened—skin, capsule muscle, tendon	Volar structures shortened—skin, volar pouch/plate, tendon, muscle, palmar aponeurosis	Collateral ligaments shortened	Intrinsic muscles shortened	Other
Loss of Flexion:					
MP	*		*		
PIP	*			*	mechanisms producing swan neck deformity
Loss of Extension:					
MP		*		*	
PIP		*	*		mechanisms producing Boutonniére deformity

ing grip strength. Males can normally squeeze hard enough to produce over 300 mm of mercury pressure and females just under 300 mm of mercury pressure. Pinch strength is tested by a pinch meter, which evaluates both lateral and pulp pinch. Table 6.4 displays average pinch strength for males and females.

Special tests may be used to isolate a particular structure with suspected dysfunction. A positive Finkelstein test reveals tenosynovitis of the extensor pollicis brevis and abductor pollicis longus tendon sheaths (De Quervain's disease). The therapist performs this test by instructing the patient to hold his flexed thumb into his palm, then ulnarly deviate the wrist to produce maximal tension in the involved musculotendinous structures (Fig. 6.14) (15). Sharp pain over the radial aspect of the wrist denotes a positive test.

A positive Bunnell-Littler test identifies intrinsic muscle shortening. Contractures of either the intrinsic muscles, extensor digitorum tendon, or capsule may limit PIP joint flexion. The intrinsic muscles are incriminated when a therapist passively extends the MP joint of the involved digit to stretch the intrinsic muscles, then passively flexes the PIP joint to its limit (Fig. 6.15A); he then flexes the MP joint to relax the intrinsic muscles, and PIP joint flexion increases (Fig. 6.15B) (15).

Another test incriminates the extensor digitorum tendon as limiting PIP joint flexion when the therapist passively flexes the wrist and the MP joint of the involved digit to stretch the tendon, then passively flexes the PIP joint to its limit; he then extends the

wrist and the MP joint to relax the tendon and PIP joint flexion increases. If the PIP joint extension contracture remains the same, regardless of the position of the other joints, then the lesion most likely lies in the capsule or related structures.

The therapist tests for shortening of the oblique retinacular ligament with a test similar to the Bunnell-Littler test, but performed one joint distally. Contractures of either the oblique retinacular ligament, extensor digitorum tendon, or capsule may limit DIP joint flexion. To incriminate the oblique retinacular ligament, the therapist passively extends the PIP joint to stretch this ligament, then passively flexes the DIP joint to its limit (Fig. 6.16A); he then flexes the PIP joint to relax the ligament, and if DIP joint flexion increases, the lesion lies in the ligament (Fig. 6.16B) (15). Tests which isolate the extensor digitorum tendon and the capsule as limiting DIP joint flexion are similar to those described in the preceeding paragraph.

Table 6.4.
Average Pinch Strengths for Males and Females[a]

	Males (gm)	Females (gm)
Lateral (key) pinch	7.3	4.8
Pulp pinch index	5.1	3.5
Pulp pinch middle	5.7	3.6
Pulp pinch ring	3.7	2.5
Pulp pinch little	2.3	1.7

[a]The strength of pulp and lateral pinch was tested by Swanson et al. with an electric pinch meter. Similar findings were obtained with the standard pinch meter.

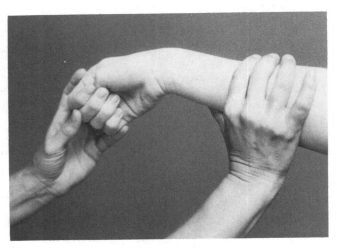

Figure 6.14.   Finkelstein test: if wrist ulnar deviation with the thumb flexed in the palm reproduces pain near the radial styloid process, the test is positive, implicating extensor pollicis brevis and abductor pollicis longus tenosynovitis (De Quervain's disease).

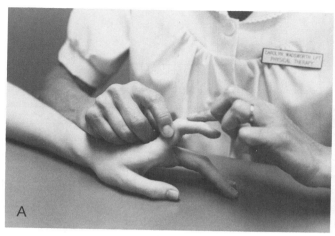 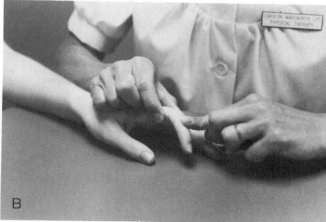

Figure 6.15.   Bunnell-Littler test: *A*, If passive PIP joint flexion is restricted when the MP joint is passively extended, but *B*, PIP joint flexion increases when the MP joint is flexed, the test is positive, implicating contracture of the intrinsic muscles.

Supporting weight on an extended wrist, as in raising oneself from a chair, is a test which may identify a lesion in the carpal area. It reproduces the pain of carpal instability, arthritis, nonunion of a scaphoid fracture, or Kienböck's disease.

Froment's sign is a positive finding associated with an ulnar nerve lesion. It is represented by thumb IP flexion during attempted lateral pinch. This occurs because a patient attempts to substitute the flexor pollicis longus muscle for the paralyzed adductor pollicis and deep head of the flexor pollicis brevis muscles.

A test of the anterior interosseous nerve, a branch of the median nerve, requires that the patient form a circle with his thumb and index finger. The flexor pollicis longus and flexor digitorum profundus muscles, which are necessary to flex the thumb IP joint and the index finger DIP joint in making a circle, are supplied by this nerve.

Testing functional movement and special tests provide a quick assessment of basic hand function and isolated structures. Although this relatively simple method is useful in gross assessment of functional capability, the examiner may need to test each individual joint and muscle more extensively, i.e., physiologic and accessory movement assessment (Fig. 6.17). First, assessment of active physiologic movement reveals a patient's general willingness and ability to move the hand. A variety of conditions, such as muscle paralysis, tendon laceration, ligamentous injury, swelling, or pain may hinder active movement. Since it is common for two or more muscles to join in producing a single joint action in the hand, steps must be taken to isolate muscle function. For example, both the flexor digitorum superficialis muscle (FDS) and the flexor digitorum profundus muscle (FDP) flex the PIP joint. To isolate FDS muscle action, the examiner passively extends all fingers except the one being

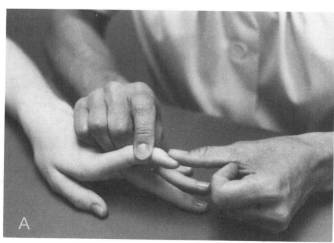 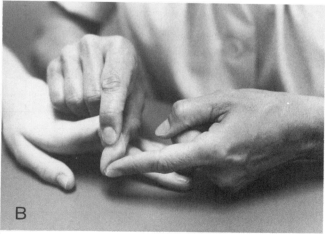

Figure 6.16.   Oblique retinacular ligament test: *A*, If passive DIP joint flexion is restricted when the PIP joint is passively extended, but *B*, DIP joint flexion increases when the PIP joint is flexed, the test is positive, implicating contracture of the oblique retinacular (Lansmeer's) ligament.

b/c/d. Physiological movement

			ACTIVE			PASSIVE				RESISTIVE	
			ROM	Symptoms	Quality	ROM	Symptoms	End-feel	Limiting Structures	Strength	Symptoms
Forearm		supination									
		pronation									
Wrist		extension									
		flexion									
		abduction									
		adduction									
Thumb	CM	extension									
		flexion									
		abduction									
		adduction									
	MP	extension									
		flexion									
	IP	extension									
		flexion									
Index	MP	extension									
		flexion									
		abduction									
		adduction									
	PIP	extension									
		flexion									
	DIP	extension									
		flexion									
Middle	MP	extension									
		flexion									
		abduction									
		adduction									
	PIP	extension									
		flexion									
	DIP	extension									
		flexion									
Ring	MP	extension									
		flexion									
		abduction									
		adduction									
	PIP	extension									
		flexion									
	DIP	extension									
		flexion									
Little	MP	extension									
		flexion									
		abduction									
		adduction									
	PIP	extension									
		flexion									
	DIP	extension									
		flexion									

Figure 6.17A.   Examination form part 5: Physiologic movement.

e. Accessory movement

		Mobility	Symptoms
Radiocarpal and midcarpal joints	dorsal glide		
	volar glide		
	radial glide		
	ulnar glide		
Ulnomeniscotriquetral "joint"			
Intercarpal joints	scaphoid		
	lunate		
	triquetrum		
	pisiform		
	trapezium		
	trapezoid		
	capitate		
	hamate		
Carpometacarpal joints	1st		
	4th		
	5th		
Intermetacarpal joints	2–3		
	3–4		
	4–5		
Metacarpophalangeal joints	1		
	2		
	3		
	4		
	5		
Proximal interphalangeal joints	1		
	2		
	3		
	4		
	5		
Distal interphalangeal joints	2		
	3		
	4		
	5		

Figure 6.17B. Examination form part 5: Accessory movement.

examined. Since the FDP tendons cannot function independently (occasionally the tendon to the index finger is independent), extension of adjacent fingers also tethers the one being tested, so PIP flexion can only be produced by FDS (Fig. 6.18) (15). Likewise, the PIP joint is extended by two muscles, the intrinsic muscles and the extensor digitorum muscle. To isolate intrinsic muscle action, the examiner instructs the patient to actively extend the MP joint, which transmits all of the force of the ED muscle to the proximal phalanx. Then the patient attempts to extend the PIP joint, which will depend solely on the action of the intrinsic muscles, since the ED muscle is tethered proximally at the MP joint (16) (Fig 6.19) Fig. 6.19 demonstrates inability to extend the PIP joint due to intrinsic muscle weakness.

The examiner records active ROM as well as symptoms and quality of movement (Fig. 6.17). When measuring the range of a joint he should position all joints proximal to it in a neutral or standard position to minimize the influence of tendon excursion. The examiner next tests passive physiologic movement and records the range of motion and symptoms as he did when testing active movement. The examiner should also pay close attention to the endfeel of joints. An osteophytic formation near joints may produce a bony limitation to motion, in contrast to a ligamentous contracture, which produces a capsular endfeel with some "give" to it. The endfeel of a volar plate tear or recurrent dorsal dislocation of a finger joint may be "empty" due to excessive instability. Empty can either be painless hypermobility (as in chronic instability of a joint) or acutely painful (such that a skilled examiner is unwilling to cause any more discomfort, even though no "endfeel" was reached).

The "constant length phenomenon" is a useful concept for isolating the site of ROM restriction when the process of elimination involves soft tissue which spans

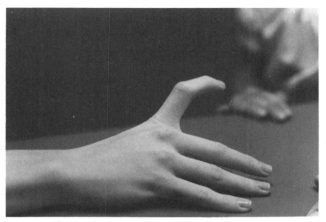

Figure 6.19.   Intrinsic muscle extension of PIP and DIP joints: if the patient can actively extend the MP joints fully (which anchors the extensor digitorum muscle) and then can actively extend the PIP and DIP joints, the intrinsic muscles are functioning. (In this picture the patient cannot extend the PIP and DIP joints).

two or more joints. For example, Dupuytren's contracture of the palmar aponeurosis tissue limits the excursion of its fibrous extensions into the fingers. The constant length of this tissue allows the MP joint to be extended only when the PIP joint is flexed, or the PIP joint to be extended only when the MP joint is flexed (Fig. 6.20). The examiner applies this same principle when testing the intrinsic muscles (Bunnell-Littler test) and long finger tendons, as described earlier.

Resistive physiologic movement testing assesses strength and symptoms associated with isometric contraction (Fig. 6.17). Standardized manual or dynamometric muscle tests provide reliable measurement of muscle strength (36, 37).

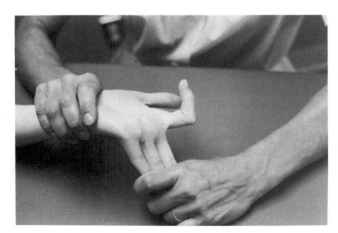

Figure 6.18.   Flexor digitorum superficialis muscle test: if the patient can flex the PIP joint while the examiner passively maintains the other fingers in complete extension, the flexor digitorum superficialis muscle is functioning.

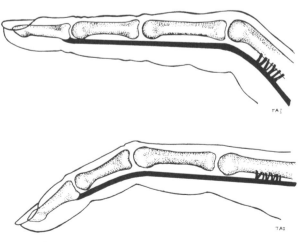

Figure 6.20.   Constant length phenomenon: if the palmar aponeurosis is tethered at the palm, it will be too short to allow extension of all the finger joints at the same time; however, if one flexes the MP joint, he can extend the PIP joint and vice versa.

Accessory movement testing lends additional information pertaining to hand function. The examiner documents joint play mobility on a scale of 0 = ankylosis to 6 = instability and describes the symptoms associated with joint play movement (Fig. 6.17) (38, 39).

Neurologic Evaluation. The neurologic evaluation provides an assessment of cervical nerve root as well as peripheral nerve lesions (Fig. 6.21). Testing key muscles, representative of each cervical root level identifies nerve root compression when positive, without performing a complete muscle test. Testing specific groups of muscles innervated by a particular peripheral nerve identifies a peripheral lesion when positive. In addition to muscle testing, evaluating sensation helps identify the site of a nerve lesion and to predict functional recovery in cases of regeneration or repair. The presence or absence of touch, pain, and temperature sensation assists lesion identification. The examiner proceeds by first demonstrating the sensory test to be performed, then asking the patient to close his eyes and report the quality and location of the tactile sensation.

The ninhydrin sweat test helps demonstrate sudomotor (sympathetic) activity. The examiner applies ninhydrin to the palm. Ninhydrin reacts with amino acids in the sweat, forming a colored tracing of perspiring areas. The noncolored areas represent the denervated part of the palm. The wrinkling test also correlates with sensory innervation. The digital pulp skin will wrinkle only if innervated, after being submerged in warm water for 5 minutes.

Two-point discrimination (2PD) tests, in addition to identifying sensory lesions, provide information for assessing functional recovery. The classic Weber 2PD test, which measures the innervation density of the slowly adapting fiber receptor system, correlates with static grip activities of the hand (29, 40). The examiner applies two blunt ends to the skin (without blanching) about 15 mm apart, then decreases the distance until only one point is felt (Fig. 6.22A). A patient who is able to make 7 out of 10 correct distinctions at a standard distance for given parts of the hand is considered

to have normal 2PD. Three mm is the standard distance for the fingertips; values for other areas of the hand, as well as functional correlations of results over 3 mm, are published in other sources (34, 40).

The moving 2PD test predicts tactile gnosis, which Dellon states is the essence of function, better than the static 2PD test (40). This test assesses the quickly adapting fiber receptor system, and is administered by moving two blunt points along the long axis of a limb or digit in a distal direction. The examiner randomly alternates one and two points of an aesthesiometer while progressively narrowing the interprong distance until a two-point limen (threshold) is reached (40). Seven out of 10 correct responses is normal when the distance is 2 mm at the fingertips (standard values increase as one moves proximally). The quickly adapting fiber receptors also mediate vibratory sensation, which is perhaps more easily tested. The examiner applies a tuning fork alternately to involved and noninvolved areas, as the patient attempts to discern whether the sensation varies or is the same (Fig. 6.22B). A 30 cycles per second (cps) tuning fork best assesses the function of Meissner afferents located in the superficial dermis, and a 256 cps tuning fork best assesses pacinian afferents in the deep dermis and subcutis (40). These tests are accurate, noninvasive, and readily accepted by patients (40). A hand which is regaining sensation progresses through the following stages: anesthetic, pinprick/30 cps vibration, moving touch, moving 2PD, static 2PD/256 cps vibration (23).

The examiner may detect central nervous system dysfunction by signs of spasticity or clonicity in the limb. If present, a physical therapist may need to perform a more detailed neurologic evaluation. Manual dexterity and coordination tests predict certain functional abilities. The detail of the tests varies from simple tasks, such as tracing, to the standardized O'Conner dexterity test and Jebson hand function test (29).

Recommendation of Other Tests. When the therapist has completed the examination, he may desire additional data to correlate and interpret the results. Whenever a fracture, with or without dislocation, is

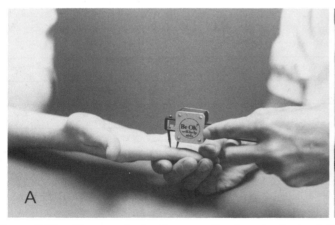
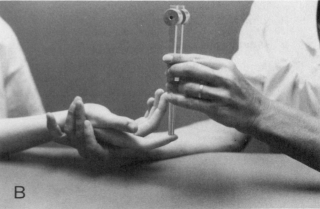

Figure 6.22.   Sensory tests. *A*, an aesthesiometer tests static or moving two-point discrimination, *B*, A 256 cps tuning fork tests vibratory perception.

4. Neurological evaluation

    a. Key muscles (strength grade 0–5)

        C6: ECRL muscle and ECRB muscle _____

        C7: ED muscle _____

        C8: FDS muscle and FDP muscle _____

        T1: Dorsal interossei muscles _____

    b. Sensibility

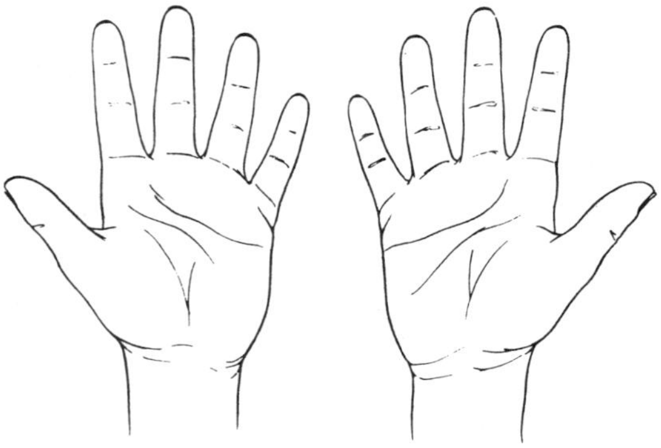

	Lacking A = light touch sensation
	B = pinprick sensation
	C = temperature discrimination
	D = sweating (ninhydrin test)
	E = two-point discrimination (constant)
	F = two-point discrimination (moving)
	G = 30 cps vibratory perception
	H = 256 cps vibratory perception (moving)

    c. Motor control: spastic _____ flaccid _____ rigid _____ clonic _____

    d. Coordination

        Trace a diagram _____   Key: C = completes task

        Button a button _____   D = completes task with

        Tie a bow _____   difficulty/discomfort

        Other _____   N = not able to complete

                                                      task

5. Recommendation of other tests

    a. Radiography _____

    b. Laboratory _____

    c. Electrodiagnostic _____

    d. Arthroscopy _____

    e. Arthrography _____

    f. Other _____

Figure 6.21. Examination form part 6: Neurologic evaluation and recommendation of other tests.

suspected, radiographic studies are necessary. Motion view radiographs often nicely depict ligamentous instability in the difficult-to-diagnose patient complaining of clicking and pain with movement (26). Also, a computerized tomographic (CT) scan may be the best method to ascertain distal radioulnar joint subluxation and dislocation because pain or plaster immobilization may preclude the optimal positioning required for radiographic diagnosis (41).

In conclusion, this section describes many of the questions, tests, and measurements which contribute to a comprehensive wrist and hand examination. The therapist uses this test data and the interpretation of results to determine the present status of a patient's condition, his specific problem(s), and his functional capabilities and impairment. Table 6.5 includes a summary of the differential diagnosis and treatment of common wrist and hand disorders.

Table 6.5.
Summary of Differential Diagnosis and Treatment of Common Wrist and Hand Disorders

Disorder	Chief Complaint	Onset	Symptom Characteristics	Static Physical Changes	Dynamic Physical Changes	Special Tests	Treatment
Arthritis a. bacterial	Rest pain, exacerbated by movement	May occur after bites, wounds, or septicemia	Local pain, swelling, and erythema; tender to palpation	Swelling of involved joints	Movement restricted by pain and swelling	Joint aspiration	Appropriate antibiotics; joint irrigation or drainage if severe; splint while acute, then early ROM and exercise
b. osteo-	Painful, nodular swelling of DIP joints	Insidious in elderly	Local pain and tenderness	Deforming bony protuberance on dorsum of DIP joints (Heberden's nodes); occasionally PIP joints	Instability of involved joints		Modalities for pain relief, such as paraffin
c. rheumatoid	Painful swelling in wrist, MP and PIP joints	Insidious: most common in women age 20 to 40	Pain, swelling, and erythema of joints, tendon sheaths inflammation; morning stiffness; exacerbations & remissions	Deformities, i.e., swan neck, MP ulnar drift, and boutonniére; described in text	Instability and muscle imbalance, e.g., intrinsic plus	RA factor, ESR, radiography; Bunnell-Littler and functional assessment	Splinting, pain management, and isometric exercise during acute flareups; active assistive and isotonic exercises later as indicated; functional training and adaptive devices; medication and/or surgery as indicated.
Carpal tunnel syndrome	Numbness, pain, or paresthesia on radial side of palm	Insidious; age 40 to 60	Sensory changes aggrevated by prolonged use of hand; worse at night	Thenar atrophy	Weakness in pinch	Phalen's test, Tinel's sign, NCV	Eliminate original cause; resting splint; surgical release followed by active exercises
DeQuervain's disease	Tenderness over radial styloid	Direct trauma or repetitive minor irritation	Pain produced by active thumb abduction or passive stretch of EPB and APL muscles	Tendon sheath swelling	Weakness of thumb abduction	Finkelstein's test	Heat; rest; hydrocortisone; surgical release of tendon sheath
Dupuytren's contracture	Palmar nodule or contracture	Insidious; most common in men age 40 to 60	Painless fibrosis of palmar aponeurosis	Flexion contractures in ring and little fingers secondary to palmar contracture		Contracture initially demonstrated by constant length principle (see text)	Prevent secondary joint contractures with exercise, US, splinting
Kienbock's disease	Wrist pain	Trauma-related; adults	Pain increased by wrist flexion and extension; lunate tender to palpation		Progressive limitation of wrist motion	Radiography	Corrective surgery
Peripheral nerve compression/ lesion	Weakness and sensory changes	Traumatic or insidious	Extent of sensory and motor loss varies according to nerve damage	Deformities, i.e., intrinsic minus, ape hand, wrist drop described in text	Weakness in specific muscles involved	Described in text for each nerve	Splinting and exercise to maintain joint position and motion during nerve regeneration; sensory and functional reeducation
Sprains	Pain; laxity	Traumatic blow, stretch or fall	Acute pain and swelling	Joint inflammation; later hypo- or hypermobility	Joint instability or contracture	Stress involved structure	Initial immobilization with gradual return to function
Tendon rupture or avulsion	Loss of movement	Sudden, forceful movement or blow	Tender to palpation, swelling, loss of movement	Drooping of involved digit; later contracture	Weakness and muscle imbalance	Described in text for individual tendons	Immobilization; surgical repair; exercise program as indicated by specific injury

WRIST AND HAND MOBILIZATION

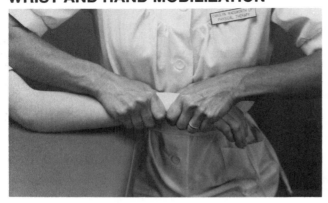

Figure 6.23.   Radiocarpal joint traction.

Patient Position: Seated with forearm resting on table and wrist extending beyond table.

Therapist Position: Seated at end of table, facing radial aspect of P's arm; S hand fixates radius and ulna; M hand grasps proximal carpals as close to joint as possible; T's arms are parallel to P's limb.

Technique: Apply traction force to carpals parallel to long axis of P's limb.

Comments: Effective for test or treatment of general hypomobility or pain as indicated; same technique is applied to midcarpal joint by moving T's M hand placement slightly distally.

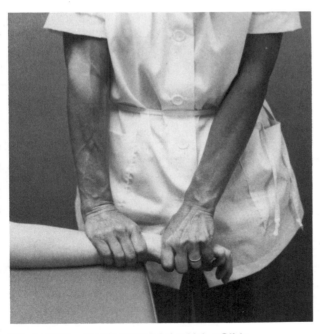

Figure 6.25.   Radiocarpal Joint Volar Glide.

Patient Position: Seated with forearm resting pronated on table and wrist extending beyond table.

Therapist Position: Standing at end of table, facing radial aspect of P's arm; S hand fixates radius and ulna; M hand grasps proximal carpals as close to joint as possible; T's arms are perpendicular to P's limb.

Technique: Apply volar force to carpals perpendicular to long axis of P's limb; maintain traction also during this technique.

Comments: Especially effective for increasing wrist extension; same technique is applied to midcarpal joint by moving T's M hand placement slightly distally.

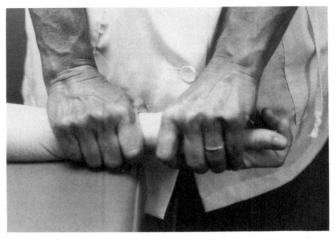

Figure 6.24.   Radiocarpal Joint Dorsal Glide.

Patient Position: Seated with forearm resting supinated on table, and wrist extending beyond table.

Therapist Position: Standing at end of table, facing ulnar aspect of P's arm; S hand fixates radius and ulna; M hand grasps proximal carpals as close to joint as possible; T's arms are perpendicular to P's limb.

Technique: Apply dorsal force to carpals perpendicular to long axis of P's limb; maintain traction also during this technique.

Comments: Especially effective for increasing wrist flexion; same technique is applied to midcarpal joint by moving T's M hand placement slightly distally.

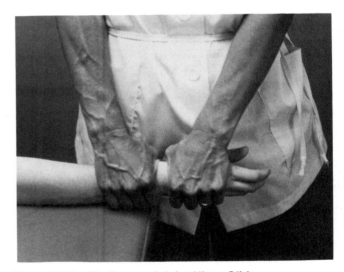

Figure 6.26.   Radiocarpal Joint Ulnar Glide.

Patient Position: Standing with forearm resting with ulnar border on table, and wrist extending beyond table.

Therapist Position: Standing at end of table, facing volar aspect of P's arm; S hand fixates radius and ulna; M hand grasps proximal carpals as close to joint as possible; T's arms are perpendicular to P's limb.

Technique: Apply ulnar force to carpals perpendicular to long axis of P's limb; maintain traction also during this technique.

Comments: Especially effective for increasing wrist radial deviation; same technique is applied to midcarpal joint by moving T's M hand placement slightly distally.

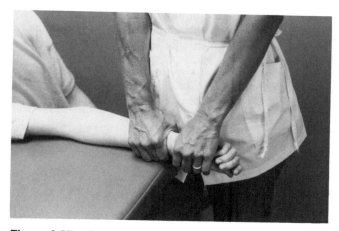

Figure 6.27.   Radiocarpal Joint Radial Glide.

Patient Position: Seated with forearm resting with radial border on table, and wrist extending beyond table.

Therapist Position: Standing at end of table, facing dorsal aspect of P's arm; S hand fixates radius and ulna; M hand grasps proximal carpals as close to joint as possible; T's arms are perpendicular to P's limb.

Technique: Apply radial force to carpals perpendicular to long axis of P's limb; maintain traction also during this technique.

Comments: Especially effective for increasing wrist ulnar deviation; same technique is applied to midcarpal joint by moving T's M hand placement slightly distally.

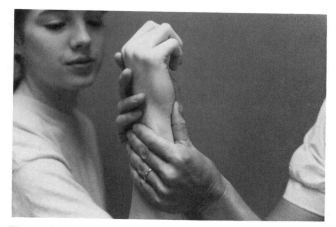

Figure 6.28.   Ulnomeniscotriquetral Joint Glide.

Patient Position: Seated with elbow on table and forearm vertical.

Therapist Position: Seated facing P; S hand grasps radial aspect of wrist and hand and maintains wrist in neutral position; M thumb rest on pisiform and index finger on dorsal ulnar head.

Technique: Compress pisiform and ulna with thumb and index finger.

Comments: Effective for increasing pronation and supination.

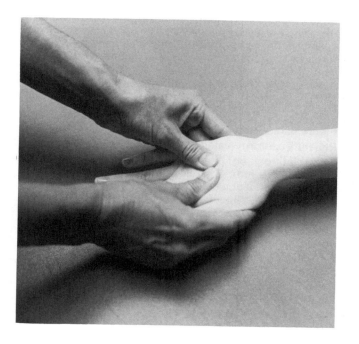

Figure 6.29.   Metacarpal Dorsal Glide (General Mobilization).

Patient Position: Seated with forearm resting pronated on table.

Therapist Position: Standing facing P; fingers grasp volarly over the thenar and hypothenar eminences and thumbs rest dorsally over metacarpals.

Technique: Press thumbs against metacarpals and pull metacarpals dorsally with finger contacts.

Comments: Especially effective for increasing intermetacarpal and carpometacarpal joint mobility. This technique may be used to produce volar glide by modifying the position so that T's fingers press into palm and thenar contacts move metacarpals volarly; this would enhance cupping of the palm.

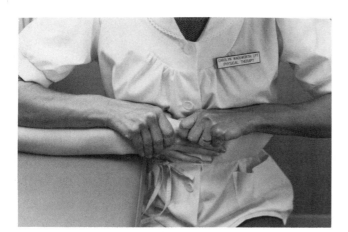

Figure 6.30. Metacarpophalangeal Joint Traction.

Patient Position: Seated with forearm resting on table.

Therapist Position: Seated at end of table, facing ventral aspect of P's arm; S hand fixates metacarpal; M hand grasps proximal phalanx as close to joint as possible; T's arms are parallel to P's limb.

Technique: Apply traction force to phalanx, parallel to long axis of P's limb.

Comments: Effective for test or treatment of general hypomobility or pain as indicated; same technique is applied to IP joints by moving T's hand placement distally.

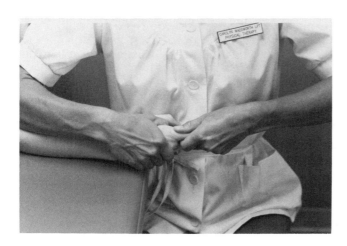

Figure 6.31. Metacarpophalangeal Joint Medial-Lateral Glide.

Patient Position: Seated with forearm resting on table.

Therapist Position: Seated at end of table, facing ventral aspect of P's arm; S hand fixates metacarpal; M hand grasps medial and lateral aspects of proximal phalanx as close to joint as possible; T's arms are parallel to P's limb.

Technique: Apply medial and lateral forces to phalanx through thumb and index finger contacts, perpendicular to long axis of P's limb; maintain traction also during this technique.

Comments: Effective for treatment of pain or restricted motion, especially abduction and adduction; same technique is applied to IP joints by moving T's hand placement distally. This technique may also be used to produce dorsal and ventral glide by modifying the position so that P's forearm is pronated on table and T imparts dorsal and ventral forces; this is especially effective for increasing extension and flexion respectively.

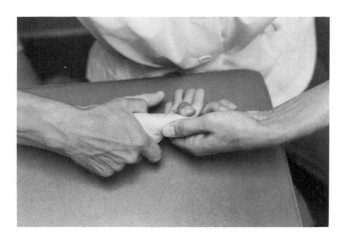

Figure 6.32. Metacarpophalangeal Joint Rotation.

Patient Position: Seated with forearm resting on table.

Therapist Position: Seated at end of table, facing ventral aspect of P's arm; S hand fixates metacarpal; M hand grasps proximal phalanx as close to joint as possible, and flexed DIP joint is fixated between middle and ring fingers to insure firm grasp; T's arms are parallel to P's limb.

Technique: Apply rotation force to phalanx through thumb and index finger contacts; maintain traction also during this technique.

Comments: Effective for treatment of pain or any restricted motion; same technique is applied to IP joints by moving T's hand placement distally.

References

1. Lockhart RD, Hamilton GF, Fyfe FW: *Anatomy of the Human Body*. Philadelphia, JB Lippincott, 1965.
2. Kapandji IA: *The Physiology of the Joints* Edinburgh, Churchill Livingstone, 1974, vol 1.
3. Kleinert HE, Hayes JE: The ulnar tunnel syndrome. *Plas Reconstr Surg* 47:21–24, 1971.
4. Koman LA, Urbaniak JR: Thrombosis of ulnar artery at the wrist. In *Symposium on Microsurgery: Practical Use in Orthopedics* Durham NC, Sept, 1977, May, 1979. American Academy of Orthopedic Surgeons. St. Louis: CV Mosby, 1979, 119–132.
5. Gross MS, Gelberman RH: The anatomy of the distal ulnar tunnel. 196:238–247, 1985.
6. Zweig J, Lie KK, Posch JL, Larsen RD: Thrombosis of the ulnar artery following blunt trauma to the hand. *J Bone Joint Surg* 51A:1191–1198, 1969.
7. Palmer AK, Werner FW: Biomechanics of the distal radioulnar joint. *Clin Orthop* 187:26–35, 1984.
8. Warwick R, Williams PC (eds): *Gray's Anatomy*, 35th British Ed. Philadelphia, WB Saunders, 1973.
9. Kauer JMG: Functional anatomy of the wrist. *Clin Orthop* 149:9–20, 1980.
10. Linscheid RL, Dobyns JH, Beckenbaugh RD, Cooney WP, Wood MB: Instability patterns of the wrist. *J Hand Surg* 8:682–686, 1983.
11. Cooney WP, Lucca MJU, Chao EYS, Linscheid RL: The kinesiology of the thumb trapeziometacarpal joint. *J Bone Joint Surg* 63A:1371–1381, 1981.
12. Weeks P, Wray C: *Management of Acute Hand Injuries*. St Louis, CV Mosby, 1973.
13. Lampe EW: Surgical anatomy of the hand. *Clin Symp* Vol #9, 1957.
14. Moore KL: *Clinically Oriented Anatomy*. Baltimore, Williams & Wilkins, 1980.
15. Hoppenfeld S: *Physical Examination of the Spine and Extremities*. East Norwalk, CT, Appleton-Century-Crofts, 1976.
16. Smith RJ: Balance and kinetics of the fingers under normal and pathological conditions. *Clin Orthop* 104:92–111, 1974.
17. Swezey RL: Dynamic factors in deformity of the rheumatoid hand. *Bull Rheum Dis* 22:649–656, 1971–72.
18. Harris C, Rutledge GL: The functional anatomy of the extensor mechanism of the finger. *J Bone Joint Surg* 54A:713–726, 1972.
19. Souter WA: The problem of Boutonniere deformity. *Clin Orthop* 104:116–131, 1974.
20. Landsmeer JM: Power grip and precision handling. *Ann Rheum Dis* 22:164–170, 1962.
21. Calliet R: *Hand Pain and Impairment*, ed 2. Philadelphia, FA Davis, 1975.
22. Cho KO: Entrapment occlusion of the ulnar artery in the hand. *J Bone Joint Surg* 60A:841–843, 1978.
23. Lister G: The Hand, Diagnosis and Indications, ed 2. New York, Churchill Livingstone, 1984.
24. Posner MA: Injuries to the hand and wrist in athletes. *Clin Orthop of North Amer* 8:593–617, 1977.
25. O'Brien ET: The sprained finger that isn't. *AFP* 23:129–137, 1981.
26. Beckenbaugh RD: Accurate evaluation and management of the painful wrist following injury: An approach to carpal instability. *Clin Orthop of North Amer* 15:289–305, 1984.
27. Morrissy RT, Nalebuff EA: Dislocation of the distal radioulnar joint: Anatomy and clues to prompt diagnosis. *Clin Orthop* 144:154–158, 1979.
28. Wadsworth C: Wrist and hand examination and interpretation. *J Orthop & Sports Phys Ther* 5:108–120, 1983.
29. Fess EE, Harmon KS, Strockland JW, Streichen JB: Evaluation of the hand by objective measurement. In Hunter JM, Schneider LH, Makin EJ, Bell JA (eds), *Rehabilitation of the Hand*, St Louis, CV Mosby, 1978, pp 70–93.
30. Hirai M, Kawai S: False positive and negative results in allen test. *J Cardiovasc Surg* 21:353–360, 1980.
31. Spinner M: *Injuries to the Major Branches of Peripheral Nerves of the Forearm*, ed 2. Philadelphia, WB Saunders, 1978.
32. Phalen GS: Carpal-tunnel syndrome. *Clin Orthop* 83:29–40, 1972.
33. Swanson AB, Goran-Hagert C, Swanson G: Evaluation of impairment of hand function. In Hunter JM, Schneider LH, Mackin EJ, Bell JA (eds), *Rehabilitation of the Hand*, St Louis, CV Mosby, 1978, pp 31–69.
34. Wynn Parry CB: *Rehabilitation of the Hand*, ed 3. Kent, England, Butterworth, 1973.
35. Stokes H: The seriously uninjured hand: Weakness of grip. *J Occup Med* 29:683–684, 1983.
36. Wadsworth C, Krishnan R, Sear M, Harrold J, Nielsen D: The Intrarater Reliability of Manual Muscle Testing and Hand-held Dynamometric Muscle Testing. Physical Therapy 64: 1342–1347, 1987.
37. Daniels L, Worthington C: *Muscle Testing*, ed 4. Philadelphia, WB Saunders, 1980.
38. Kaltenborn F: *Manual Therapy for Extremity Joints*. Oslo, Norway, Olaf Norlis Bokhandel, 1974.
39. Maitland GD: *Peripheral Manipulation*, ed 2. Kent, England, Butterworth, 1977.
40. Dellon AL: *Evaluation of Sensibility and Re-education of Sensation in the Hand*. Baltimore, Williams & Wilkins Co, 1981.
41. Mino DE, Palmer AK, Levinsohn EM: The role of radiography and computerized tomography in the diagnosis of subluxation and dislocation of the distal radioulnar joint. *J Hand Surg* 8:23, 1983.

CHAPTER

7

THE HIP

CLINICAL ANATOMY AND MECHANICS OF THE HIP

The hip joint links the lower limb with the pelvis. It is a multiaxial articulation between the femoral head and the acetabulum. The lower limb's two basic functions, weight support and locomotion, strongly influence hip joint morphology (1). The hip must be relatively stable for weightbearing, and yet it must still provide the mobility necessary for gait and functional positions of the leg.

Osteology

Pelvis. The two innominate bones and sacrum join in forming a bony ring, the pelvis. The pelvis holds and protects the viscera, and provides a base of origin for the thigh musculature. The pelvis also supports the weight of a seated individual and transmits this weight to the lower limbs when an individual stands.

Arch-like construction enhances the pelvis's role in weightbearing and weight transmission. The sacrum forms the keystone of this arch, and strong pillars of bone between the sacroiliac joints and the acetabulae serve as its piers (2). Anteriorly, the pubic bones offer additional support, functioning both as buttresses resisting the medial thrust of the femora and tie beams securing the ilia against the downward force of the sacrum (Fig. 7.1). Since the pubic bones don't directly comprise the weightbearing portion of the arch, fractures of the pubic rami do not disrupt the arch as long as the SI joints are stable; therefore, early ambulation is permitted (3,4).

The large innominate (hip) bone displays an irregular shape. Expanded portions of bone radiate superiorly and inferiorly from its constricted center. The three segments comprising the innominate bone initially are separated by cartilage, but later fuse at a Y-shaped epiphysis in the acetabulum (Fig. 7.2). The superior segment, the ilium, contains the upper two-fifths of the acetabulum and the fan-shaped portion of bone above it. The iliac crest marks the upper border of the ilium, and is superficial so that one may palpate

its entire length. The crest coincides with the level of the L4-5 interspace. The anterior point of the crest, the anterior superior iliac spine, is an easily identified bony landmark, and offers attachment for the inguinal ligament and sartorius muscle. The posterior superior iliac spine is not as prominent, but is marked by a skin dimple. It represents the location of the sacroiliac joint.

The inferior component of the innominate bone, the ischium, forms the posterior-lateral two-fifths of the acetabulum and the lower portion of the pelvis. The arrangement of the three components of the ischium is as follows: the ischial body joins the ilium, the ischial tuberosity juts inferiorly, and a short column of bone terminates anteriorly into an inferior ramus. The pubis, the smallest component of the innominate bone, contributes the anterior one-fifth of the acetabulum. Its body faces medially, to articulate with its opposing member at the symphysis pubis, and its superior and inferior rami contribute to the rims of the obturator foramen.

The acetabulum, a cup-shaped indentation on the lateral side of the innominate bone, forms the socket of the hip joint. Slightly less than a hemisphere in depth, it provides inherent bony stability to the hip, yet the necessary range of motion (3,5). The articular surface of the acetabulum consists of a lunate strip around the periphery of the cavity. Inferiorly, a gap in the articular surface, the acetabular notch, provides an inlet for the vessels supplying the acetabulum. The articular surface surrounds a nonarticular area, the acetabular fossa, which is filled with fat, synovium, and the ligamentum teres. The acetabulum faces laterally, inferiorly, and anteriorly; this orientation has implications regarding joint congruity that are discussed later.

The medial aspect of the ilium displays the smooth shallow iliac fossa anteriorly, which the iliacus muscle occupies. Posterior to the iliac fossa is the roughened iliac tuberosity, to which the interosseous and dorsal sacroiliac ligaments attach. The auricular surface, just inferior to the tuberosity, articulates with the sacrum in a synovial joint. The pelvic surface of the ilium extends inferior and anterior to the iliac fossa, contributing to the wall of the lesser pelvis.

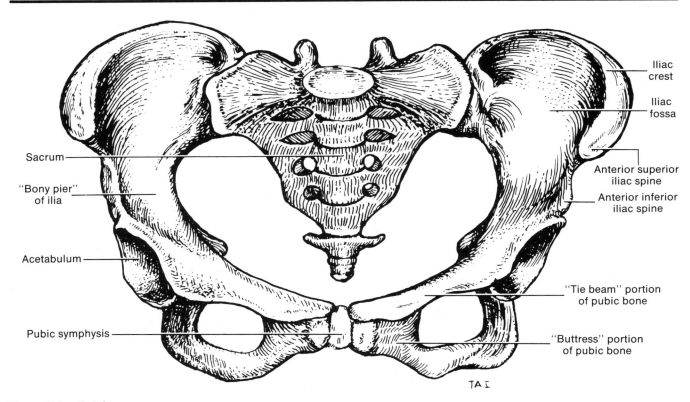

Figure 7.1.   Pelvis.

Iliac crest
Iliac fossa
Anterior superior iliac spine
Anterior inferior iliac spine
"Tie beam" portion of pubic bone
"Buttress" portion of pubic bone
Sacrum
"Bony pier" of ilia
Acetabulum
Pubic symphysis

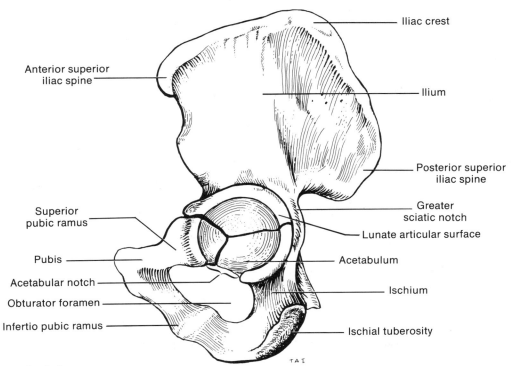

Figure 7.2.   Innominate bone.

Iliac crest
Anterior superior iliac spine
Ilium
Posterior superior iliac spine
Greater sciatic notch
Lunate articular surface
Acetabulum
Ischium
Ischial tuberosity
Superior pubic ramus
Pubis
Acetabular notch
Obturator foramen
Infertio pubic ramus

Femur. The femur, the longest bone in the body, contributes to man's striding gait. The strongest bone as well, it withstands substantial forces from muscle contraction and weight transmission (2). In an anatomical position, the two femurs extend obliquely from the pelvis medially toward the knee, bringing the legs closer to the midline where they can best support the body.

The femoral shaft assumes a nearly cylindrical shape, while the ends of the femur adopt configurations to meet the specific functional needs of the hip and knee joints. The proximal end terminates in an ellipsoid-shaped head, equivalent to two-thirds of a spheriod (1,6). The femoral head joins the shaft via the femoral neck (Fig. 7.3). An intertrochanteric line marks the junction of the neck and shaft anteriorly, and an intertrochanteric crest marks it posteriorly. The neck's narrow circumference prevents impingment upon the acetabulum, allowing a greater ROM. The neck axis runs obliquely—superiorly, medially, and anteri-

orly—from the shaft. Since both the femoral head and the acetabulum face anteriorly, the superior anterior portion of the femoral head is exposed and does not contact the acetabulum during erect standing (1). In the adult, the neck forms an angle of 125° with the shaft in the frontal plane (angle of inclination Fig. 7.3A), and 15° anteriorly with the shaft in the horizontal plane (angle of anteversion Fig. 7.3B). The length and angle of the femoral neck facilitate range of motion of the hip and allow greater leverage for the muscles inserting distal to the neck. The configuration of the neck, however, subjects it to greater shear force and renders it more susceptible to fracture (7). Also, excessive angles of inclination or anteversion may increase the risk of hip dislocation. A diminished angle of inclination, coxa vara, shortens the limb and reduces the leverage and strength of the gluteus medius muscle, and may produce a Trendelenburg limp.

The femoral neck, interposed between the head and shaft, is similar in configuration to an oblique strut

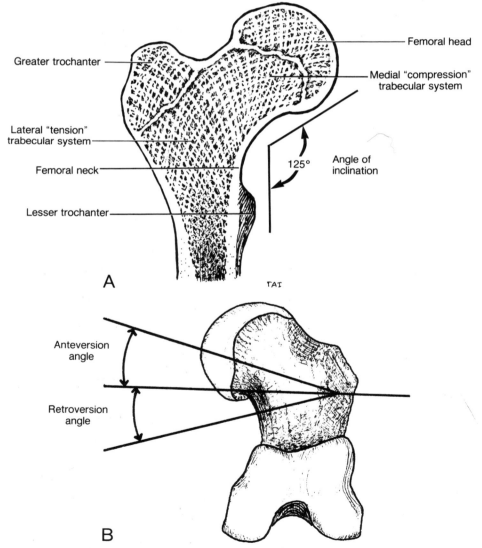

Figure 7.3.   *A*, Cross-section of the femur. *B*, Femoral neck–shaft relationships.

between vertical and horizontal beams. It serves as a lever arm to transmit the body weight and to prevent shear. The trabecular arrangement of lamellae within the femoral head and neck corresponds to functional demands placed upon this area (Fig. 7.3). A medial "compression" trabecular system arises from the cortex of the upper shaft and inferior part of the neck, and fans our vertically to terminate on the cortical bone of the superior aspect of the head. A lateral "tension" (arcuate) trabecular system arises from the cortical bone on the lateral aspect of the femoral shaft and passes medially to terminate in the inferior portion of the femoral head.

The greater trochanter projects laterally at the junction of the femoral neck and shaft (Fig. 7.3). One may palpate it a hand's breadth below the iliac crest, where it marks the level of the femoral head that lies medially. Many of the gluteal muscles insert into the greater trochanter. The lesser trochanter, too deep to be palpated, lies at the posteromedial junction of the shaft and the neck. The iliopsoas muscle inserts onto it.

Arthrology

The hip is a ball-and-socket joint, permitting motion in three planes: flexion and extension in the sagittal plane, abduction and adduction in the frontal plane, and rotation in the transverse plane. Circumduction results from a combination of these cardinal plane movements. Accessory movement is minimal, but passive force can produce a small amount of gliding and traction.

Hip flexion reaches 90° actively with the knee extended, 120° actively with the knee flexed, and up to 145° passively with the knee flexed. Hip extension reaches 10° actively with the knee flexed, 20° actively with the knee extended, and 30° passively with knee extended. (Clinically, anterior tilt of the pelvis will appear to enhance hip extension, so stabilization is essential during examination.) Abduction may reach up to 45° actively. (Some individuals achieve a much greater ROM through training.) Adduction, when combined with either flexion or extension, reaches 30° actively. Medial rotation from 30–50° is possible actively or passively. Lateral rotation reaches from 45–60° actively or passively, the range increasing as the hip flexes and relaxes the iliofemoral and pubofemoral ligaments.

The acetabulum is the concave member of the hip joint. Only the outer, lunate surface of the acetabulum articulates with the femur, and is covered by articulate cartilage (Fig. 7.4). The cartilage is broadest superiorly where the pressure of the body weight falls in the erect position, and narrowest anteriorly. A fibrocartilaginous collar, the acetabular labrum, surrounds the acetabulum, deepening the cavity and embracing the femoral head (Fig. 7.4).

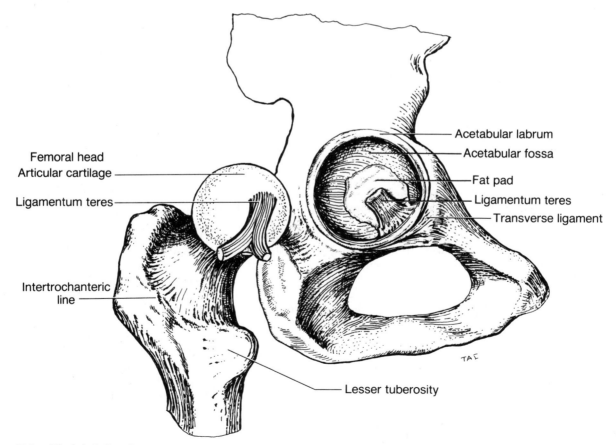

Figure 7.4. Hip joint structures.

The labrum attaches around the acetabular rim, but ceases at the acetabular notch. A transverse ligament joins the ends of the labrum and converts the notch into a foramen through which neurovascular structures enter the joint.

The femoral head is the convex member of the hip joint. Articular cartilage completely covers the head except for a small area, the fovea, to which the ligamentum teres attaches (Fig. 7.4). The articular surfaces of the femur and acetabulum are relatively extensive, although somewhat irregular, the contact area changing with the position of the joint (3). Since the hip is a weightbearing joint, the articular surfaces are more prone to degenerative changes. Due to the large forces transmitted through the hip, a small defect in either surface may seriously impair its function. Hip dysfunction may indirectly affect the posture and movement of numerous other joints (7).

In contrast to the mobility of the ball-and-socket shoulder joint, stability characterizes the hip. Factors that lend stability include close conformity of the articular surfaces, the acetabular labrum encircling the femoral head, strong capsular ligaments that become taut in extension, and negative atmospheric pressure in the joint. Although the inherent design of the hip joint favors stability, it still allows a certain amount of mobility. In addition to joint motion per se, the suppleness of the acetabular labrum, the length and obliquity of the femoral neck, and lumbar spine flexibility all contribute to the total range of lower limb movement.

In the evolutionary process, assuming an erect posture tilted the pelvis posteriorly relative to the femur, causing the ligaments of the hip joint to become coiled around the femoral neck (1). They become more taut as extension increases, pulling the joint surfaces together in a position of maximum stability. Conversely, flexion relaxes the ligaments and promotes instability. A relatively mild force upon the flexed and adducted hip may produce posterior dislocation of the hip (7).

The close-packed position of the hip, contrary to most other joints, occurs in two positions: either 90° of flexion and slight abduction and lateral rotation (1), or complete extension, internal rotation, and abduction (5). The "rest" position of the hip, in which the capsule is totally slack, is 10° flexion, 10° abduction, and 10° external rotation. Often a patient assumes a "rest" position to accommodate swelling. Assuming a rest position may be one of the only clinical indications of hip joint inflammation; otherwise the depth of this joint obscures signs of inflammation. In the later stages of arthritis, muscle spasm and capsular contracture alter the rest position, so that a patient assumes a posture of flexion, **adduction**, and external rotation; this position is the classic capsular pattern of the hip (8).

The cylindrical joint capsule resembles a sleeve running between its attachment around the peripheral surface of the acetabular labrum and transverse ligament, to its insertion near the base of the femoral neck.

Anteriorly it extends to the intertrochanteric line, but posteriorly it covers only one-half of the neck; hip flexion and adduction may cause the femoral head to protrude posteriorly and inferiorly where the capsule is deficient. The capsule is thickest anteriorly and superiorly where it has ligamentous reinforcement. Fractures of the femur may occur totally within the area of the capsule, partially within the capsule, or outside of the capsule. The intracapsular type of fracture heals poorly for reasons discussed later.

The large synovial membrane of the hip joint extends from the femoral head articular margin and covers the part of the neck lying within the capsule. It lines the interior surface of the capsule, the acetabular labrum, the fat pad, and vessels in the acetabular fossa; it attaches to the acetabular articular margin.

Powerful ligaments, named for the bony regions to which they are attached, strengthen the capsule of the hip. The iliofemoral ligament, the strongest ligament in the body, stems as an inverted Y from the lower part of the anterior inferior iliac spine (AIIS) to the trochanteric line of the femur (Fig. 7.5). It is capable of preventing posterior tilt of the pelvis during erect standing, even in the absence of muscle contraction, in the so-called "balancing on the ligaments" maneuver. It also helps limit extension of the hip joint.

The ischiofemoral ligament spirals from its posterior attachment along the ischium and acetabulum over the posterior aspect of the femoral neck to insert into the inner surface of the greater trochanter (Fig. 7.5). It reinforces the posterior capsule and limits excessive medial rotation, abduction, and extension (1). The pubofemoral ligament arises from the pubis and inserts into the anterior surface of the trochanteric fossa. It reinforces the medial-inferior capsule and limits excessive abduction, lateral rotation, and extension.

The ligamentum teres arises from the transverse ligament and acetabular notch, and runs along the floor of the acetabular fossa to the fovea where it inserts into the femur (Fig. 7.4). This ligament does not contribute to support of the joint; however, it sometimes carries an artery which supplies the femoral head. A strong band of circular fibers, the orbicular ligament, constricts the narrowest part of the femoral neck. This ligament reinforces the capsule and helps prevent hip dislocation.

Eighteen or more bursae exist in the hip region, but only three appear to have clinical significance. The iliopsoas (iliopectineal) bursa lies between the psoas muscle and the anterior joint capsule. It frequently communicates with the joint cavity, and thus excess fluid from trauma or arthritis may spill into it. The combined motions of hip flexion and adduction, or excessive extension, can compress the inflamed bursae and elicit pain (6). The trochanteric (gluteal) bursa lies between the greater trochanter and the gluteus maximus. This large bursa is commonly the site of calcium deposits or tubercular involvement. Gluteal bursitis is painful during any movement of the hip. The ischiogluteal bursa lies superficially over the ischial

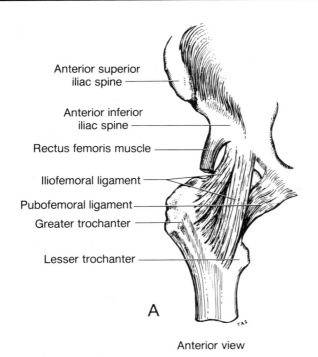

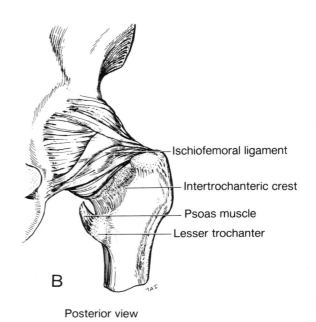

Anterior superior iliac spine

Anterior inferior iliac spine

Rectus femoris muscle

Iliofemoral ligament

Pubofemoral ligament

Greater trochanter

Lesser trochanter

A

Anterior view

Ischiofemoral ligament

Intertrochanteric crest

Psoas muscle

Lesser trochanter

B

Posterior view

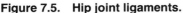

Figure 7.5. Hip joint ligaments.

tuberosity. ''Weaver's bottom'' became a synonym for ischiogluteal bursitis, which affects persons whose occupations involve prolonged sitting, and/or flexion and extension of the hip.

Mechanics

The hip's roles in locomotion and posture require the combined actions of many powerful muscles. Frequently the muscles assist in producing more than one type of movement. Due to extensive coverage elsewhere (1, 2, 7), muscle origins, insertions, and actions will not be reviewed. Instead, a brief description of the pertinent features of muscles acting upon the hip is presented.

The iliopsoas is the most powerful hip flexor, but is assisted by the "long flexors" which include the rectus femoris, pectineus, adductor longus, gracilis, tensor fascia lata and sartorius muscles. The rectus femoris muscle contracts strongly in kicking; adolescents occasionally avulse its insertion, the AIIS, during a forceful kick. The gluteus maximus muscle, the most powerful muscle in the body, extends the hip (1). The hamstring muscles assist hip extension and are active during walking, whereas the gluteus maximus muscle is more active in running and jumping (1). The short lateral rotators (piriformis, obturator internus, obturator externus, superior and inferior gemelli, and quadratus femoris muscles), work as a unit and are stronger than the medial rotators (tensor fascia lata, gluteus medius, gluteus minimus and gracilis muscles). The gluteus medius, gluteus minimus, tensor fascia lata, and sartorius muscles combine actions to produce hip abduction. The abductors must contract to stabilize the pelvis in order for a person to balance on one leg; otherwise the pelvis drops on the other side. The gracilis, pectineus, adductor magnus, adductor brevis, and adductor longus muscles, with some assistance from the hamstrings, adduct the hip.

As in other joints, the efficiency of the hip musculature largely depends upon the position of the joint. For example, when the joint is flexed, the extensor muscles are under tension and can achieve maximum contraction. Likewise, the position of the knee affects the muscles crossing both the hip and knee joints. Thus the starting position of runners, in order to achieve greatest efficiency, is maximal flexion of the hip, followed by extension of the knee.

The muscles in the hip region may have different actions, depending upon the joint position. The quadratus femoris muscle, for instance, will assist flexion when the hip is in an extended position, but will assist extension when the hip is in a flexed position.

Neurology

Ventral rami of the first four lumbar nerves form the lumbar plexus. The plexus gives off the iliohypogastric, ilioinguinal, and genitofemoral nerves, and muscular branches to the quadratus lumborum, psoas minor, psoas major, and iliacus muscles. Its terminal divisions include the lateral cutaneous nerve of the thigh, the obturator nerve, and the femoral nerve. The obturator nerve supplies the gracilis, obturator externus, adductor brevis, adductor longus, adductor magnus, and sometimes pectineus muscles. The femoral nerve supplies the sartorius, quadriceps femoris and sometimes pectineus muscles. The femoral nerve also gives off three cutaneous branches—the intermediate anterior cutaneous nerve of the thigh, the medial anterior cutaneous nerve of the thigh, and the saphenous nerve.

Ventral rami of the 4th and 5th lumbar nerves and the first four sacral nerves form the sacral plexus. The nerves entering into the sacral plexus converge into the sciatic nerve that exits from the greater sciatic foramen, deep to the piriformis muscle, where swelling of the muscle or posterior hip dislocations commonly impinge upon it (4, 9). In the posterior thigh, the sciatic nerve divides into the common peroneal and tibial nerves. Branches of the sacral plexus include the superior gluteal nerve to the gluteus medius, gluteus minimus, and tensor fascia lata muscles, the inferior gluteal nerve to the gluteus maximus muscle, the nerve to the piriformis muscle, the posterior femoral cutaneous nerve, the nerve to the quadratus femoris and gemellus inferior muscles, and the nerve to the obturator internus and gemellus superior muscles. The muscular branches of the sciatic nerve supply the hamstring and adductor magnus muscles.

Hilton's law states that a joint receives its proprioceptive and pain fibers from the same nerves that supply the muscles moving the joint. This law applies to the hip joint. Twigs from the femoral nerve supply the anterior portion of the capsule, the nerve to the quadratus femoris muscle supplies the posterior portion, the obturator nerve supplies the inferior portion, and the superior gluteal nerve supplies the superior portion. (7).

When evaluating a patient who complains of hip pain, it is important to rule out pain referred from the lumbar spine. According to Cyriax, pain in the buttock usually has a lumbar origin, whereas pain in the anterolateral area of the thigh originates from the hip (8). Hip pathology commonly refers pain along the L3 dermatome.

Angiology

The external iliac artery bifurcates into the femoral and profunda femoral arteries. The profunda femoral artery gives origin to two major branches, the medial and lateral circumflex arteries, which provide the major source of blood to the proximal femur (10). The retinacular arteries branch off the medial and lateral circumflex arteries and course along folds in the articular capsule, supplying the trochanteric region, femoral neck, and femoral head (Fig. 7.6).

The obturator artery also supplies the femoral head through its acetabular branch, which sends a small twig to run with ligamentum teres (this source is somewhat inconsistent) (Fig. 7.6). In addition to the obturator artery retinacular arteries also supply the femoral head and neck; they branch from the metaphyseal vessels off of the femoral nutrient artery and ascend through the medullary cavity. This pattern of arterial distribution, in which the femoral neck and head are dependent upon the long vulnerable retinacular arteries and relatively distant metaphyseal supply, predisposes the femoral head to more vascular disorders than any other bone in the body (5). Trauma may sever the proximal end of the bone from its tenuous blood supply.

Branches from the superior gluteal artery supply the upper portion of the acetabulum and fibrous capsule. The inferior gluteal artery supplies the inferior and posterior portions of the acetabular rim and adjacent capsule.

The long and superficial great saphenous vein and the deep femoral and iliac veins provide the venous drainage of the hip.

HIP EXAMINATION

History

An examiner initiates a hip examination by acquiring identifying data (Fig. 7.7). A patient's age and gender may reveal the likelihood of certain patholo-

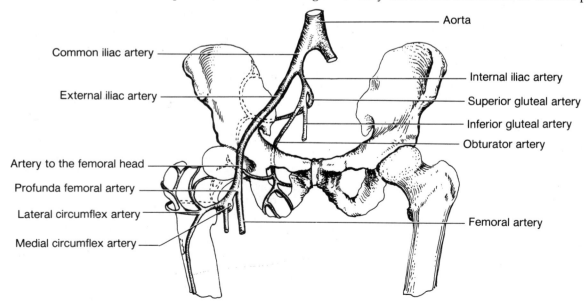

Figure 7.6. Arteries supplying the hip.

A. HISTORY

  1. Identifying Data

    Name _____ Age _____ Gender _____ Date _____

    Provisional diagnosis _____ Precautions _____

    Chief complaint _____

    Dominant side R _____ L _____ Prior condition of involved part _____

  2. Present Episode or Illness

    a. Description of symptoms

      1) location: //// = pain
                ==== = paresthesia
                °°°° = numbness
                xxxx = other _____

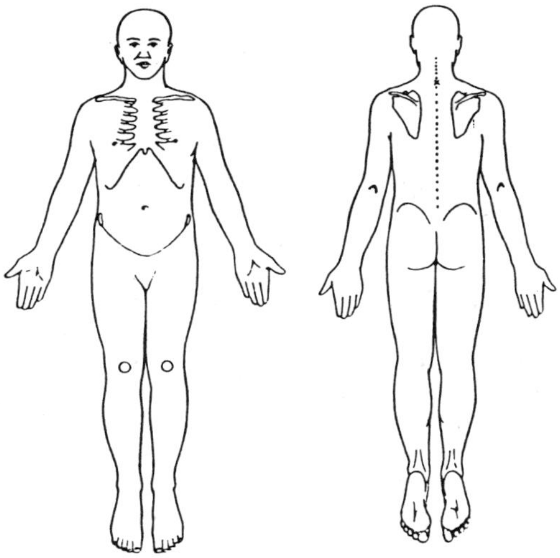

      2) severity:

      _____
      none   worst

      3) impairment:

      _____
      annoying   completely disabling

      4) nature:

        cramping _____ aching _____

        shooting _____ burning _____

        throbbing _____ tingling _____

        stabbing _____ sore _____

        other _____

      5) behavior:

        constant _____ intermittent _____ duration _____

        occurs when _____ elicited by _____

        aggravated by _____ relieved by _____

        24-hour pattern _____

        highly irritable _____ mildly irritable _____ not irritable _____

      6) joint characteristics: catches _____ , locks _____ , swells _____ , gives way _____ , dislocates _____ ,

        other _____

Figure 7.7. Examination form part 1: History.

gies common to his group. Congenital hip dysplasia is present in infancy and more common in females: Legg-Calvé-Perthes disease typically occurs between ages 3 and 12 and is 4 times more frequent in males. Slipped capital femoral epiphysis presents more often in males between 10 and 15 years of age. Adult males sustain the highest incidence of traumatic dislocations and fractures (5). Elderly females are frequent victims of osteoporotic fractures and osteoarthritis. The chief complaint of a patient with a hip disorder usually includes one or more of the following: pain, decreased motion, weakness, joint deformity, or gait disturbance (6).

The examiner next requests a specific description of the present episode or illness. The patient should indicate his symptoms on a body chart, using the given key (Fig. 7.7). The patient frequently experiences pain arising from the spine or sacroiliac joints in the posterior hip region, whereas he most commonly feels pain arising from the hip joint in the anterior thigh (3, 6). The synovial lining of the hip joint is often the source of hip pain, which is characteristically dull and throbbing in nature, varies with fluctuations of inflammation, and is worse at night or after periods of immobilization (3). Bursitis manifests as tenderness and inflammation localized around the involved bursa. Behavior of symptoms associated with a particular activity may reflect aggravating factors, i.e., long distance cycling may precipitate or aggravate ischial bursitis, and lateral hip rotation and squatting may elicit a piriformis muscle syndrome.

The examiner should also explore the background and associated findings of the present episode or illness (Fig. 7.8). According to Tronzo, the most common etiology of hip dysfunction is trauma, followed in order by congenital disorders, developmental disorders, and infectious conditions (5). Therefore, the mechanism of injury frequently becomes a part of the history. A direct blow or impact from a fall, or an indirect torsion force through the femur, are the mechanisms for many femoral neck fractures. A posteriorly directed force through the long axis of a flexed and adducted femur produces a posterior dislocation, the most common type of traumatic hip dislocation. Hip fracture or dislocation severely disables an individual so that he refuses to bear weight or move the limb. Swelling and bleeding within the hip joint capsule are difficult to detect clinically because of its depth, but sometimes synovial fluid escapes into the more superficial iliopsoas bursa or extravasated blood surfaces in the thigh.

Relevant past and family history may reveal predisposition toward hormonally influenced disturbances or certain types of arthritis (Fig. 7.8). Also, the degenerative changes a patient experiences in his later years often stem from mechanical alterations initiated earlier by conditions such as congenital hip dysplasia or Legg-Calvé-Perthes disease. The patient's life-style can disclose activities that adversely stress the hip, such as yoga and aerobics. Investigation of current medications and recent radiographs completes the history. The therapist integrates this information from the history in preparation for the physical examination.

Physical Examination

Inspection.   A patient's posture often signifies hip pathology (Fig. 7.9). Some causes of pelvic obliquity include scoliosis, hip abduction or adduction contractures, and leg length discrepancy. A patient will not bear weight equally on both lower limbs when, for instance, they are of unequal length, or this activity produces hip pain. Excessive anterior pelvic tilt (lumbar lordosis) compensates for hip flexion contracture(s) in conditions such as osteoarthritis. Absence of the normal lumbar lordosis may suggest paravertebral muscle spasm (11). Disruption of the normal femoral head-neck-shaft relationships by disorders such as slipped capital femoral epiphysis or coxa vara can affect the level of the trochanters. The proper trochanteric position is just distal to a line joining the anterior

superior iliac spine and the ischial tuberosity (Néla-ton's line) (5).

Congenital hip dislocation typically produces asymmetric gluteal folds, as well as a shortened limb on the involved side. A toeing-out posture or laterally rotated limb could be indicative of retroversion of the femoral neck, whereas toeing-in compensates for anteversion. A patient with an acute femoral neck fracture often lies with the limb laterally rotated; following acute posterior dislocation, the limb is medially rotated (12).

The depth of the hip joint itself renders it difficult to inspect for changes in shape. The examiner, however, may assess many of the more superficial pelvic structures for deformity or assymetry in contour. Localized swelling characterizes bursitis or muscle spasm. Disuse atrophy typically affects the gluteal muscles in patients with arthritis. The examiner measures the distance between the anterior superior iliac spine (ASIS) and the medial malleolus as indicative of true leg length.

The postural changes described in the preceeding paragraphs may also serve as indirect clinical signs of deformity. Likewise, gait deviations provide clues for indirect assessment. An antalgic gait, or painful limp, is characterized by an attempt to decrease loading on the painful hip, by decreasing stance time, and by tilting the trunk toward the affected side. Unequal timing clues the examiner to an antalgic gait. A Trendelenburg gait, produced by hip joint instability or gluteus medius weakness, incorporates a pelvic drop with a lateral shift of the shoulders to the normal (dropped) side, for which a patient often compensates by lurching toward the affected side (3, 11). This compensation maneuver may increase stance time on the affected side. A shortened limb produces a gait with trunk tilting to the affected side, but timing remains even. The gait of a patient with an ankylosed hip is characterized by excessive lumbar and body motion, which compensate for the decreased ROM. A patient with a weak gluteus maximus muscle extends the body posterior to the hip axis, which represents an extensor thrust gait.

The examiner notes skin changes or lesions that may be associated with hip pathology. He also describes the aids or assistive devices a patient requires.

Palpation.   Through palpation it is possible to detect superficial inflammation and localized tenderness about the hip. The examiner palpates the skin, subcutaneous tissue, and musculotendinous units in a systematic fashion (Fig. 7.9). He next locates the iliopectineal, trochanteric, and ischiogluteal bursae anteriorly, laterally, and posteriorly respectively. Palpation may also reveal asymmetry between bony landmarks which was not observable upon inspection. The examiner routinely assesses the level of anterior superior iliac spines, iliac crests, greater trochanters, posterior superior iliac spines, and ischial tuberosities (Fig. 7.10). The hip joint itself is not accessible to palpation; however, the symphysis pubis and SI joints are. A tender sym-

b. Background and associated findings

Date of present injury _____ or onset _____ insidious _____

Dates of hospitalization _____ and/or other health care

Treatments; dates; results _____

_____

Status of condition: acute _____ or chronic _____

constant _____ or intermittent _____

better _____ or worse _____

Nature and mechanism of injury or events precipitating present episode _____

_____

Results of injury (if applicable): deformity (describe) _____

corrected _____ disability (type and cause) _____

loss of motion (specify) _____ when occurred _____

loss of strength (specify) _____ when occurred _____

swelling (specify) _____ when occurred _____

bleeding (specify) _____ when occurred _____

3. Relevant Past History and Family History

History of similar condition: dates _____ nature _____

_____

Treatment _____

Other relevant illnesses or disorders _____

General health status _____

Health problems of immediate family _____

4. Life-style

Occupation _____ ADL _____

Regular (3 times/week minimum) physical activities requiring: strength _____ agility _____ endurance _____

flexibility _____ other _____

What patient does to promote wellness _____

Patient's concept of cause of condition _____

Patient's concept of functional and/or cosmetic deficit(s) _____

Anticipated goals _____

5. Other

Current medications _____

Recent radiographs _____

6. Therapist's Interpretation and Plans for Objective Exam _____

_____

Figure 7.8. Examination form part 2: History continued.

B. PHYSICAL EXAMINATION

1. Inspection

   a. Posture (standing)

   pelvic obliquity _____ more weight on R ____ L ____ equal ____

   anterior pelvic tilt _____ posterior pelvic tilt _____

   level of trochanters _____ gluteal folds _____

   Nelaton's line _____ to (R) trochanter; _____ to (L) trochanter

   lateral rot. R leg ____ L leg ____ medial rot. R leg ____ L leg ____

   b. Shape

   deformity (describe) _____ asymmetry _____

   swelling or masses _____ atrophy _____

   leg length R _____ L _____

   c. Use

   gait deviations: antalgic ____ Trendelenburg ____ shortened limb ____ ankylosed ____

   extensor thrust ____ other _____

   sit and rise from chair/plinth _____

   d. Skin

   color ____ condition ____ lesions ____ scars ____

   e. Aids

   cane ____ crutches ____ walker ____ wheelchair ____

2. Palpation (note location and nature of abnormality)

   a. Skin and subcutaneous tissue: tenderness ____ temperature ____ swelling ____ decreased mobility ____

   trigger points ____ other _____

   b. Muscles and tendons: tenderness ____ temperature ____ spasm ____ loss of continuity ____

   decreased mobility ____ other _____

   c. Iliopectineal bursa: tenderness ____ temperature ____ swelling ____

   Trochanteric bursa: tenderness ____ temperature ____ swelling ____

   Ischiofemoral bursa: tenderness ____ temperature ____ swelling ____

   d. Bones and joints: tenderness ____ temperature ____ swelling ____ bony prominences ____

   e. Arteries and nerves: femoral pulse ____ sciatic n. ____

Figure 7.9. Examination form part 3: Inspection and palpation.

physis pubis is one symptom of osteitis pubis (13). (Sacroiliac findings are discussed in Chapter 3.) One may palpate the femoral artery pulse just inferior to the center of the inguinal ligament. The sciatic nerve lies midway between the greater trochanter and ischial tuberosity, and is best palpated when the patient is side lying with the hip flexed. A herniated lumbar disc, piriformis muscle spasm, or nerve trauma produce tenderness upon palpation of the sciatic nerve (11).

Movement Assessment. Functional active movement may disclose certain hip pathologies (Fig. 7.11). A waddling gait symbolizes bilateral congenital hip dislocation or conditions with bilateral gluteal weakness. An antalgic limp characterizes osteoarthritis.

Limited hip movement may characterize various contractures. Both Legg-Calvé-Perthes disease and slipped capital femoral epiphysis present as a painful limitation of abduction and medial rotation, plus an antalgic gait.

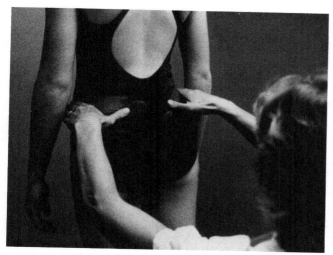

Figure 7.10. Inspection of pelvis and hips: examiner is posterior to patient for assessing alignment of iliac crests, sacroiliac joints, and other bony landmarks.

Active, passive, and resisted physiologic movements more specifically implicate or rule out symptomatic structures. Loss of motion in a capsular pattern, i.e., no medial rotation nor extension and limited abduction and flexion, is indicative of arthritis (8). Restriction or weakness of other motions will signal various inert or contractile tissue lesions. Assessment of accessory movement reveals the status of joint surface movement, although it is normally small in this relatively stable joint.

Special passive tests include the Ortolani and Barlow tests for congenital hip dislocation (Fig. 7.11). To perform the Ortolani test, the examiner places an infant supine with knees and hips flexed to 90°. He abducts the legs and presses the hip anteriorly with the fingers placed posteriorly over the joint; a relocating click designates a positive test (Fig. 7.12). The Barlow test is performed in the same position, but opposite manner, dislocating the hip by adducting and pressing it posteriorly.

To detect a hip flexion contracture, the examiner performs a Thomas test. This is done by placing the patient supine with the opposite knee flexed to his chest to stabilize the pelvis and eliminate lumbar lordosis; then the examiner extends the leg being tested as far as possible, measuring the range of extension (Fig. 7.13).

An Ober test, for contracture of the iliotibial band, commences with the patient side lying on the opposite leg; the examiner abducts the leg being tested, then slightly extends it (Fig. 7.14). Normally, the leg drops into adduction when released, but a contracture prevents this from occurring.

A Patrick, or fabere, test may indicate pathology either in the hip or SI joint, depending on the location of symptoms. The examiner positions the leg of a supine patient into flexion, abduction, and external rotation, then moves it into extension, while he stabilizes the pelvis over the opposite ASIS (Fig. 7.15). Inguinal pain and limited range signify hip involvement, whereas posterior pelvic pain may imply SI pathology.

Neurologic Evaluation. The examiner assesses strength of the iliopsoas muscle as the key muscle representing the L2 neurologic level (Fig. 7.16). No key reflexes are present in the hip region. The examiner performs sensory testing as described in Chapter 2, and records the results on the accompanying form (Fig. 7.16). A posterior hip dislocation or piriformis muscle syndrome may compress the sciatic nerve, producing sensory changes. Swelling of the iliopectineal bursa may impinge upon the femoral nerve. The examiner completes motor and coordination tests as indicated.

Recommendation of Other Tests. The examiner determines if other tests are necessary based upon the data obtained thus far. When he has obtained all of the necessary information, he is prepared to interpret the examination and recommend patient disposition. Table 7.1 includes a summary of the differential diagnosis and treatment of common hip disorders.

3. Movement assessment

   a. Functional active movement

      gait _____

      up and down stairs _____

      squat _____

      knee to chest _____

      don and remove shoes _____

Key: C = completes task

     D = completes task with difficulty/discomfort

     N = does not complete task

b/c/d. Physiological movement

	ACTIVE			PASSIVE			RESISTIVE	
	ROM	Symptoms	Quality	ROM	Symptoms	Endfeel	Strength	Symptoms
flexion								
extension								
abduction								
adduction								
lateral rotation								
medial rotation								

e. Accessory movement

	Mobility	Symptoms
lateral traction		
caudal femoral glide		
dorsal femoral glide		
ventral femoral glide		

f. Special tests

	+	−	Comments
Ortolani test			
Barlow test			
Thomas test			
Ober test			
Patrick test			

Figure 7.11. Examination form part 4: Movement assessment.

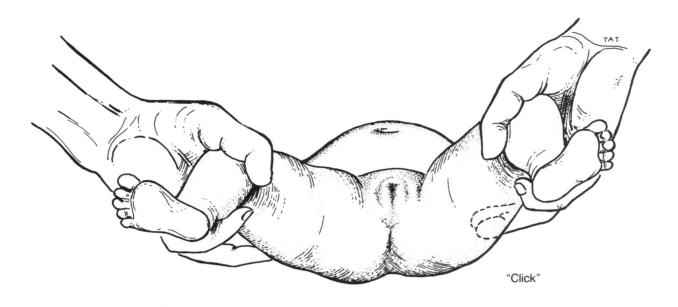

Figure 7.12. Ortolani test: if a newborn's hip can be dislocated by flexion, adduction, and pressing in a posterior direction, then relocated by abduction and anterior pressure, producing a click, the test is positive, implicating congenital hip dislocation.

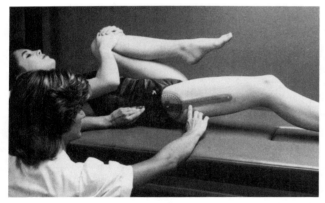

Figure 7.13. Thomas Test: if stabilizing the pelvis by full passive flexion of the uninvolved hip and knee prevents the involved hip from extending to a rest position on the plinth, the test is positive, implicating a hip flexion contracture.

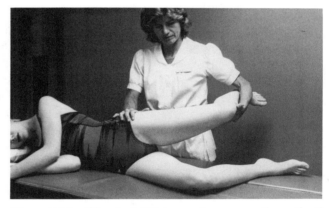

Figure 7.14. Ober test: if the examiner moves the patient's hip into abduction and extension, then releases his hold, and the leg doesn't drop into adduction, the test is positive, implicating contracture of the iliotibial band.

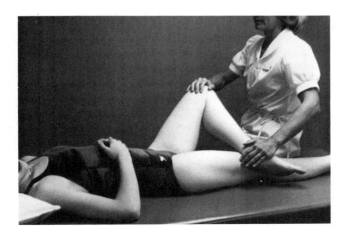

Figure 7.15. Patrick (fabere) test: if the patient cannot flex, abduct, externally rotate, then extend his hip to allow placement of his lateral malleolus on the opposite knee, the test is positive, implicating hip disease, if it reproduces inguinal pain, or sacroiliac joint dysfunction, if it reproduces posterior sacral pain.

4. Neurological evaluation

   a. Key muscles (strength grade 0–5)

      _____ L2 iliopsoas muscle

   b. Key reflexes—none at hip

   c. Sensibility

Key: lacking   A = light touch sensation
B = sharp/dull discrimination
C = temperature discrimination
D = proprioception

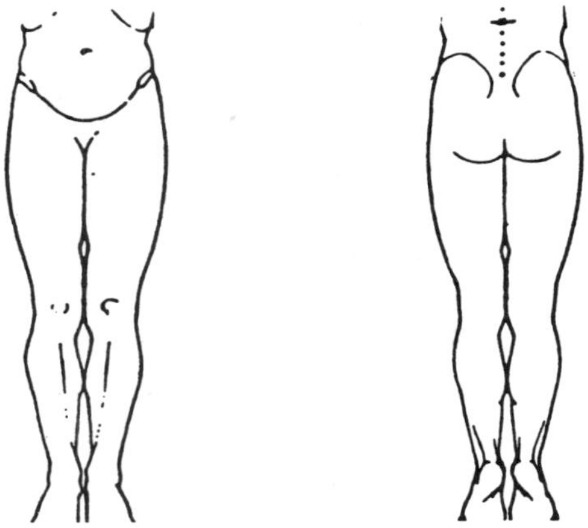

   d. Motor control: spastic _____ flaccid _____ rigid _____ clonic __

   e. Coordination

      knee and hip flex./ext.

      (supine) _____

Key: C = completes task

D = completes task with

     difficulty/discomfort

N = does not complete

     task

5. Recommendation of other tests

   a. Radiography _____

   b. Laboratory _____

   c. Electrodiagnostic _____

   d. Arthroscopy _____

   e. Arthrography _____

   f. Other _____

Figure 7.16. Examination form part 5: Neurologic evaluation and recommendation of other tests.

Table 7.1.
Summary of Differential Diagnosis and Treatment of Common Hip Disorders

Disorder	Chief Complaint	Onset	Symptom Characteristics	Static Physical Changes	Dynamic Physical Changes	Special Tests	Treatment[a]
Bursitis a. iliopsoas b. ishiogluteal c. trochanteric	Local tenderness to pressure over: a. anterior hip b. ischial tuberosity c. greater trochanter	a. May develop from hip joint inflammation b. Related to irritating activity such as prolonged sitting c. May stem from excessive adduction or hip muscle imbalance	a,b,c local pain and tenderness	a,b,c Local swelling	Symptoms increased by: a. extreme hip flexion or extension and adduction in flexion b. walking, climbing, or sitting c. hip medial and lateral rotation and adduction or resisted abduction	Tenderness to palpation: a. inguinal area; signs of femoral nerve compression b. ischial tuberosity c. greater trochanter	a,b,c joint aspiration and fluid culture; ice for acute pain relief; anti-inflammatory drugs; rest from aggravating activities; later moist heat, diathermy or ultrasound; eliminate cause when possible.
Congential hip dislocation/displasia	None in newborn; gait deviations in older child	In utero; predisposing factors are interuterine crowding, excessive capsular laxity, and genetic influence	Hip weakness, balance and gait difficulties	Limb shortening; asymmetrical skin folds; postero-superior prominence of proximal femur	Trendenenburg gait; decrease abd. ROM and weak hip abductors	Ortolani; Barlow; radiographic	If recognized in newborn, splint in abduction and flexion (Pavlik harness); later manage symptoms or surgical correction
Legg-Calvé-Perthes Disease	Groin and anterior thigh pain	Insidious onset between 3–12 years of age; male:female = 4:1; 12% bilateral	Antalgic limp	Disuse atrophy of hip and thigh muscles	Painful limitation of abduction and medial rotation	Radiographic changes	Splint in abduction and medial rotation to center femoral head during biologic remodeling; surgical osteotomy; maintain ROM
Osteoarthritis	Hip pain and stiffness	Insidious onset, common in elderly or those with mechanical alternations of hip	Pain in groin, anterior thigh, and knee increased after prolonged activity or prolonged rest	Hip flexion contracture, compensated by lumbar lordosis	antalgic limb; loss of abduction, medial rotation, and extension	Capsular pattern; osteophytes and joint space narrowing on x-ray	Reduce load on hip by weight loss, assistive devices, or osteotomy; increase strength and ROM via nonloading exercises (swim, bicycle) joint mobilization; arthroplasty
Piriformis syndrome	Posterior hip and sacral pain	Insidious or overuse syndrome related to contracture or hypertrophy of piriformis muscle	Severe pain increased by sitting, squatting,. or lateral rotation of hip; radiates to posterior thigh	Lateral rotation contracture	Limited medial rotation	Sensation and blood supply to perineum and genitalia may be decreased by pressure on sacral plexus and internal iliac vessels	Stretching to relieve contracture; contract-relax technique; forceful osteopathic manipulation; surgical release of piriformis muscle
Slipped capital femoral epiphysis	Hip pain and tenderness	Onset between 10–16 yrs; male:female = 3:1; 30% bilateral a. acute—following relatively mild or moderate trauma, a patient is unable to weightbear; severe pain b. chronic (75% cases) insidious development of limp, with no pain, or intermittent discomfort	Vague hip and anterior thigh pain (may radiate to knee)	Decreased abduction and medial rotation; shortened limb	Trendelenburg gait	Hip tender to palpation; radiographic diagnosis necessary	Surgical reduction and stabilization with pins; NWB for 6 weeks; rehab. includes maintaining strength and ROM

[a]ROM, range of motion.

HIP MOBILIZATION

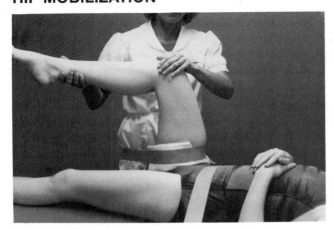

Figure 7.17.   Lateral Hip Joint Traction.

Patient Position: Supine with pelvis stabilized by strap; hip and knee flexed 90°.

Therapist Position: Standing at P's side; hands stabilize knee and ankle; mobilizing belt around T's hips controls P's proximal femur.

Technique: Use body weight to impart force in a lateral direction; T's hands move simultaneously with belt.

Comments: Effective as test or treatment for any painful limitation or hypomobility.

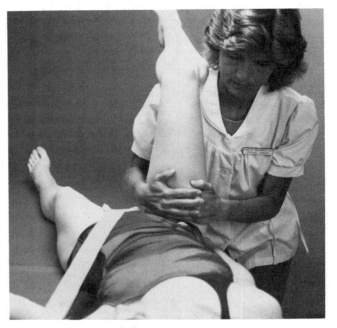

Figure 7.18.   Caudal Femoral Glide, 90° Flexion.

Patient Position: Supine with pelvis stabilized by strap; leg rests on T's shoulder.

Therapist Position: Standing facing P's head; clasped hands grasp upper thigh as close to hip joint as possible.

Technique: Use body weight to impart force in a caudal-lateral direction (parallel to femoral neck).

Comments: Effective as test or treatment for any painful limitation or hypomobility.

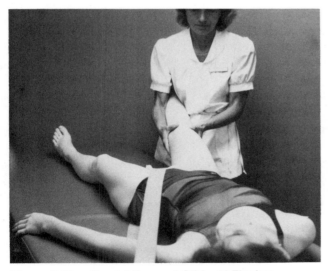

Figure 7.19.   Caudal Femoral Glide, 0° Flexion.

Patient Position: Supine with pelvis stabilized by strap.

Therapist Position: Standing facing P's head; hands grasp distal femur.

Technique: Use body weight to impart force in a caudal-lateral direction (parallel to femoral neck).

Comments: Effective as test or treatment for any painful limitation or hypomobility.

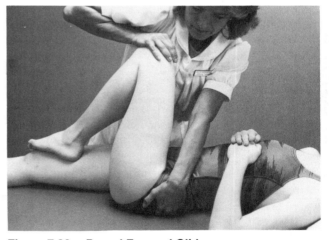

Figure 7.20.   Dorsal Femoral Glide.

Patient Position: Supine; hip flexed and adducted.

Therapist Position: Standing at P's opposite side; S hand fixates pelvis; M hand rests on knee.

Technique: Use chest contact upon M hand to apply dorsal-lateral force through the long axis of femur.

Comments: Especially effective for increasing flexion.

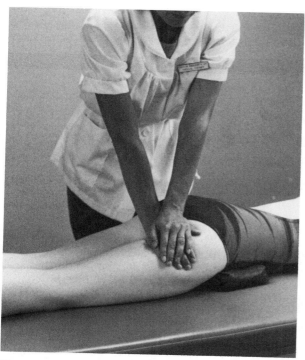

Figure 7.21.   Ventral Femoral Glide.
Patient Position: Prone with sandbag slightly raising and stabilizing pelvis.
Therapist Position: Standing at P's opposite side; overlapped hands rest on dorsal proximal femur.
Technique: With arms parallel to force, use body weight to apply ventral force to femoral head.
Comments: Especially effective for increasing extension.

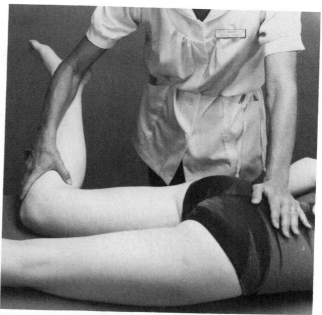

Figure 7.22.   Lateral Femoral Rotation.
Patient Position: Supine with hip slightly abducted and laterally rotated until ASIS lifted from table; knee flexed 90°.
Therapist Position: Standing at P's opposite side; S hand and forearm fixate lower leg; M hand on pelvis of involved side.
Technique: Press pelvis ventrally (rotate opposite to lateral rotation of hip).
Comments: General, physiologic technique, effective for increasing lateral hip rotation; use with caution or modify if knee instability exists.

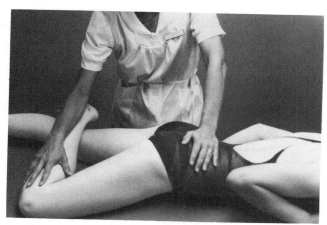

Figure 7.23.   Medial Femoral Rotation.
Patient Position: Supine with hip slightly abducted and medially rotated until opposite ASIS lifted from table; knee flexed 90°.
Therapist Position: Standing at P's side; S hand and forearm fixate lower leg; M hand on pelvis of involved side.
Technique: Press pelvis ventrally (rotate opposite to medial rotation of hip).
Comments: General, physiologic technique, effective for increasing medial hip rotation; use with caution or modify if knee instability exists.

References

1. Kapandji IA: *The Physiology of the Joints*, Edinburgh, Churchill Livingstone, 1974, vol 2.
2. Warwick R, Williams PL (eds): *Gray's Anatomy*, 35th British Edition. Philadelphia, WB Saunders, 1973.
3. Lee DMG: *Disorders of the Hip*. Philadelphia, JB Lippincott, 1983.
4. Muckle DS (ed): *Femoral Neck Fractures and Hip Joint Injuries*. New York, John Wiley & Sons, 1977.
5. Tronzo RG: *Surgery of the Hip Joint*, ed 2. New York, Springer-Verlag, 1984, vol 1.
6. D'Ambrosia RD: *Musculoskeletal Disorders—Regional Examination and Differential Diagnosis*. 2nd ed. Philadelphia, JB Lippincott, 1986.
7. Lockhart R, Hamilton GF, Fyfe FW: *Anatomy of the Human Body*. Philadelphia, JB Lippincott, 1959.
8. Cyriax J: *Textbook of Orthopaedic Medicine*. London, Baillière Tindall, 1982.
9. Hallin RP: Sciatic pain and the piriformis muscle. *Postgrad Med* 74:69–72, 1983.
10. Katz JF: *Management of Hip Disorders in Children*. Philadelphia, JB Lippincott, 1983.
11. Hoppenfeld S: *Physical Examination of the Spine and Extremities*. East Norwalk, CT, Appleton-Century-Crofts, 1976.
12. Salter RB: *Textbook of Disorders and Injuries of the Musculoskeletal System*, ed 2. Baltimore, Williams & Wilkins, 1983.
13. Lloyd-Smith R, Clement DB, McKenzie DC, Taunton JE: A survey of overuse and traumatic hip and pelvic injuries in athletes. *The Physician & Sportsmedicine* 13:131–141, 1985.

CHAPTER 8

THE KNEE

CLINICAL ANATOMY AND MECHANICS OF THE KNEE

The knee is the largest and most complex joint in the body. It includes a compound condylar joint (two tibiofemoral articulations) and a sellar joint (patellofemoral articulation). These joints occupy a common articular cavity (1). The fibula does not participate in the knee joint.

The knee suffers derangement of stability and function more frequently than any other joint, and is a common site of osteoarthritis. Factors that contribute to knee joint pathology include superficial anatomical exposure, functional demands of weightbearing activities, and stress from its location between the body's two longest levers, i.e., the femur and tibia.

Osteology

Femur. The oblique alignment of the femoral shaft relative to the lower leg produces an obtuse angle (opening laterally) at the knee. This normal angulation, physiological valgus, approximates 170–175° (Fig. 8.1). Angles of greater or lesser magnitude fall into the pathologic categories termed genu varus and genu valgus respectively.

In addition to the knee's bony angulation, another angle of clinical significance is the Q angle. It is the angle between the line of the quadriceps muscle pull and the line of insertion of the patellar tendon. Clinicians measure it by centering a goniometer over the patella, with one arm directed toward the anterior superior iliac spine (ASIS) and the other toward the tibial tuberosity; the acute angle between a proximal extension of the line through the tibial tuberosity and the line through the ASIS is the Q angle (Fig. 8.1). Many authorities in knee mechanics consider Q angles in excess of 20° to contribute to abnormal patellofemoral forces or patellar dislocation (2, 3).

The distal end of the femoral shaft expands into a large, convex, U-shaped articular surface for transmission of weight to the tibia. An intercondylar fossa (notch) separates the medial and lateral femoral condyles, forming the "U" (Fig. 8.2). The lateral is the stronger of the condyles, more aligned with the femoral shaft, and more involved in weight transmission (1). The medial condyle is curved with a medial convexity; it projects more distally to compensate for femoral obliquity and to provide a horizontal joint surface.

The articular surface of the femoral condyles extends anteriorly as the trochlear groove, which supports the patella. Medial and lateral projections deepen the concavity of the trochlear groove, and maintain the patella in its proper position. The more prominent lateral projection counteracts the stronger lateral dislocating forces of the extensor mechanism.

Tibia. The proximal end of the tibia flares out into a plateau which projects posteriorly relative to the shaft. A bifid nonarticulating intercondylar eminence divides the tibial articular surface into medial and lateral condyles which resemble concave gutters (Fig. 8.2). The lateral condyle is flatter and circular; the medial has a larger surface, is more concave, and is oval. The intercondylar eminence serves as a pivot for the slight rotation that occurs during knee flexion. During extension, it locks into the intercondylar fossa of the femur to enhance bony stability.

A tibial tuberosity protrudes from the proximal anterior surface of the tibia. It is the point of insertion of the infrapatellar tendon. A lateral tibial (Gerdy's) tubercle projects from the anterolateral tibial surface, marking the iliotibial tract insertion. An articular facet for the head of the fibula occupies the posterolateral part of the tibial condyle, just distal to the tibial plateau.

Patella. The patella is the largest sesamoid bone in the body, and lies within the quadriceps mechanism. It is a flat, triangular bone with an inferiorly directed apex. A longitudinal ridge divides its articular surface, creating medial and lateral facets. These facets articulate with the femoral patellar surface, while the ridge fits into the femoral trochlear groove. An odd facet occupies the extreme medial border of the patella; it contacts the femur only after 90° of knee flexion. The patella offers protection to the knee joint, and functions as a mobile lever which increases the mechanical advantage of the quadriceps tendon. It serves as a bearing surface to prevent forward shear

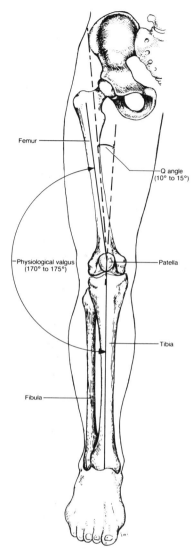

Figure 8.1. Lower limb.

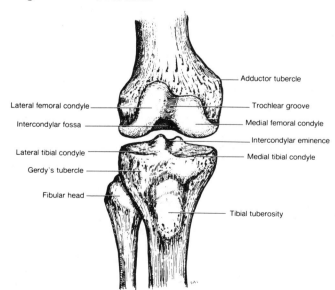

Figure 8.2. Bones of the knee.

of the femur upon the tibia. It also represents a fulcrum for static and dynamic stabilization forces (2).

Arthrology

Capsule and Synovial Membrane. The capsule of the knee joint is weak or absent in some areas, but thickened by ligamentous and tendinous reinforcements in others. Proximally, the capsule attaches to the femur around the articular margins of the condyles, except for a small area laterally where the popliteus tendon crosses the joint. An anterior extension of the capsule onto the femur forms the suprapatellar pouch. The capsule extends distally to attach to the periphery of each meniscus, and again the popliteus tendon breaches its lateral attachment. From its meniscal attachments the capsule continues to the adjacent articular margins of the tibia. This part of the capsule between the menisci and tibia is the coronary ligament. The pain and effusion associated with meniscal injury most likely result from tearing peripheral meniscal attachments to the capsule, as the central meniscus itself is avascular and aneural.

An opening in the anterior capsule allows the patella to communicate with the knee joint (Fig. 8.3). Medial and lateral capsular ligaments strengthen the capsule on both sides. Posteriorly, where the capsule inserts into the superior border of the articular surfaces of the femoral condyles, two condylar plates thicken the capsule, and separate the heads of the gastrocnemius muscle from the condyles. The oblique popliteal ligament reinforces the capsule posteromedially, and the arcuate ligament reinforces it posterolaterally. Also, the cruciate ligaments, which are intracapsular but extrasynovial, lie adjacent to the posterior invagination of the capsule and serve to reinforce this portion of the capsule.

The synovial membrane of the knee joint is more complex and extensive than that of any other joint in the body. It lines the joint capsule except posteriorly, where it passes anterior to the cruciate ligaments, excluding them from the joint cavity. At the superior border of the patella the membrane lines the suprapatellar pouch beneath the quadriceps muscle. The articularis genu muscle prevents this pouch from being pinched in the joint. Another outpouching of synovial membrane posterior to the lateral meniscus, the subpopliteal recess, separates the popliteus tendon from the lateral femoral and tibial condyles.

During embryonic development, three separate pouches fuse to form the synovial lining of the knee joint. Seams remaining at the fusion points are termed plicae (3). Plica synovialis suprapatellaris, infrapatellaris, and mediopatellaris are the three main synovial pleats of the knee joint (4). Occasionally, the joint surfaces impinge the plicae, producing one type of internal derangement of the knee.

The capacity of the joint is maximal at 25° of knee flexion. In this position, the joint fluid is under least tension, so it is the position of comfort that a patient with a knee joint effusion assumes.

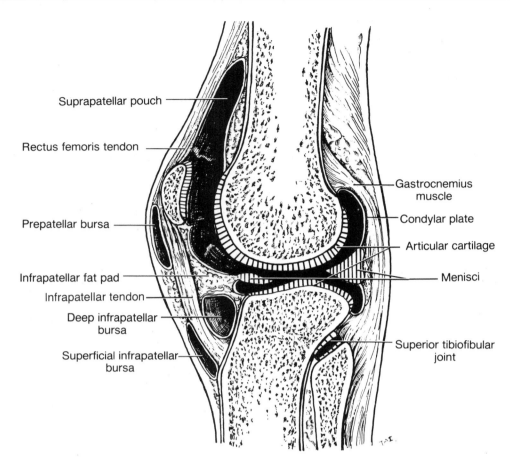

Suprapatellar pouch

Rectus femoris tendon

Prepatellar bursa

Infrapatellar fat pad

Infrapatellar tendon

Deep infrapatellar
bursa

Superficial infrapatellar
bursa

Gastrocnemius
muscle

Condylar plate

Articular cartilage

Menisci

Superior tibiofibular
joint

Figure 8.3.   Cross-section of the knee joint.

Bursae and Fat Pads.   Numerous bursae occupy the knee region, many of which are subject to bursitis (Fig. 8.3). The most significant and constant of the bursae include:

1. Prepatellar—a relatively large, superficial bursa that lies between the skin and the patella;
2. Superficial infrapatellar—a smaller bursa that separates the skin from the area of insertion of the infrapatellar tendon;
3. Deep infrapatellar—encased by fat, this bursa lies between the proximal tibia and the infrapatellar tendon;
4. Gastrocnemius—two bursae, each separates the medial and lateral heads of the gastrocnemius muscle origin from the joint capsule; both usually communicate with the joint; the medial bursa also communicates with the semimembranosus bursa lying just superficial to it (effusion of the medial gastrocnemius and the semimembranosus bursae is a Baker's cyst).
5. Semimembranosus—bursa that lies between the semimembranosus tendon and the medial head of the gastrocnemius muscle;
6. Pes anserine—bursa that eases pressure upon the tibial collateral ligament from the common insertion of the sartorius, gracilis, and semitendinosus tendons.

Several fat pads line the knee. The infrapatellar fat pad is the largest; it separates the infrapatellar tendon from the joint capsule and serves as a cushion to the front of the knee joint (4). The other major fat pads at the knee include the anterior and posterior suprapatellar and the popliteal. Some of these fat pads occupy space within the synovial cavity, and thus reduce the amount of synovial fluid that is necessary to fill the joint.

Ligaments.   In general, the collateral ligaments function to provide medial-lateral stability and support for the knee (Fig. 8.4). They also prevent excessive external rotation of the tibia. They offer greatest support when the knee is extended, a position in which all of their fibers become taut; conversely, they offer least support in flexion, when only the anterior fibers of the medial collateral ligament are taut.

The medial (tibial) collateral ligament (MCL) binds the medial femoral epicondyle and the medial tibial condyle. Its posterior fibers blend with the joint capsule and medial meniscus; however, its anterior margin lies free where a bursa separates it from the medial meniscus and capsule (4, 5). The lateral (fibular) collateral ligament (LCL) connects the lateral femoral epicondyle to the head of the fibula. The popliteus tendon completely separates the fibular collateral ligament from the lateral capsule and meniscus (Fig. 8.4).

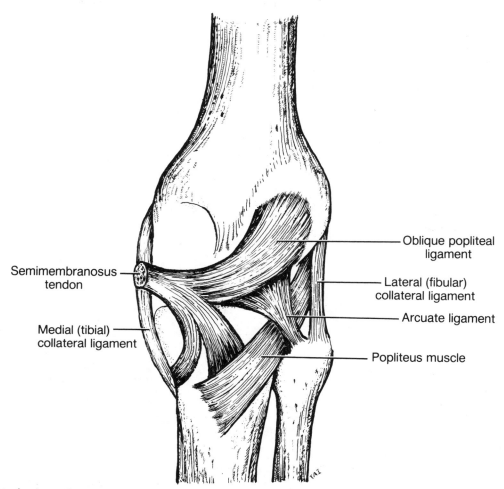

Semimembranosus tendon

Oblique popliteal ligament

Lateral (fibular) collateral ligament

Arcuate ligament

Medial (tibial) collateral ligament

Popliteus muscle

Figure 8.4. Posterior knee ligaments.

Anatomists refer to a substantial thickening in the medial portion of the joint capsule as the medial capsular ligament. This ligament attaches to the periphery of the medial meniscus, binding it firmly to the femur, and somewhat more loosely to the tibia (5). According to Houghston, a tear in these meniscotibial fibers alone can produce a positive anterior drawer sign (6). A similar thickening in the lateral joint capsule is the lateral capsular ligament. The posteromedial capsule thickens into a ribbon-like structure, the posterior oblique ligament, which enhances medial stability (7).

The oblique popliteal ligament (of Winslow) stems from an expansion of the semimembranosus tendon. It runs obliquely proximal-laterally to attach to the lateral femoral condyle (Fig. 8.4). It partially blends with, and supports, the posterior capsule.

The Y-shaped arcuate ligament stems from its base on the fibular head to arch over the popliteus tendon and blend with the posterior capsule (Fig. 8.4). The patellofemoral ligaments are thickenings of the anterior capsule. They extend from the middle of the patella to the medial and lateral femoral condyles. They help stabilize the patella in the trochlear groove.

The cruciate ligaments provide anterior-posterior, as well as medial-lateral stability at the knee. They also prevent excessive medial rotation of the tibia, and serve to maintain contact between the articular surfaces of the knee joint. Since some of the fibers of both cruciates are always in a state of tension during flexion and extension, these ligaments provide stability in any position of the knee.

Each cruciate ligament receives its name from its point of tibial origin. The anterior cruciate ligament (ACL) emerges from the anterior intercondylar eminence of the tibia and runs posterolaterally to the lateral femoral intercondylar notch (Fig. 8.5). It is the main structure that resists anterior tibial displacement, although the MCL reinforces it (8, 9). Because the MCL serves as a secondary restraint, the results of an anterior drawer test (anterior tibial displacement) may be somewhat equivocal; however, Hastings produced a 2–6 cm anterior tibial displacement by isolated lesioning of the ACL (7). Functionally, the ACL consists of two parts, although structurally the fibers of both parts are continuously attached throughout the ligament. The anteromedial band is primarily responsible for preventing anterior dislocation, and the posterolateral band for preventing hyperextension. Stress tests demonstrate that the ACL has the same tensile strength as the medial collateral ligament, and one-half the

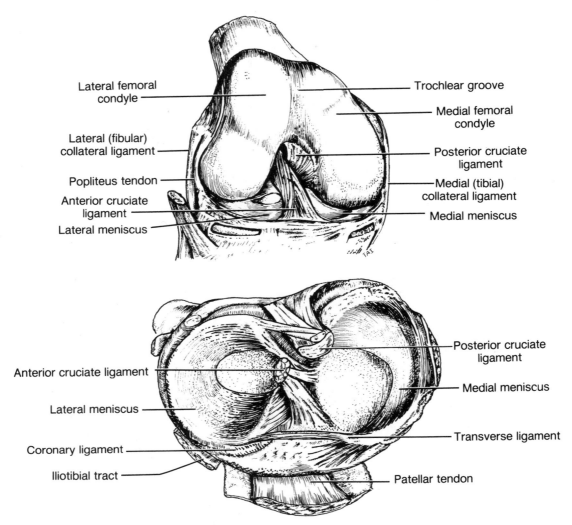

Figure 8.5. Internal structures of the knee joint.

strength of the posterior cruciate ligament (PCL) (10). The ACL is maximally taut between 0–20° of flexion and also between 70–90° of flexion.

The PCL is the main stabilizer of the knee. It runs from the posterior intercondylar tibial eminence, passing medial to the ACL, to insert into the medial femoral intercondylar notch (Fig. 8.5). It is the strongest of the knee ligaments (5). It prevents posterior displacement of the tibia, limits excessive medial rotation of the tibia, and provides medial-lateral stability, especially in knee extension. An intact PCL alone will provide medial-lateral stability in extension (6).

Menisci. Two menisci occupy each knee joint. These fibrocartilaginous discs are wedge-shaped, and are thicker around their outer rim than in the center. Their superior surfaces are concave, whereas their inferior surfaces are flat. The geometric shape of each meniscus coincides with the tibial surface upon which it rests: the medial meniscus is semi-lunar and broader posteriorly; the lateral is almost circular (Fig. 8.5)

The periphery of each meniscus attaches to the capsule; the inside edge remains free. Capsular fibers at their anterior and posterior horns attach the menisci to the femur and tibia. Menisco-patellar fibers join the menisci with the patella. A transverse ligament joins the menisci to one another (Fig. 8.5). The semimembranosus tendon attaches to the posterior edge of the medial meniscus through a fibrous expansion. The popliteus tendon attaches to the lateral meniscus and blends with the lateral condyle (5, 11).

The menisci perform various functions, including: improving articular surface congruity, protecting the capsular wall from impingement, improving joint lubrication by assisting synovial fluid circulation, assisting in force distribution, and sharing in weight-bearing. The wedge shape of the medial meniscus is a major factor preventing anterior subluxation of the medial tibial plateau on the femur (12, 13). Also, the semimembranosus muscle attachment to the medial meniscus and oblique popliteal ligament acts as a dynamic restraining unit (12).

During knee flexion and extension, the menisci move with the tibia upon the femur. During rotation, they follow the displacement of the femoral condyles on the tibial condyles (for example, with tibial lateral rotation, the lateral meniscus moves anteriorly, while the medial moves posteriorly) (14). Their location between the moving joint surfaces, however, renders the menisci vulnerable to trauma, especially when the knee is loaded in flexion and rotation (5). The medial meniscus sustains injury more frequently than the lateral meniscus for various reasons. Its posterior horn receives greater shear, and its close attachments to the capsule render it less mobile and incapable of moving away from compressive forces. Most likely, the lateral meniscus often escapes injury because it has a looser capsular attachment, and is under dynamic control of the popliteus muscle, which retracts it posteriorly during knee flexion, preventing impingement between the joint surfaces (5).

Mechanics

The knee functions as a modified hinge joint. Flexion and extension are its primary motions, and limited rotation is possible when the knee is flexed. Its ingenious mechanical composition allows the knee to achieve two mutually exclusive functions 1. stability in extension, which is necessary to sustain the forces of weightbearing, and 2. mobility in flexion, which is essential for activities such as running, cutting, and adaptation of the foot to the ground (11).

The knee acquires stability from its surrounding capsule, ligaments, muscles, menisci, and joint surfaces. Extension tightens the capsule and ligamentous structures, which in turn approximate the articular surfaces of the femur and tibia that "lock," creating a position of maximum stability (close-packed position). Flexion produces laxity in the capsular and ligamentous structures so that contact between the articular surfaces decreases. In flexion, the tibial intercondylar eminence moves free of the femoral intercondylar notch, thus permitting rotation, and sacrificing stability for mobility. Since the collateral ligaments become taut with lateral rotation, they prevent excessive motion in that direction. The cruciate ligaments are taut with medial rotation, and thus prevent excessive medial rotation.

Physiologic knee motion varies depending upon hip position, body build, etc. Flexion and extension occur in a sagittal plane around an axis that corresponds to the point of intersection of the cruciate ligaments. During flexion, this axis shifts posteriorly (7). Average range of active knee motion is 120° of flexion (hip extended), 140° of flexion (hip flexed), 30° of medial, and 40° of lateral rotation (knee flexed 90°). For a knee to be truly functional, however, accessory motion must accompany physiologic motion. Accesory motion is necessary to accommodate the anatomical configuration of the articular surfaces and ligamentous structures, as well as to satisfy the biomechanical requirements of a knee. For example, since the anterior-posterior circumference of the femoral condyles is twice that of the tibial condyles, simple rolling alone is precluded during flexion and extension; the femur must also glide on the tibia as flexion increases (7, 11) (Fig. 8.6).

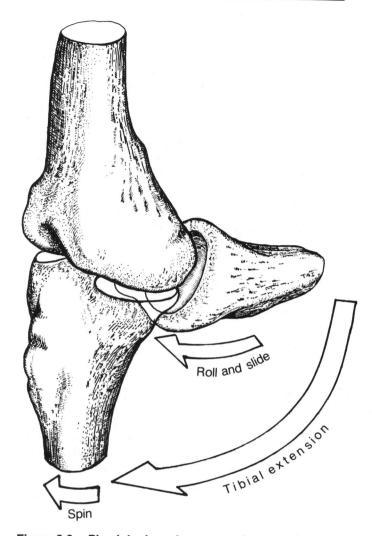

Figure 8.6. Physiologic and accessory knee motion.

The medial condylar surface of the femur is larger than the lateral. During extension the lateral surface is "used up" first and the tibia must then rotate laterally around the lateral femoral condyle to complete its extension (1, 5, 14). This synchrony of knee extension with lateral tibial rotation (the "screw home" mechanism) is critical to knee function (Fig. 8.6). Knee rehabilitation incorporates the concepts that one must restore lateral rotation in order to achieve complete extension, and one must restore extension in order to assure ultimate stability.

Accessory motions that accompany physiologic knee extension with the femur stationary are: anterior glide of the tibia on the femur, lateral rotation of the tibia on the femur, cephalic movement of the fibula, and cephalic movement of the patella.

Patellofemoral (PF) joint mechanics play an important role in knee function. As flexion progresses from 0°, the patella first contacts the femur with its inferior margin at 10–20°; at 45° the midsection of the patella contacts the femur; at 90° the superior area meets the femur; at 135° the odd facet touches the femur (15).

The entire articular surface of the patella never makes complete contact with the femoral condyles, but the contact area does increase with flexion. This increased contact area helps to distribute the patellofemoral joint forces which increase with weightbearing flexion, e.g., squatting. Extension decreases patellofemoral compression forces (as the contact area also decreases) if the leg is unloaded or nonweightbearing, e.g., extending the knee while sitting. Extending the knee from nonweightbearing flexion when the foot is loaded with weights, however, produces sufficient quadriceps muscle tension to increase patellofemoral compression forces. Because the patellofemoral contact area is decreasing, these forces are not well distributed. Patients with patellofemoral syndrome, therefore, should not lift weights from a flexed to an extended position, nor should they exercise the knee into a fully flexed range where patellofemoral compression is the greatest. Instead, they should perform isometric quadriceps muscle setting or terminal knee extension exercises (15, 17, 18). (Exceptions are patients with ACL pathology also, who should not exercise in terminal extension because the ACL is maximally stressed at 0°–20° of flexion.)

The muscles acting upon the knee serve as powerful motors, and equally importantly, serve as dynamic stabilizers of the knee joint. Anteriorly, the quadriceps femoris muscle incorporates the vastus medialis, vastus lateralis, vastus intermedius, and rectus femoris muscles which insert by a common tendon into the tibial tuberosity. It is a very powerful muscle and functions to extend the knee; in addition, it externally rotates the leg (4). No one component of the muscle is dominant in terminal extension (17). The quadriceps femoris muscle also counteracts posterior, varus, and valgus stresses upon the leg. The rectus femoris muscle, the only biarticular muscle among the group, extends the knee, and assists in hip flexion or flexion of the pelvis when the thigh is stabilized. The vastus medialis obliqus fibers contribute to patellar alignment. The quadriceps femoris muscle generates its maximum torque around 60° of knee flexion (16, 17).

A clinical condition, extensor lag, occurs when the quadriceps femoris muscle is not able to fully extend the leg. The following factors may be responsible:

1. The quadriceps femoris muscle exerts its poorest leverage in the last 10° of extension;
2. Muscle power decreases as the muscle shortens;
3. Pain following trauma to the knee may inhibit muscle contraction;
4. Contracture of the joint capsule, ligaments, or adhesion of the quadriceps femoris muscle to the femur, may limit range of motion.

Medially, the tendons of the sartorius, gracilis, and semitendinosus muscles cross the knee and enter into a common insertion, the pes anserine. The semimembranosus muscle joins the pes anserine muscles to medially rotate the leg and counteract valgus stress. The popliteus muscle also assists in medial rotation.

The hamstring muscles flex the knee. They occupy the posterior thigh, and include the biceps femoris, semitendinosus, and semimembranosus muscles. These muscles counteract knee hyperextension and anterior stress upon the leg, and substitute for a deficient ACL. The gracilis and sartorius muscles assist the hamstring muscles in flexing the knee. The tensor fascia latae muscle becomes a knee flexor once the knee has started to flex, placing it behind the knee joint axis. The popliteus muscle also assists in initiating flexion by unscrewing the locked, extended knee. When the foot is planted, the gastrocnemius muscle provides minor assistance in knee flexion. The biarticular hamstrings, in addition to their action at the knee, extend and adduct the hip.

The biceps femoris muscle and iliotibial tract traverse the lateral aspect of the knee. They laterally rotate the leg and counteract varus stress. The popliteus muscle, which originates on the lateral femoral condyle and inserts on the posterior medial edge of the tibia, reinforces the posterolateral aspect of the joint and resists varus and posterior stress on the leg.

Neurology

Muscle Innervation. Innervation of muscles acting upon the knee is as follows: the femoral nerve (L2,3,4) supplies the quadriceps femoris, sartorius, and articularis genu muscles; the superior gluteal nerve (L4,5,S1) supplies the tensor fasciae lata muscle; the obturator nerve (L2,3,4) supplies the gracilis muscle; the sciatic nerve (L4,5,S1,2,3) supplies the biceps femoris, semitendinosus, and semimembranosus muscles; the tibial nerve (L4,5,S1,2,3) supplies the popliteus muscle.

Sensation. The L3, L4, and L5 dermatomes cross the anterior part of the thigh and knee, while the S1 and S2 dermatomes cross the posterior area. The peripheral sensory nerves branch from the obturator, femoral, tibial, and common peroneal nerves.

Innervation of the synovial joint of the knee is as follows: branches of the femoral nerve through the saphenous nerve, and nerves to the vasti muscles supply the suprapatellar pouch, the infrapatellar fat pad, and the anteromedial and anterolateral regions; branches of the tibial nerve supply the posterior, medial, and lateral regions; branches of the common peroneal nerve supply the anterolateral region and the infrapatellar fat pad; the recurrent articular branch of the peroneal nerve supplies the infrapatellar fat pad; and the obturator nerve supplies the upper posteromedial region, the anteromedial region, and the infrapatellar fat pad.

Reflexes. Nerves emanating from the L3-4 levels mediate the patellar tendon reflex.

Angiology

The popliteal artery, a continuation of the femoral artery, vascularizes the knee joint. It begins at the adductor hiatus, and terminates at the lower border of the popliteus muscle, where it bifurcates into the anterior and posterior tibial arteries. Palpation of the popliteal pulse is difficult because it lies so deeply, but may be facilitated by flexing the knee to reduce the tension of the posterior capsule. The popliteal artery has five branches in the area of the knee: the medial and lateral superior genicular arteries, the middle genicular artery, and the medial and lateral inferior genicular arteries. A descending branch of the lateral femoral circumflex artery and the recurrent branch of the anterotibial artery also provide some blood supply.

The great (long) and small (short) saphenous veins, and the deep veins, which accompany the arteries and their branches, drain blood from the leg. Valve arrangement in perforating veins prevents blood flow from deep to superficial. If the valves become incompetent, muscle contraction may force blood in the deep veins into the superficial system, resulting in dilatation and varicosities.

The inner portion of the menisci is avascular, but the outer third is vascularized by the middle and inferior genicular branches through capillary loops at the capsular attachment, and from the fringes of the adjacent synovial membrane. Regeneration of the cartilage can occur only from the vascular fibroareolar tissue around the periphery of the meniscus.

The middle genicular branch of the popliteal artery also supplies the cruciate ligaments. Traumatic disruption of the cruciates interrupts the blood supply and induces ligament atrophy, increasing the difficulty of obtaining a clinically viable and vascularized graft or repair.

Knee Examination

History. The examiner first requests the patient to provide identifying data (Fig. 8.7). A patient's age and gender assist diagnosis of pathologies which typically affect certain groups. For example, in males, patellar subluxation occurs most often in a younger, athletic population, whereas in females it occurs in the 4th and 5th decades as part of a degenerative condition (19). A patient's dominant side may relate to the forces imposed upon the knee. The prior condition of the knee is also relevant, because a large number of knee problems involve chronic laxity, degeneration, and accumulation of ongoing stresses.

The patient next describes the symptoms stemming from his present episode or illness. Leg pain associated with musculotendinous lesions, stress fractures, bony reactions, or vascular disorders is usually localized and easy to identify (20). There are numerous specific knee lesions which also produce localized symptoms. Pain localized over the tibial tubercle is the predominant symptom of Osgood-Schlatter's disease (19, 21). Iliotibial band syndrome manifests as pain just proximal to the lateral joint line, where the band irritates the lateral femoral condyle. Popliteus tendinitis produces pain posterior to the lateral collateral ligament, just above the joint line (22). Posterior tibialis tendinitis and periostitis, commonly referred to as

shin splints, present as pain over the medial distal two-thirds of the tibial shaft (18, 23). In contrast to shin splints, anterior compartment syndrome causes pain over the lateral anterior tibial shaft (18, 23).

Symptom nature and behavior are representative of some disorders. Dull, retropatellar aching which is worse after prolonged sitting in a cramped, flexed position characterizes patellofemoral joint syndrome. Since knee flexion increases patellofemoral joint forces, it enhances symptoms of chondromalacia and other extensor mechanism disorders. A reactive synovitis usually manifests as swelling aggravated by activity that subsides with rest. The examiner should ascertain a knee's tolerance of walking, running, starting, stopping, cutting, and landing from a jump. Less intense activities will aggravate a highly irritable joint, whereas a mildly irritable joint responds only after repeated, vigorous activities. Pain which continues in spite of activity cessation, and afflicts a patient throughout the night, may be indicative of a stress fracture.

The examiner must probe into the onset and background of the present condition (Fig. 8.8). He must determine whether the condition is acute, chronic, or perhaps reappears with overuse. In the event of an injury, the mechanism of trauma is especially useful in identifying the involved structures at the knee. The hip, knee, and foot positions, combined with the direction and magnitude of stress, allow the therapist to reasonably differentiate knee ligament or meniscal injury.

One must not overlook the potential seriousness of indirect (noncontact) injury. Running, twisting, and landing from a jump are common causes of muscle strains and bruises, and the source of more than three-fourths of ACL ruptures (24, 25). The examiner asks the patient to describe any deformity, disability, etc., resulting from an injury, and the timeframe within which it occurred. Seventy-five percent of patients who sustain an ACL rupture can't walk normally for at least 2 weeks (25). Severe trauma produces effusion, but if the trauma is sufficient to rupture the joint capsule, much of the fluid will leak into the adjacent areas. One should not be misled, therefore, into ruling out major joint trauma based upon minimal effusion.

When discussing past history, a therapist should confirm preexisting lesions or an old injury that may predispose to reinjury. Congenital or acquired deformity, laxity, or mechanical imbalance can become symptomatic with increased physical activity. The patient's response to previous treatment may clue the examiner to the severity and nature of the condition.

A life-style assessment should review occupational demands as well as recreational activities. The examiner should analyze strenuous sport participation as a source of potential mechanical stress of the knee.

Radiographs are necessary to confirm fractures, changes in joint space, reactive bony lesions, etc. They are also useful in diagnosing certain conditions with typical radiographic findings, such as Osgood-Schlatter's disease, which involves apophyseal separation and fragmentation.

A. HISTORY

1. Identifying Data

Name _____ Age _____ Gender _____ Date _____

Provisional diagnosis _____ Precautions _____

Chief complaint _____

Dominant side R _____ L _____ Prior condition of involved part _____

2. Present Episode or Illness

a. Description of symptoms

1) location: / / / / = pain
               = = = = = paresthesia
               ° ° ° ° = numbness
               xxxx   = other _____

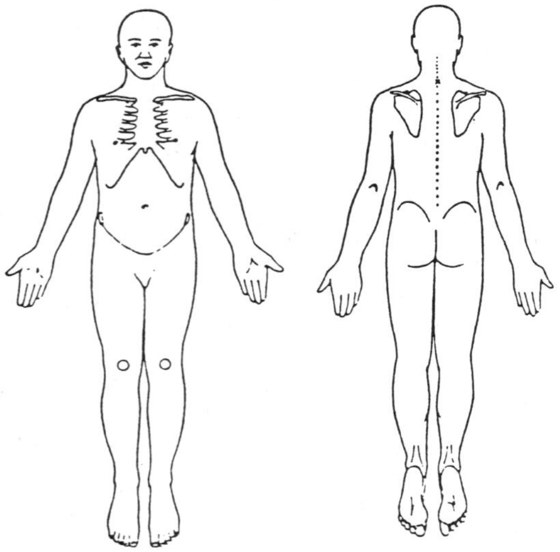

2) severity:

_____
none   worst

3) impairment:

_____
annoying   completely disabling

4) nature:

cramping _____ aching _____

shooting _____ burning _____

throbbing _____ tingling _____

stabbing _____ sore _____

other _____

5) behavior:

constant _____ intermittent _____ duration _____

occurs when _____ elicited by _____

aggravated by _____ relieved by _____

24-hour pattern _____

highly irritable _____ mildly irritable _____ not irritable _____

6) joint characteristics: catches _____ , locks _____ , swells _____ , gives way _____ , dislocates _____ ,

other _____

Figure 8.7. Examination form part 1: History.

The therapist analyzes data from the patient's history in order to plan and prepare for the physical examination that follows.

Physical Examination

Inspection. Postural evaluation in a frontal plane may reveal genu varus or valgus deformities (Fig. 8.9).

The Q-angle represents the frontal plane alignment of the extensor mechanism. With the quadriceps mus-

cle contracted, the Q-angle normally approximates 10° (19) (Fig. 8.10).

Femoral torsion may cause deviation of the patella's anterior surface from its normal frontal plane alignment. Tibial torsion may disrupt normal patellar alignment between the 1st and 2nd toes. Excessive medially displaced patellae are labeled "squinting," and excessive laterally displaced patellae are labeled "frog's eye" patellae.

b. Background and associated findings

Date of present injury _____ or onset _____ insidious _____

Dates of hospitalization _____ and/or other health care

Treatments; dates; results _____

_____

Status of condition: acute _____ or chronic _____

constant _____ or intermittent _____

better _____ or worse _____

Nature and mechanism of injury or events precipitating present episode _____

_____

Results of injury (if applicable): deformity (describe) _____

corrected _____ disability (type and cause) _____

loss of motion (specify) _____ when occurred _____

loss of strength (specify) _____ when occurred _____

swelling (specify) _____ when occurred _____

bleeding (specify) _____ when occurred _____

3. Relevant Past History and Family History

History of similar condition: dates _____ nature _____

_____

Treatment _____

Other relevant illnesses or disorders _____

General health status _____

Health problems of immediate family _____

4. Life-style

Occupation _____ ADL _____

Regular (3 times/week minimum) physical activities requiring: strength _____ agility _____ endurance _____

flexibility _____ other _____

What patient does to promote wellness _____

Patient's concept of cause of condition _____

Patient's concept of functional and/or cosmetic deficit(s) _____

Anticipated goals _____

5. Other

Current medications _____

Recent radiographs _____

6. Therapist's Interpretation and Plans for Physical Exam _____

_____

Figure 8.8. Examination form part 2: History continued.

B. PHYSICAL EXAMINATION

1. Inspection

   a. Posture

frontal

	Varus		Valgus		Q-Angle		Femur		Tibia		Patella			
											R		L	
R	L	R	L	R	L	R	L	R	L	Stand	Sit	Stand	Sit

sagittal

hyperextension		flexion contracture		patella baja		patella alta	
R	L	R	L	R	L	R	L

   leg length (R) _____ (L) _____

   b. Shape

   deformity (describe) _____ asymmetry _____

   swelling or masses _____ atrophy _____

   circumference: joint line R _____ L _____ ; 4 cm prox. R _____ L _____ ; 8 cm prox. R _____ L _____

   c. Use

   sitting knee extension from 90° _____

   stand and squat _____

   gait deviations _____

   d. Skin

   color _____ condition _____ lesions _____ scars _____

   e. Aids

   assistive device _____ orthosis _____ support _____ other _____

   purpose _____

2. Palpation (note location and nature of abnormality)

   a. Skin and subcutaneous tissue: tenderness _____ temperature _____ swelling _____ decreased mobility _____

   trigger points _____ other _____

   b. Muscles and tendons: tenderness _____ temperature _____ spasm _____ loss of continuity _____

   decreased mobility _____ other _____

   c. Tendon sheaths and bursae: tenderness _____ temperature _____ swelling _____ crepitus _____ other _____

   d. Bones and joints: tenderness _____ temperature _____ swelling _____ bony prominences _____ other _____

   e. Arteries and nerves: popliteal artery _____ Tinel sign (infrapatellar branch of saphenous nerve) _____

   common peroneal nerve _____

Figure 8.9.   Examination form part 3: Inspection and palpation.

Sagittal plane deviations include hyperextension (genu recurvatum), knee flexion contracture, patella baja, and patella alta. Normally, the proximal patellar pole aligns with the anterior femur. If it lies more proximal, patella alta exists; if more distal, patella baja. Patella alta often exposes the infrapatellar fat pad, revealing a double hump at the knee, or the "camel sign."

Bony deformity, soft tissue lesions, synovial proliferation, and fluid accumulation are some of the conditions that alter a knee's shape. A knee assumes a position of 20° flexion to accommodate maximal effusion such as that which often accompanies internal derangement (26). Minimal swelling may be more difficult to detect; sometimes its only manifestation is obliteration of the identation medial to the patellar

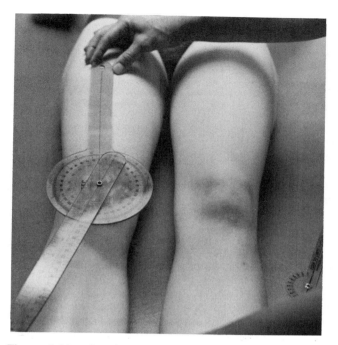

Figure 8.10.   Q angle measurement: if the acute angle between a line which bisects the patella and tibial tuberosity and a line which bisects the patella and ASIS is greater than 20°, there may be excessive lateral force on the patella.

tendon insertion. To record knee joint effusion objectively, the examiner makes circumferential (anthropometric) measurements at the joint line, and at given distances from the joint line (Fig. 8.9).

While sitting, the patient extends his knee from 90°, which may demonstrate vastus medialis obliquus muscle dysplasia or abnormal patellar alignment (19). The patient's ability to stand, squat, and walk reveals the general level of knee function.

Skin color and condition demonstrate signs of trauma, inflammation, vascular disturbances, etc. Aids may be used prophylactically or during rehabilitation.

Palpation.   One generally proceeds by palpation of superficial to deep structures. Starting at the front of the knee, the examiner feels the skin and subcutaneous tissues, then progresses around the medial side, and next the lateral side (Fig. 8.9). Superficial tenderness to palpation adjacent to the patellar tendon may stem from infrapatellar fat pad injury, a significant source of knee joint pain. Irritation of the plica that extends from the infrapatellar fat pad to the superior medial edge of the patella produces tenderness deep to the medial patellar border. Scarring or adhesions of the deep infrapatellar bursa or extensor retinaculae produces local pain and fixes the patella distally. Patellar tendinitis (jumper's knee) is painful at the patellar tendon insertion. Anterior compartment syndrome imparts warmth over the tibial shaft along with a hard and intractable feel in the subcutaneous tissues and muscles (23).

The pes anserine expansion may be painful over the anterior medial aspect of the tibia. Bursal swelling,

such as Baker's cyst on the posteromedial knee surface, is easily palpated when the bursa is a superficial one.

Point tenderness along the joint line is indicative of a meniscal or capsular tear. Ligamentous tear or avulsion also produces local pain and swelling at the site of injury. The examiner may palpate the MCL from its origin distal to the femoral adductor tubercle to its insertion 2½ inches distal to the joint line. He may palpate the LCL from the lateral femoral condyle to the fibular head, which he facilitates by having the patient cross his involved leg over his uninvolved leg. The tibial tubercle is tender and swollen in Osgood-Schlatter's disease. A ballotable patella rebounds when it is compressed, then released, signifying joint effusion. Patellofemoral crepitation may accompany chondromalacia or osteitis dessicans. A Tinel sign, resulting from neuroma of the infrapatellar branch of the saphenous nerve, may be elicited by tapping over the medial side of the tibial tubercle (26). This nerve may be cut during a medial meniscectomy. The common peroneal nerve crosses the fibular head in a superficial and palpable position.

Movement Assessment.   Through functional active movement, the examiner attempts to reproduce the injury position and mechanism or to elicit symptoms (Fig. 8.11). Pain, instability, weakness, or stiffness may limit a patient's ability to walk, run, squat, kneel, jump, hop, twist, and negotiate stairs. Since the knee is a weightbearing joint that frequently encounters these functional stresses, it is important that they be simulated during examination. Passive NWB tests often aren't forceful enough to reproduce a patient's symptoms. For example, patellofemoral joint forces reach three times body weight with walking, four and one-half times body weight with a stair climbing, and seven times body weight with rising from a chair; the examiner would have difficulty imparting these forces passively.

The examiner tests physiologic movement, as Chapter 2 describes, to help differentiate the source of the problem. The quality and quantity of movement, and related symptoms, often suggest contractile or inert structure lesions. Likewise, the amount of accessory movement and related symptoms assist problem identification. The examiner tests accessory movement using techniques described in the joint mobilization section of this chapter.

Clinicians have devised a number of special passive tests for knee examination (Fig. 8.11). Many rely on the detection of clinical laxity to identify or rule out ligamentous lesions. One must use caution when interpreting the results of these tests because secondary ligamentous restraints may impart stability during a clinical laxity test when the primary ligament is actually torn or injured. Such a false-negative test occurs because the testing force is not great enough to produce instability which may occur under the higher forces of functional activity (8,16,25).

An anterior drawer test assesses anterior displacement of the tibia on the femur (Fig. 8.12). The patient

3. Movement assessment

a. Functional active moment

walk _____	jump _____	
run _____	hop _____	
squat _____	twist _____	
kneel _____	stairs _____	

Key: C = completes task

D = completes task with difficulty/discomfort

N = not able to complete task

b/c/d. Physiological movement

	ACTIVE			PASSIVE			RESISTIVE	
	ROM	Symptoms	Quality	ROM	Symptoms	Endfeel	Strength	Symptoms
flexion								
extension								
lateral rot.								
medial rot.								

e. Accessory movement

	Mobility	Symptoms
tibiofemoral traction		
dorsal tibial glide		
ventral tibial glide		
caudal patellar glide		

f. Special tests

	+	−	Comments
Anterior drawer test tibia neutral			
tibia laterally rot.			
tibia medially rot.			
Lachman test			
Posterior drawer test			
Godfrey (sag) test			
Apley test			
McMurray test			
Valgus stress test knee extended			
knee flexed 30°			
Varus stress test knee extended			
knee flexed 30°			
Apprehension test			
Helfet sign			
Pivot shift test			
Lateral rot./recurv. test			

Figure 8.11. Examination form part 4: Movement assessment.

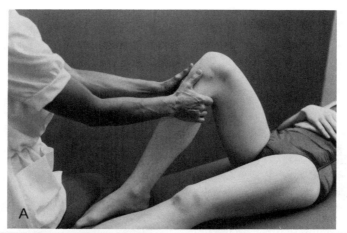

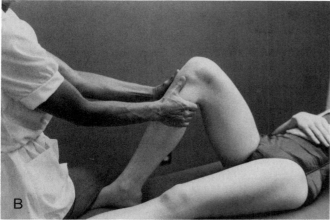
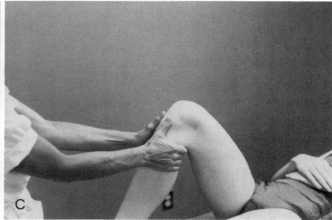

Figure 8.12. Anterior drawer test. *A,* If anterior stress with the tibia in neutral rotation produces anterior subluxation of the tibia, the test is positive, implicating laxity or tear of the anterior cruciate ligament and possibly the collateral ligaments. *B,* If the test is positive with the tibia laterally rotated, it implicates anteromedial rotary instability involving the medial collateral and capsular ligaments, and possibly the anterior cruciate ligament. *C,* If it is positive with the tibia medially rotated, it implicates anterolateral rotary instability involving the anterior cruciate ligament and posterolateral joint structures.

lies supine, with his hip and knee flexed so that his foot rests upon the table. The examiner stabilizes his foot by sitting on it, and places his thumbs on the joint line and fingers around the leg posteriorly. He attempts to draw the tibia anteriorly. Laxity with neutral tibial rotation implicates the ACL and possibly the collateral ligaments; in lateral tibial rotation, it implicates the medial collateral and capsular ligaments and possibly the ACL; in medial rotation, it implicates the ACL and posterolateral joint structures (27).

A Lachman test similarly assesses anterior tibial displacement; however, the knee is flexed only 15° (Fig. 8.13). This position reduces the mechanical advantage of the hamstring muscles and thus lessens the possibility of a false-negative test from substitution or stabilization by the hamstring muscles. The Lachman test also allows the posterior horns of the menisci to clear the femoral condyles, eliminating another source of a false-negative test.

A posterior drawer test assesses posterior tibial displacement on the femur (Fig. 8.14). In the same position as an anterior drawer test, the examiner presses the tibia posteriorly. Acute laxity implicates the PCL and the posterior capsular structures, whereas chronic laxity implicates a PCL rupture perhaps with stretching of the posterior capsular structures. A Godfrey (sag) test also assesses posterior tibial displacement by allowing gravity to sublux a PCL deficient joint (Fig. 8.15).

An Apley test may reveal either meniscal or ligamentous injury. The patient lies prone with his knee flexed 90°, then the examiner applies compression through the foot to the knee while medially and laterally rotating the tibia (Fig. 8.16*A*). If this maneuver produces clicking or pain at the joint line, it could be indicative of a meniscal tear. The examiner then repeats the test, applying traction to the knee through distraction of the foot while medially rotating the tibia (Fig. 8.16*B*). If this produces pain at the joint line, there could be lateral or medial colateral ligament involvement.

A McMurray test may reveal a tear of the posterior horn of the medial meniscus. With the patient supine, the examiner lifts the leg and flexes the knee, and

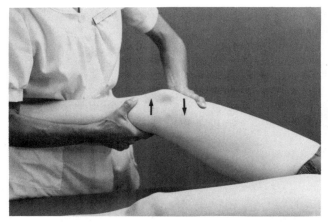

Figure 8.13.   Lachman test: if anterior stress on the tibia with the knee flexed 15° produces anterior subluxation of the tibia, the test is positive, implicating laxity or tear of the posterior cruciate ligament.

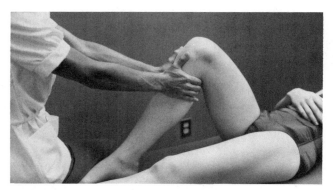

Figure 8.14.   Posterior drawer test: if posterior stress on the tibia produces posterior subluxation of the tibia, the test is positive, implicating laxity or tear of the posterior cruciate ligament and perhaps the posterior joint capsule.

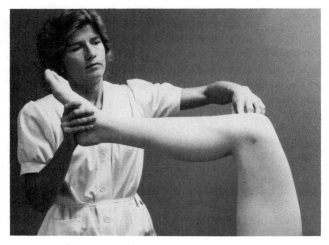

Figure 8.15.   Godfrey (sag) test: if the patient's leg is suspended by supporting the foot, with 90° hip and knee flexion, and the proximal tibia "sags" posteriorly, the test is positive, implicating laxity or tear of the posterior cruciate ligament and perhaps the posterior joint capsule.

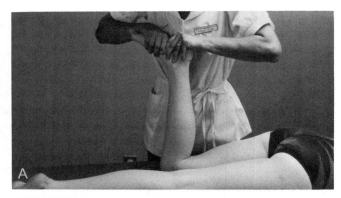

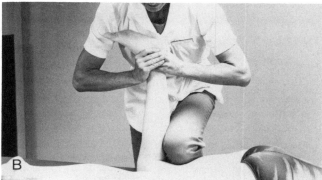

Figure 8.16.   Apley tests. *A,* If compression and simultaneous rotation with the knee flexed 90° produces clicking or pain, the test is positive, implicating tear of a meniscus. *B,* If distraction with medial or lateral rotation with the knee flexed 90° produces pain, the test is positive, implicating laxity or tear of the lateral or medial collateral ligaments, respectively.

laterally rotates the tibia by grasping the foot (Fig. 8.17). The examiner uses his other hand to impart a valgus stress on the knee, and to palpate the medial joint line, as he slowly extends the knee. A click or pain at the medial joint line indicates a positive test for meniscal injury.

Valgus and varus stress tests evaluate the integrity of the collateral, capsular, and posterior cruciate ligaments. Most clinicians grade this instability by measuring the joint line separation as follows: less than 5 mm greater than the uninjured knee is a grade I (mild) instability; 5–10 mm greater than the uninjured knee is a grade II (moderate) instability; over 10 mm greater than the uninjured knee is a grade III (severe) instability.

The examiner first applies valgus stress with the knee in 30° of flexion (Fig. 8.18). The patient lies supine as the examiner supports his leg with one hand and applies force with the other arm perpendicular to the limb over the lateral side of the knee. Gapping or pain at the medial joint line may indicate involvement of the medial collateral and capsular ligaments. If positive, the examiner repeats this test with the knee at 0° (Fig. 8.19). Positive findings in this position implicate the PCL along with the medial ligaments.

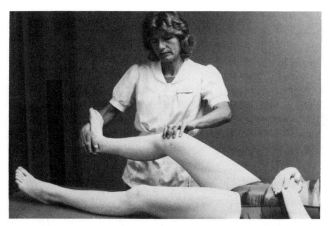

Figure 8.17.   McMurray test: if slowly extending a knee with valgus stress from a flexed and laterally rotated position produces a click or pain at the medial joint line, the test is positive, implicating a tear of the posterior horn of the medial meniscus.

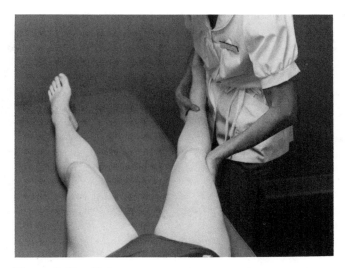

Figure 8.19.   Valgus stress test at 0°: if valgus stress at 0° knee extension produces pain and/or gapping at the medial joint line, the test is positive, implicating laxity or tear of the medial collateral, capsular, and posterior cruciate ligaments.

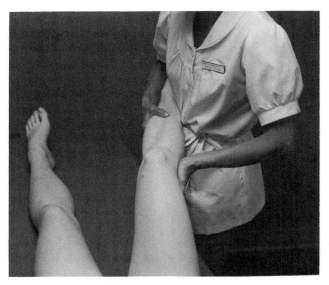

Figure 8.18.   Valgus stress test at 30°: if valgus stress at 30° knee extension produces pain and/or gapping at the medial joint line, the test is positive, implicating laxity or tear of the medial collateral and capsular ligaments.

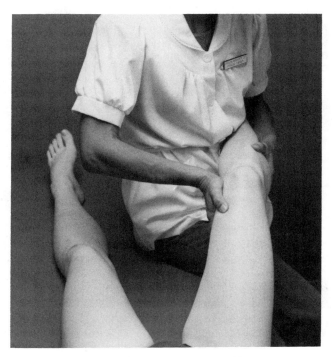

Figure 8.20.   Varus stress test at 30°: if varus stress at 30° knee extension produces pain and/or gapping at the lateral joint line, the test is positive, implicating laxity or tear of the lateral collateral and capsular ligaments.

A varus stress test utilizes the same positions, except that the examiner imparts force over the medial side of the knee (Fig. 8.20). Positive findings at 30° of flexion may indicate involvement of the lateral collateral and capsular ligaments, and at 0° the PCL as well (Fig. 8.21).

An apprehension test assesses patellar stability within the trochlear groove. With the patient supine and leg relaxed, the examiner attempts to laterally displace the patella (Fig. 8.22). If this elicits the patient's symptoms, or apprehension of a possible subluxation, the test is positive.

A Helfet test indicates whether the tibia laterally rotates during extension. The examiner marks a central point on the patient's patella, which should align with the tibial tuberosity while sitting with the knee flexed. A 0° extension the point should lie medial to the tuberosity, but if the tibia doesn't rotate, the point will remain aligned (Fig. 8.23).

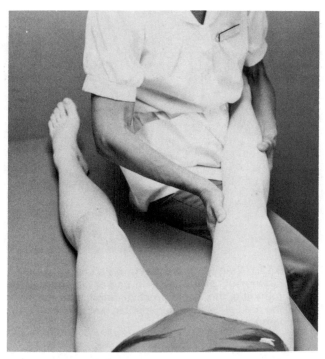

Figure 8.21. Varus stress test at 0°: if varus stress at 0° knee extension produces pain and/or gapping at the lateral joint line, the test is positive, implicating laxity or tear of the lateral collateral, capsular, and posterior cruciate ligaments.

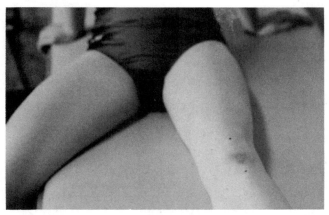

Figure 8.23. Helfet test: if the tibial tuberosity maintains vertical alignment with a central point on the patella when the knee is extended, the test is positive, implicating lack of lateral tibial rotation (no "screw home" motion).

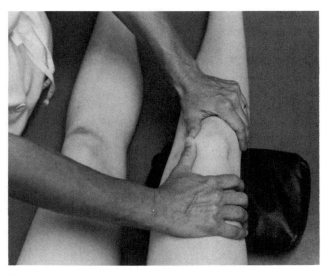

Figure 8.22. Apprehension test: if passive lateral pressure on the patella produces a fear or sensation of subluxation in a patient, the test is positive, implicating pathology of patellofemoral stabilizing structures associated with chronic patellar subluxation or dislocation.

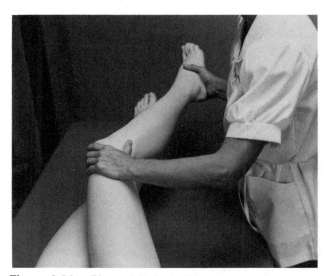

Figure 8.24. Pivot shift test: if knee extension, valgus stress, and medial tibial rotation with anterior pressure on the fibula produce anterolateral subluxation of the tibia, which is then reduced (signaled by a "clunk") at about 15° as the knee is passively flexed, the test is positive, implicating anterolateral rotary instability with laxity or tear of the anterior cruciate ligament and posterolateral structures.

A pivot shift test may depict anterolateral rotary knee instability. The patient lies supine, as the examiner lifts his leg with his knee extended. The examiner then attempts to anteriorly sublux the lateral tibial plateau by medially rotating the tibia through his hand, holding the foot and imparting a valgus and anterior stress through his hand resting upon the lateral side of the knee (Fig. 8.24). As the examiner slowly flexes the knee, a palpable clunk around 15° signifies relocation in the presence of anterolateral rotary instability

resulting from laxity or tear of the ACL and posterolateral structures.

A lateral rotation-recurvatum test may depict anteromedial rotary instability. As the patient lies supine, the examiner lifts his leg through his big toe, maintaining knee extension (Fig. 8.25). If the tibia laterally rotates, the test is positive, implicating involvement of the arcuate complex, posterior capsule, PCL, or ACL.

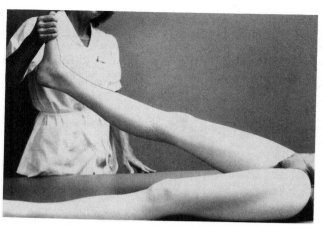

Figure 8.25. Lateral rotation-recurvatum test: if, when an examiner lifts a patient's leg by the big toe with the knee extended, the knee hyperextends and the tibia laterally rotates, the test is positive, implicating laxity or tear of the arcuate complex, posterior capsule, and posterior cruciate ligament, or the anterior cruciate ligament.

Neurologic Evaluation. Two muscles acting upon the knee represent key nerve root levels (Fig. 8.26). The quadriceps muscle receives its primary innervation from L3, and the gastrosoleus muscle from S1-2. The knee jerk reflex represents the L3-4 levels. Nerve root levels L3–S2 convey sensation to various aspects of the knee, via the obturator, femoral, tibial, and common peroneal nerves. A central nervous system lesion may cause generalized spasticity, flaccidity, rigidity, or clonicity involving the knee. A local injury may produce involuntary muscle spasm or inhibition which alters knee function. The examiner assesses coordination through heel to knee touching on command, and reciprocal lower limb flexion and extension.

Recommendation of Other Tests. Other tests contribute to clinical findings to complete the examination. Early arthroscopic examination may show ACL, meniscal, and other ligamentous damage. Table 8.1 includes a summary of the differential diagnosis and treatment of common knee disorders.

4. Neurological evaluation

   a. Key muscles (strength grade 0–5): L3 = quadriceps femoris muscle _____

                                 S1–S2 = gastrocsoleus muscle _____

   b. Key reflexes: L3–4 = knee jerk _____

   c. Sensibility

                                                   Key: lacking A = light touch sensation
                                                                     B = sharp/dull discrimination
                                                                     C = temperature discrimination
                                                                      D = proprioception

   d. Motor control: spastic _____ flaccid _____ rigid _____ clonic _____

   e. Coordination

      Heel to knee on command _____

      Reciprocal knee and hip flex./ext. (supine) _____

                                                    Key: C = completes task
                                                                      D = completes task with difficulty/
                                                                                    discomfort
                                                                      N = not able to complete task

5. Recommendation of other tests

   a. Radiography _____

   b. Laboratory _____

   c. Electrodiagnostic _____

   d. Arthroscopy _____

   e. Arthrography _____

   f. Other _____

Figure 8.26. Examination form part 5: Neurologic evaluation and recommendation of other test.

Table 8.1.
Summary of Differential Diagnosis and Treatment of Common Knee Disorders

Disorder	Chief Complaint	Onset	Symptom Characteristics	Static Physical Changes	Dynamic Physical Changes	Special Tests	Treatment[a]
Bursitis	Pain and swelling	Acute following moderate trauma such as kneeling	Localized pain and tenderness to palpation	Swelling over involved bursa	Pain may limit flexion or inhibit walking	Soft tissue calcification seen radiographically in chronic cases	Ice, rest, gradual resumption of ROM; use protective knee pads to prevent
Chondromalacia Patella	Knee pain, catching, giving way	Common in physically active teens; predisposed by recurrent patellar dislocation	Retropatellar aching increased by descending stairs, prolonged sitting, squatting, running	Transient swelling after exercise	Guarded activity due to sensation of insecurity	Pain and crepitus with patellar compression against femur; radiograph may reveal spurs	Anti-inflammatory medication; avoid running and squatting while pain exists; quad sets, SLR, and terminal extension PRE; surgical shaving of articular surface
Ligamentous injury a. ACL b. LCL c. MCL d. PCL	a–d. Pain or pop; decreased function	a. Acute trauma, producing hyperextension or lateral tibial rotation b. Sudden forceful adduction of tibia or knee dislocation c. Forceful abduction of tibia or lateral tibial rotation when knee flexed or hyperextended d. Hyperflexion or hyperextension; sudden posterior blow to tibia	a–d. Symptoms vary according to extent of tear; localized pain; joint effusion or hemarthrosis	a–d. Initial swelling	a–d. Guarded activity due to pain and instability; decreased ROM due to swelling and spasm	a. Anterior drawer, Lachman, pivot shift, lateral rotation—recurvatum b. Varus stress at 30° and 0°; Apley distraction c. Valgus stress at 30° and 0°; anterior drawer in lateral rotation, lateral rotation—recurvatum; Apley distraction d. Posterior drawer; Godfrey; varus and valgus stress at 0° (must be accompanied by tear of MCL or LCL)	a–d. Grade I: cold, compression, rest; heat and mobilization in 48 hrs. Grade II: cold, compression, rest; NWB ambulation, modalities for pain relief; isometric exercises progressing to PRE. Grade III: acute surgical repair or reconstruction; follow rehabilitation protocols cited in references
Meniscal injury a. medial b. lateral	a and b. local tenderness; locking and catching	a. Sudden extension, lateral rotation and abduction with knee flexed, tibia laterally rotated and foot fixed b. Sudden extension, medial rotation, and adduction with knee flexed, tibia medially rotated and foot fixed	a and b. Joint line tenderness; knee gives way when step on uneven ground	a and b. Synovial effusion	a and b. Transient impingement; locking	a and b. Apley compression; McMurray	a and b. Reduce immediately if locked; ice then heat in 48 hrs; aspiration; arthroscopic or surgical meniscectomy, followed by PRE and functional rehab
Osgood-Schlatter's disease	Pain and tenderness over anterior knee	Insidious in adolescents; traction epiphysitis or avulsion of tibial tuberosity	Pain with resisted extension or kneeling	Swelling over tibial tuberosity	Antalgic limp; decreased knee flexion	Radiographic evidence of bone fragmentation and epiphyseal separation	Quad sets, SLR, and hamstring stretch; avoid aggravating activities; salicylates; spontaneous improvement in 1–2 yrs
Patellar dislocation/subluxation	Anteromedial knee pain	More common in females; predisposed by acute injury or congenital abnormality of extensor mechanism	Knee gives way when twist or turn; pain over medial patella and lateral femoral condyle	Mild effusion or hemarthrosis	Guarded due to sensation of giving away	Apprehension	Relocate; immobilize 6–8 weeks; quad sets and SLR; PRE emphasizing VMO; surgical stabilization

[a]ACL, anterior cruciate ligament; LCL, lateral collateral ligament; MCL, medial collateral ligament; PCL, posterior cruciate ligament; ROM, range of motion; SLR, straight leg raising; PRE, progressive resistive exercise; NWB, nonweightbearing; VMO, vastus medialis obliquus.

KNEE MOBILIZATION

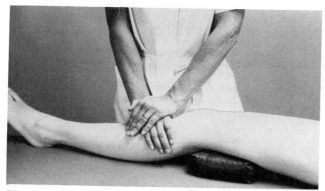

Figure 8.27. Dorsal Tibial Glide, 0° flexion.
Patient Position: Supine with sandbag slightly raising and stabilizing femur.
Therapist Position: Standing at patient's side; overlapped hands rest on ventral proximal tibia.
Technique: With arms parallel to force, use body weight to apply dorsal force to proximal tibia.
Comment: Especially effective for increasing flexion.

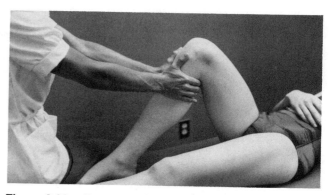

Figure 8.28. Dorsal Tibial Glide, 90° flexion.
Patient Position: Supine with 90° knee flexion, 45° hip flexion; foot resting on table.
Therapist Position: Seated facing patient's head; stabilize patient's foot under thigh; both hands grasp proximal tibia with thenar contract ventrally.
Technique: With arms parallel to force, use body weight to apply dorsal force to proximal tibia. (Similar to posterior drawer test).
Comment: Especially effective for increasing flexion, when flexion already surpasses 90°.

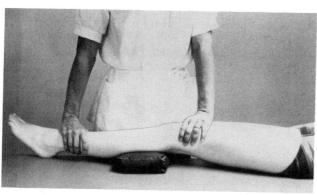

Figure 8.29. Dorsal Femoral Glide (Ventral Tibial Glide), 0° flexion.
Patient Position: Supine with sandbag slightly raising and stabilizing tibia.
Therapist Position: Standing at patient's side; S hand fixates distal tibia; M hand rests on distal femur.
Technique: With arms parallel to force, use body weight to apply dorsal force to distal femur.
Comment: Especially effective for increasing extension when patient lacks end range.

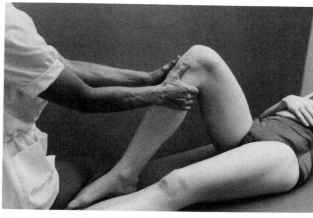

Figure 8.30. Ventral Tibial Glide, 90° flexion.
Patient Position: Supine with 90° knee flexion, 45° hip flexion; foot resting on table.
Therapist Position: Seated facing patient's head; stabilize patient's foot under thigh; both hands grasp proximal tibia with finger contact posteriorly.
Technique: With arms parallel to force, use body weight to apply ventral force to proximal tibia (similar to anterior drawer test).
Comment: Especially effective for increasing extension when there is major restriction.

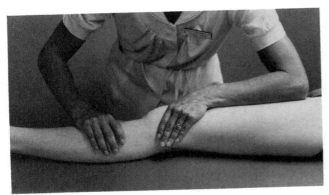

Figure 8.31. Caudal Patellar Glide.

Patient Position: Supine (knee may be flexed at various degrees and stabilized with sandbag).

Therapist Position: Standing at patient's side; S hand restrains lower leg; M hand web space contacts superior aspects of patella.

Technique: With M forearm parallel to force, glide patella caudally.

Comment: Especially effective for increasing knee flexion when patellar restriction exists; avoid dorsal compression of patella into femur.

References

1. Warwick R, Williams PL (eds): *Gray's Anatomy*, 35th British Edition. Philadelphia, WB Saunders, 1973.
2. Malek MM, Mangine RE: Patellofemoral pain syndromes: A comprehensive and conservative approach. *J Orthop Sports Phys Ther* 2:108–116, 1981.
3. Blackburn TA, Craig E: Knee anatomy: A brief review. *Phys Ther* 60:1556–1564, (1980).
4. Helfet AJ: *Disorders of the Knee*, ed 2. Philadelphia, JB Lippincott, 1982.
5. Welsh RP: Knee joint structure and function. *Clin Orthop* 147:7–14, 1980.
6. Hughston JC, Andrews JR, Cross MJ, Moschi A: Classification of knee ligament instabilities part I. The medial compartment and cruciate ligaments. *J Bone Joint Surg* 58A:159–172, 1976.
7. Hastings DE (ed): *Progress in Orthopedic Surgery, The Knee: Ligament and Articular Cartilage Injuries.* New York, Springer-Verlag, 1978, vol 3.
8. Butler DL, Noyes FR, Grood ES: Ligamentous restraints to anterior-posterior drawer in the human knee. *J Bone Joint Surg* 62A:259–270, 1980.
9. O'Donoghue D: Diagnosis and treatment of injury to the anterior cruciate ligament. *J Orthop Sports Phys Ther* 2:100–107, 1981.
10. King S, Butterwick DJ: The anterior cruciate ligament: A review of recent concepts. *J Orthop Sports Phys Ther* 8:110–122, 1986.
11. Kapandji IA: *The Physiology of the Joints*, ed 2, vol 2. Edinburgh, Churchill Livingstone, 1974.
12. Hughston JC, Andrews JR, Cross MJ, Moschi A: Classification of knee ligament instabilities part II. The lateral compartment. *J Bone Joint Surg* 58A:173–179, 1976.
13. Levy IM, Torzilli PA, Warren RF: The effect of medial meniscectomy on anterior-posterior motion of the knee. *J Bone Joint Surg* 64A:883–888, 1982.
14. Cailliet R: *Knee Pain and Disability*. Philadelphia, FA Davis, 1973.
15. Hungerford DS, Lennox DW: Rehabilitation of the knee in disorders of the patellofemoral joint: Relevant biomechanics. *Orthop Clin North Amer* 14:397–402, 1983.
16. Grood ES, Wilfredo JS, Noyes FR, Butler DL: Biomechanics of the knee-extension exercise. *J Bone Joint Surg* 66A:725–734, 1984.

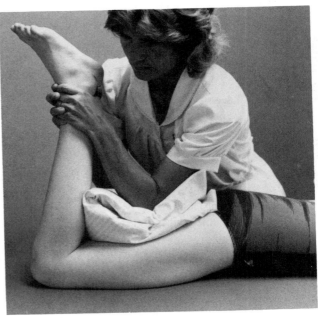

Figure 8.32. Tibiofemoral Joint Traction.

Patient Position: Prone with knee flexed.

Therapist Position: Standing at patient's side; overlapped hands grasp leg just proximal to malleoli; therapist's M elbow supported on pillow over patient's thigh.

Technique: Maintain hand position while flexing patient's knee to impart traction force on tibia.

Comment: Effective as test or treatment for any painful limitation or hypomobility.

17. Wild JR Jr, Franklin TD, Woods GW: Patellar pain and quadriceps rehabilitation: An EMG study. *Amer J Sports Med* 10:12–15, 1982.
18. Brody DM: Running injuries. *Clin Symp* 32(4), 1980.
19. Hughston JC, Walsh WM, Puddu G: Patellar subluxation and dislocation. *Saunders Monographs in Clinical Orthopedics*. Philadelphia, WB Saunders, 1984, vol 5.
20. Jackson DW: Shinsplints: An update. *Physician Sports Med* 10:51–61, 1978.
21. Antich TJ, Lombardo SJ: Clinical presentation of Osgood-Schlatter disease in the adolescent population. *J Orthop Sports Phys Ther* 7:1–4, 1985.
22. Apple DF: End-stage running problems. *Clin Sports Med* 4:657–670, October 1985.
23. Galstad LA: Anterior tibial compartment syndrome. *Athletic Training* 3:139–142, 1979.
24. Granna WA, Schelberg-Karnes E: How I manage deep muscle bruises. *Physician Sports Med* 11:123–127, 1983.
25. Noyes FR, Pekka AM, Matthews DS, Butler DL: The symptomatic anterior cruciate-deficient knee. Part I: The long-term functional disability in athletically active individuals. *J Bone Joint Surg* 65A:154–161, 1983.
26. Davies GJ, Larsen R: Examining the knee. *Physician Sports Med* 4:49–67, 1978.
27. Ellison AE: Skiing injuries. *Clin Symp* 29(1), 1977.

CHAPTER 9

THE ANKLE AND FOOT

CLINICAL ANATOMY AND MECHANICS OF THE ANKLE AND FOOT

The ankle and foot comprise the terminal segment of a kinetic chain responsible for propulsion and balance. This segment must attenuate weightbearing forces, support and propel the body, and maintain equilibrium. The following section describes the structure and function of this intriguing unit that serves both as a semi-rigid base and a dynamic lever.

Osteology

Tibia and Fibula.　The tibia transmits most of the body weight to the foot. The proximal surface of the tibia, the tibial plateau, supports the femur. Just distal to the plateau, the tibia narrows to a shaft. An oval facet indents the tibia posterolaterally and provides an articular surface where the fibula joins the tibia in the superior tibiofibular joint (Fig. 9.1). This facet varies in its orientation between horizontal and oblique; the more horizontal, the greater its surface area and capacity for rotary mobility (1).

From a cylindrical shaft, the tibia expands at its distal end where several features contribute to ankle function (Fig. 9.1). A broad, slightly concave, distal surface conforms to and rests upon the talus. A medial projection, the medial malleolus, bears a comma shaped facet that grips the medial side of the talus. The fibular notch, a shallow fossa, marks the lateral distal aspect of the tibia and articulates with the fibula at the inferior tibiofibular joint. A posterolateral projection, the "third malleolus," has little functional significance, but is sometimes fractured along with the medial and lateral malleoli in what constitutes a trimalleolar fracture.

The fibula is a long, slender bone with great tensile strength. Its slightly expanded proximal end, the fibular head, possesses a single facet that contacts the tibia at the superior tibiofibular joint. Its bulbous distal end also articulates with the tibia. The fibula projects distally as the lateral malleolus, that grips the lateral side of the talus (Fig. 9.1). Although the fibula is not directly involved in weight transmission, it plays a vital role in ankle stability through the lateral malleolus. Both the lateral and medial malleoli closely approximate the talus throughout the range of dorsiflexion and plantarflexion (2, 3). The more posterior and distal position of the lateral malleolus, however, limits eversion within the mortice and reduces the incidence of eversion ankle sprains. Consequently, 85% of ankle ligament injuries result from inversion sprains (4).

Rearfoot.　The talus links the leg with the foot (Fig. 9.1). Comprised of a superior body (dome), a neck, and an anterior head, the talus forms the keystone of the foot's longitudinal arch. The tibia and fibula encase the talar body in the close-fitting ankle mortise articulation. The body is widest anteriorly, so that dorsiflexion of the ankle wedges it between the tibia and fibula. Two articular areas mark the inferior surface of the talus. These areas articulate with the calcaneus at the subtalar joint. A groove between these two inferior articular surfaces provides a space, the sinus tarsi, through which major nutrient vessels pass. The talar neck projects anterior and 15° medial to the talar body (Fig. 9.2). Anterior to its neck, the talus terminates in a relatively large, convex head. No muscles or tendons insert onto the talus, but a number of ligaments attach to it.

The calcaneus is the largest and most frequently injured tarsal bone. Three facets on its superior surface articulate with the talus at the subtalar joint. A groove through this articular surface forms the floor of the sinus tarsi. A medial, shelf-like projection, the sustentaculum tali, supports the talus. The lateral side of the calcaneus bears a peroneal tubercle which provides a pulley for the peroneus longus tendon, and separates it from the peroneus brevis tendon. The flattened anterior surface of the calcaneus articulates with the cuboid.

Midfoot.　The naviculum transmits weight from the talus to the cuneiforms. Its posterior, concave surface articulates with the talus, and its anterior, convex surface articulates with the cuneiforms (Fig. 9.2). A large tubercle on its medial aspect is an easily identified, palpable bony landmark.

The cuboid articulates posteriorly with the calcaneus, anteriorly with the 4th and 5th metatarsals, and medially with the naviculum and 3rd cuneiform. A

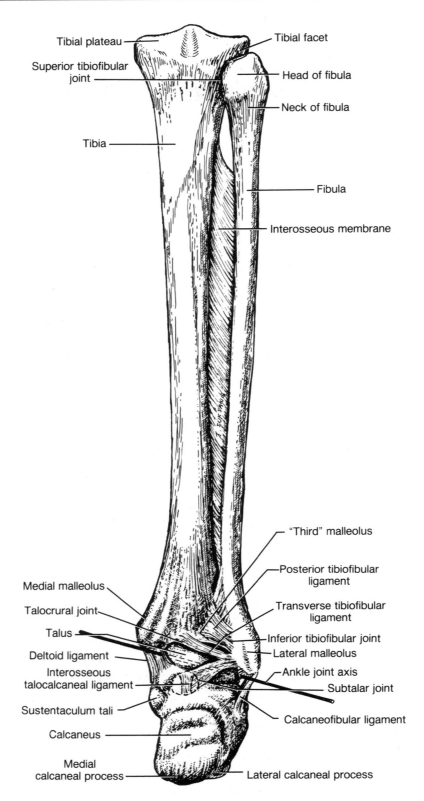

Figure 9.1.   Bones and ligaments of the leg and ankle, posterior view.

groove on its lateral surface contains the peroneus longus tendon.

The three wedge-shaped cuneiforms articulate posteriorly with the naviculum, anteriorly with the first three metatarsals, and laterally with one another and the cuboid.

Forefoot. The metatarsals are the major stabilizers of the foot (5). Like the metacarpals, they resemble miniature long bones, possessing elongated shafts, expanded concave bases, and distal convex heads. The first metatarsal is shortest and thickest, and does not participate in the common articulation joining the bases of the other metatarsals. The articular surfaces of the metatarsal heads extend dorsally to accommodate the range of toe extension that exceeds flexion. The phalanges also display shafts, concave bases, and convex heads (Fig. 9.2). They correspond in number and arrangement to the phalanges of the hand, but are much shorter.

Practitioners often divide the foot longitudinally into rays. The 1st ray includes the 1st cuneiform, and 1st metatarsal; the 2nd ray includes the 2nd cuneiform and metatarsal; the 3rd ray includes the 3rd cuneiform and metatarsal; the 4th and 5th rays only include the respective metatarsals.

Bony Arches of the Foot. The arrangement of the tarsals and metatarsals forms intersecting arches that distribute weight, absorb shock, and allow the foot to adapt to uneven ground. Some compare this arched framework to an architectural vault supported by the 1st metatarsal head, 5th metatarsal head, and calcaneus (4, 6). All of the metatarsal heads, however, bear an approximately equal load, except the 1st, which carries double the load of the others (7). There is a 1:1

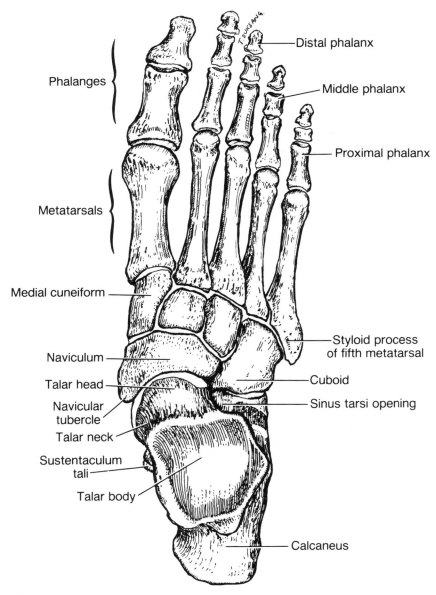

Figure 9.2. Bones of the foot.

ratio of weight distribution between the calcaneus and the metatarsal heads in erect standing. The medial longitudinal arch between the 1st metatarsal head and calcaneus contributes to propulsion and shock absorption. The lateral longitudinal arch between the 5th metatarsal head and calcaneus provides balance and support. The transverse arch between the metatarsal heads allows the foot to adapt to the ground. The plantar aponeurosis, the beam action of the metatarsals, and joint congruity support the fully loaded foot at rest so that muscle action is not necessary (5, 8).

Arthrology

Steindler described the lower limb as a kinetic chain: a series of links free to move on each other but also capable of combining into a rigid column to support the body. The chain is "open" when the distal link is free to move, i.e., the distal link moves on the proximal link. The chain is "closed" when the distal link is fixed, i.e., the proximal link moves on the distal link (7). The joints of the ankle and foot function differently in open and closed chain situations.

Tibiofibular Joints.   The tibia and fibula articulate with one another at both their proximal and distal ends (Fig. 9.1). Proximally, the junction of the fibular facet with the inferior posterolateral rim of the tibial condyle comprises the superior tibiofibular joint. It is a plane synovial joint between two relatively flat surfaces, which permits three movements: anterior-posterior glide, superior-inferior glide, and rotation (1). These motions accommodate knee and foot positions, and dissipate torsional ankle stresses as well as lateral tibial bending (9). Ligamentous fibers descending from the tibia strengthen the superior tibiofibular joint capsule anteriorly and posteriorly.

An interosseous membrane binds the tibia and fibula throughout their lengths. Distally, an interosseous tibiofibular ligament and anterior and posterior tibiofibular ligaments unite the bones at the inferior tibiofibular joint, a syndesmosis with no articular cartilage. Ankle joint stability requires some rigidity in this syndesmosis, yet ankle function depends on a slight amount of movement. During ankle dorsiflexion, the fibula moves laterally, superiorly, and rotates medially; during plantarflexion, it moves in the opposite direction (6).

Talocrural Joint.   The tibia and fibula form a mortise which embraces the talar dome in a uniaxial joint. The talocrural (ankle) joint axis approximates a line passing just distal to the tips of the malleoli, which diverges slightly posterior to the frontal plane, as well as downward from a medial to a lateral direction (Fig. 9.1). The primary talocrural joint movements are dorsiflexion in a range of 20–30° and plantarflexion in a range of 30–50°. Functional range for walking is much less, however, requiring only 10° of dorsiflexion and 20° of plantarflexion (8, 10). People more commonly lack the 10° of necessary dorsiflexion than the 20° of plantarflexion, leading to compensatory mechanisms, such as early heel off, with potential pathomechanics. The joint axis inclination causes some foot abduction with dorsiflexion and adduction with plantar flexion (10). Dorsiflexion is the close-packed position of the joint in which there is maximal joint surface congruency and ligamentous tension.

The structures sustaining the ankle mortise include the interosseous tibiofibular ligament, the anterior and posterior tibiofibular ligaments, the joint capsule, and medial and lateral ligament systems attaching to the malleoli (8). The capsule attaches proximally to the borders of the tibial and fibular articular surfaces and

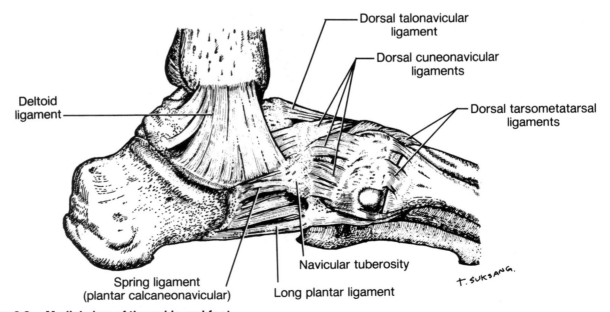

Deltoid ligament

Spring ligament (plantar calcaneonavicular)

Long plantar ligament

Navicular tuberosity

Dorsal talonavicular ligament

Dorsal cuneonavicular ligaments

Dorsal tarsometatarsal ligaments

T. SUKSANG.

Figure 9.3.   Medial view of the ankle and foot.

malleoli. Distally, the capsule attaches to the margins of the talar trochlear surface, except anteriorly, where it extends onto the anterior neck of the talus (11). The capsule is thinnest anteriorly and posteriorly, whereas strong collateral ligaments reinforce each side. A large deltoid ligament provides medial support for both the talocrural and subtalar joints (Fig. 9.3). It originates on the medial malleolus and splays distally as slips attaching to the naviculum, talus, and calcaneus. Due to the strength of the deltoid ligament, eversion stress often fractures the malleolus rather than tears the ligament (12).

Three ligaments provide lateral ankle stability (Fig. 9.4). They are stressed individually by different ankle positions. The anterior talofibular ligament resists inversion maximally when the ankle is plantarflexed. The calcaneofibular ligament provides maximal resistance to inversion in dorsiflexion. The posterior talofibular ligament resists anterior dislocation of the leg on the foot, and is the strongest of the lateral ligaments.

Subtalar Joint.   Facets on the inferior talar surface articulate with facets on the superior calcaneal surface in the subtalar joint. These articulations move in unison about a common axis in this hinge-like joint. Its

oblique axis passes from a posterior, lateral, plantar point to an anterior, medial, dorsal point (Fig. 9.5*A*). Relative to the cardinal planes, the axis' position is 42° from the transverse plane and 16° from the midline of the foot (3, 10, 13). Since the subtalar joint axis traverses all three cardinal planes, its movement is triplanar, although this hinge-like joint has only a single axis. Its triplanar movements include pronation, which is combined eversion, abduction, and dorsiflexion of the calcaneus (and foot) on the talus (and leg), and supination, which is inversion, adduction, and plantarflexion (Fig. 9.5*B*). These movements occur in an open kinetic chain when there is no resistance to foot movement. No accurate clinical mechanism for measuring subtalar supination and pronation exists (10). The frontal plane component of subtalar joint motion determines the amount of calcaneal inversion and eversion that can be measured. The inversion range of approximately 20° is normally twice as great as the eversion range of approximately 10°.

During weightbearing (closed kinetic chain), friction and ground reaction forces prevent free forefoot movement, therefore the talar and calcaneal relationships change. Calcaneal eversion along with talar adduction and plantarflexion comprises subtalar

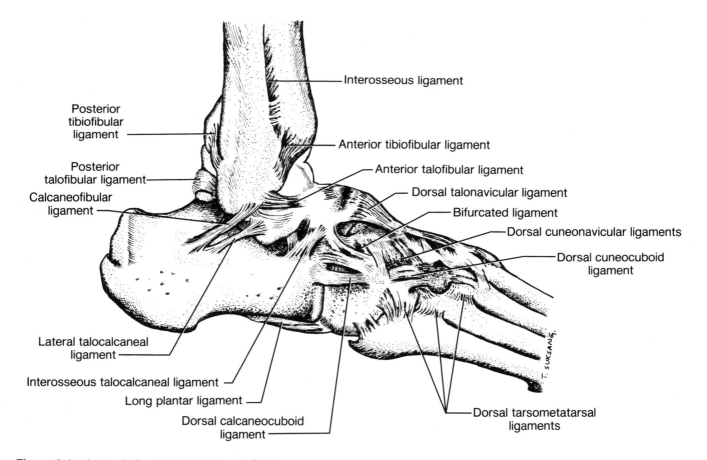

Figure 9.4.   Lateral view of the ankle and foot.

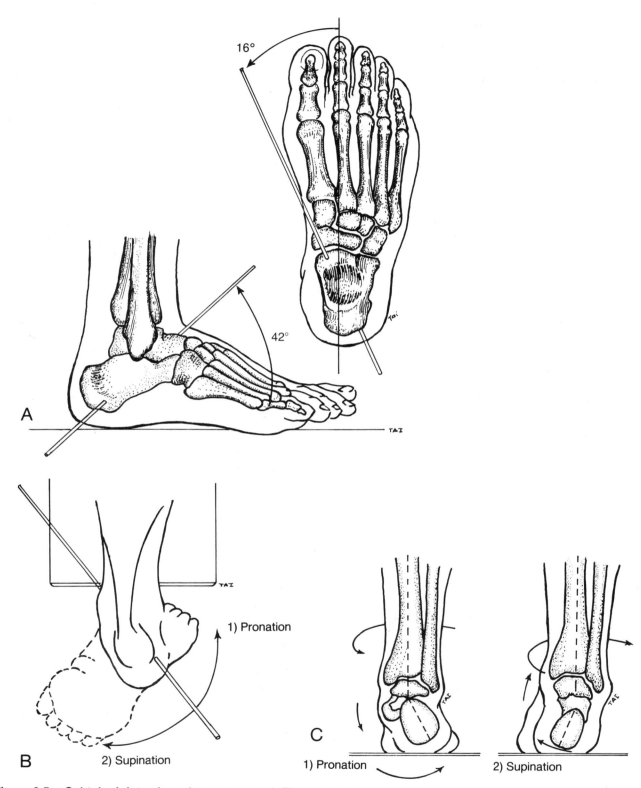

Figure 9.5. Subtalar joint axis and movements. *A,* The subtalar joint axis is 42° from the transverse plane and 16° from the foot's midline, so the axis, as well as movement, is triplanar (does not lie in any cardinal plane). *B,* In an open kinetic chain motion occurs between the proximal segment (talus) and distal segment (calcaneus), producing: 1) pronation: abduction, eversion, and dorsiflexion of the foot, or 2) supination: adduction, inversion, and plantarflexion of the foot. *C,* In a closed kinetic chain motion occurs between the talus and calcaneus, producing: 1) pronation: adduction and plantarflexion of the talus with eversion of the calcaneus and foot and 2) supination: abduction and dorsiflexion of the talus and inversion of the calcaneus and foot.

pronation (Fig. 9.5C). Calcaneal inversion, with talar abduction and dorsiflexion, comprises supination.

The subtalar joint absorbs transverse plane rotation of the lower extremity during the stance phase of gait (13). One may illustrate this function by simply standing on both feet and rotating the body to the left; the left lower extremity rotates laterally and the left subtalar joint supinates. Simultaneously, the right lower extremity rotates medially and the right subtalar joint pronates. Body rotation to the right would reverse subtalar joint motion in this example. The subtalar joint also serves to absorb shock at heel strike; during pronation the talus plantarflexes, which functionally shortens the extremity (10).

Short, powerful ligaments unite the talus and calcaneus. The interosseous talocalcaneal ligament is one of the major ligaments that resists the severe stresses imposed upon this joint. It two fibrous bands occupy the sinus tarsi (Fig. 9.1). This ligament tightens during supination, and thus provides additional stability in this position. The lateral and posterior talocalcaneal ligaments, along with ligaments of the talocrural joint which span the talus, also enhance subtalar joint stability (Fig. 9.4).

Midtarsal Joint.   The midtarsal (transverse, Chopart's) joint includes both the talonavicular and calcaneocuboid articulations. Although the two articulations have separate joint cavities, they move in unison. The midtarsal joint has two independent axes of motion, each of which is oblique to the cardinal planes and about which triplanar motion occurs (10, 13) (Fig. 9.6). The longitudinal midtarsal joint axis lies 15° from the transverse plane and 9° from the midline of the foot. The oblique midtarsal joint axis lies 52° from the transverse plane and 57° from the midline of the foot. Motion about each axis can be independent of the other, but is dependent on the foot's position of pronation or supination. Pronation moves the axes into parallel alignment. This "unlocks" the midtarsal joint and allows mobility with relatively little skeletal stability. Supination causes the axes to diverge and creates a rigid skeletal structure that is necessary for maximum stability at heeloff (13). The longitudinal axis primarily allows eversion and inversion of the forefoot, whereas the oblique axis allows dorsiflexion and abduction or plantarflexion and adduction (10).

Sturdy ligaments spanning the plantar surface of the midtarsal joint absorb stress, maintain the longitudinal arch, and assist supination (5, 14). The spring ligament (plantar calcaneonavicular), located at the apex of the medial longitudinal arch, runs between the sustentaculum tali and the naviculum (Fig. 9.3). It supports the talar head and is crucial to foot stability. Laxity of the spring ligament allows the naviculum and calcaneus to separate, creating a space into which the talus may slip, with resulting flatfoot. The plantar calcaneocuboid (short plantar) ligament spans the plantar surface of the calcaneus and attaches to the cuboid. The long plantar ligament also originates on the calcaneus and runs distally to insert on the cuboid and bases of the 2nd, 3rd, 4th, and 5th metatarsals. It

is essential to arch support. Superficially, the plantar aponeurosis runs from the medial calcaneal tuberosity to the metatarsal heads, dividing into digital slips that blend with the plantar metatarsophalangeal ligaments and skin overlying the ball of the foot.

Dorsally, the bifurcated ligament forms the keystone of the transverse arch. It arises from the anterior sinus tarsi floor and bifurcates into bands that insert into the naviculum and cuboid (Fig. 9.4). The dorsal talonavicular ligament connects the talar neck with the naviculum.

Anterior Tarsal and Tarsometatarsal Joints.   There is little movement between the individual tarsals and metatarsals, but their collective movement can enhance either the foot's stability or flexibility. A common joint cavity connects the cuboid, naviculum, three cuneiforms, and 2nd and 3rd metatarsal bases. The 1st cuneiform and 1st metatarsal articulation has a separate cavity, as does the cuboid articulation with the 4th and 5th metatarsals. Interosseous, dorsal, and plantar ligaments strengthen all of these small joints.

Firm proximal articulations allow only minimal movement of the three middle metatarsal rays in a dorsoplantar direction (70). The 1st and 5th rays, however, have a greater range of dorsoplantar movement as well as slight inversion and eversion, allowing them to adapt to the ground. The first ray moves about an axis that is oriented 45° to the frontal and sagittal planes. The axis passes from a point posterior, medial, and dorsal to a point anterior, lateral, and plantar. Its primary movements include combined dorsiflexion and inversion, and combined plantar flexion and eversion. In a neutral position, the 1st metatarsal head lies in the same plane as the other metatarsal heads; when the other metatarsals dorsiflex, the 1st should be able to move an equal distance above and below their transverse plane. Plantarflexion of the first ray is necessary for propulsion; lack of plantarflexion is a frequent cause of sesamoiditis and plantar keratoma (10).

Metatarsophalangeal Joints.   The metatarsals articulate with the proximal phalanges in condyloid, biaxial joints. Normal locomotion requires that their range of dorsiflexion (60–90°) be greater than plantarflexion (40–50°). Since locomotion demands minimal lateral mobility, their range of abduction and adduction has lost clinical significance. A line connecting the 2nd and 5th metatarsal heads forms an angle of 62° with the midline of the foot (Fig. 9.6). This line constitutes a functional axis, the metatarsal break, which accounts for a passive supination shift as weight is transferred onto the metatarsal heads (8).

Collateral, plantar, and deep transverse ligaments support the metatarsophalangeal (MP) joints, and a dorsal hood reinforces their dorsal aspect. The plantar ligaments (equivalent to the hand's volar plates) are continuous with the plantar aponeurosis, so that toe dorsiflexion tenses the fascia and stabilizes the foot's longitudinal arch.

Normal ambulation requires a minimum of 60–65° of 1st MP joint dorsiflexion (extension). This range of motion is also necessary to transform the foot into a

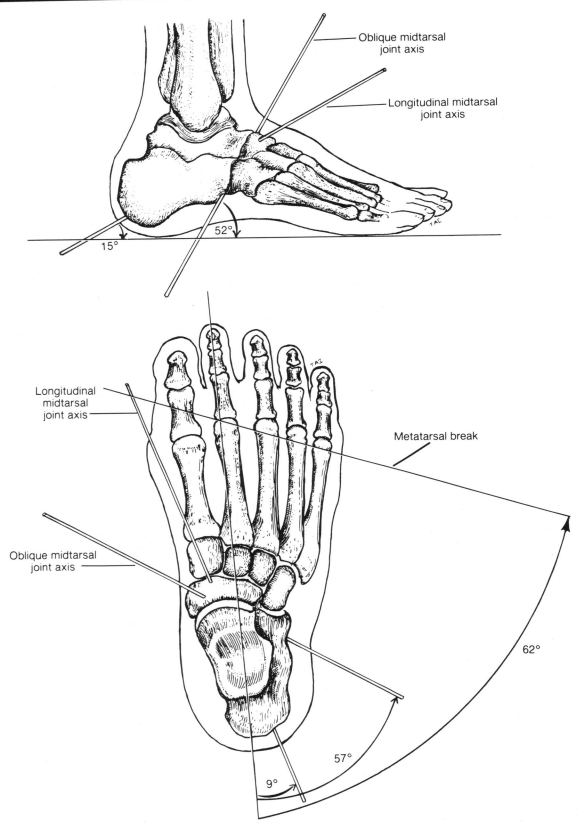

Figure 9.6.   Midtarsal joint axes and movements. The longitudinal axis is 15° from the transverse plane and 9° from the foot's midline. The oblique axis is 52° from the transverse plane and 57° from the foot's midline. Forefoot eversion and inversion occur primarily around the longitudinal axis; dorsiflexion and abduction, or plantarflexion and adduction occur primarily around the oblique axis.

rigid lever during gait (15). Dorsiflexion tenses the plantar aponeurosis, which approximates the rearfoot and forefoot, and enhances subtalar joint supination (5, 14). This facilitates the peroneus longus muscle's ability to stabilize the first ray for normal push-off during gait (10, 15). First MP joint dorsiflexion also improves the mechanical advantage of the flexor hallucis longus muscle, allowing it to stabilize the hallux and to plantarflex the foot during gait.

Interphalangeal Joints. The interphalangeal (IP) joints are hinges that permit flexion and extension as primary motions, and minimal abduction, adduction, and rotation as accessory motions. Collateral and plantar ligaments support these joints.

Proper IP joint function is necessary for normal locomotion. Upon forefoot loading, the short toe flexor and lumbrical muscles hold the PIP joints slightly plantarflexed and the DIP joints slightly dorsiflexed to ensure firm contact of the toe plantarpads with the ground. Thus, the toes maintain a stable base for the extrinsic toe muscles which propel the limb (7).

Bursae. The largest bursae in the foot occur about the calcaneus, and the heads of the 1st and 5th metatarsals. The three calcaneal bursae of clinical significance are located: between the Achilles tendon and skin; between the posterior calcaneus and Achilles tendon; between the plantar surface of the calcaneus and the subcutaneous tissue of the heel. Subcutaneous bursae may form in any area upon which excessive friction occurs.

Mechanics

One can divide the extrinsic ankle and foot muscles into four groups according to the functions they perform. Posteriorly, the gastrocnemius, soleus, and plantaris muscles plantarflex the foot. Laterally, the peroneus longus and brevis muscles pronate and evert the foot, and reinforce the lateral ligaments of the ankle. Medially, the tibialis posterior, flexor digitorum longus, and flexor hallucis longus muscles invert the foot, flex the toes, and reinforce the deltoid ligament. Anteriorly the extensor hallucis longus, extensor digitorum longus, tibialis anterior, and peroneus tertius muscles dorsiflex the foot, and extend the toes.

Four layers of intrinsic muscles occupy the plantar surface of the foot. The most superficial layer includes the abductor hallucis, flexor digitorum brevis, and abductor digiti minimi muscles. The next layer contains the quadratus plantae (accessorius) and lumbrical muscles. The 3rd layer includes the flexor hallucis brevis, adductor hallucis, and flexor digiti minimi muscles. The dorsal and plantar interosseous muscles comprise the 4th and deepest layer. The origins, insertions, and actions of these muscles are covered extensively elsewhere (11, 16).

The importance of ankle and foot functional biomechanics emerges during the weightbearing (stance) phase of locomotion (Fig. 9.7). Actions within a closed kinetic chain occur during this phase that comprises 60% of the gait cycle. The foot moves through ranges of supination and pronation to assist movement, stabilize joints, and reduce forces within the foot and lower leg (5).

The three intervals that comprise the stance portion of the gait cycle include heel strike to foot flat (15% of total cycle), foot flat to heel off (30%), and heel off to toe off (15%) (3). At the onset of stance, the supinated subtalar joint causes the lateral side of the heel to strike the ground (7). This lateral contact produces a valgus thrust which initiates calcaneal eversion and subtalar

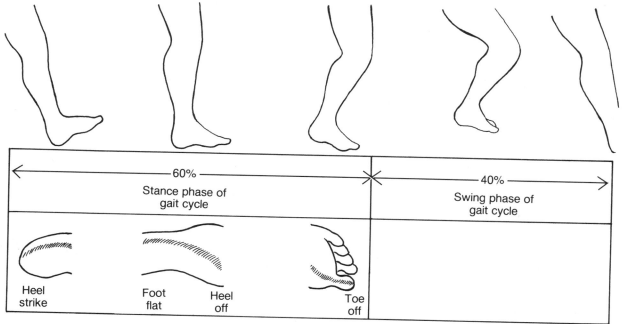

Figure 9.7. Ankle and foot participation in the gait cycle (hatched areas indicate areas of greatest weightbearing).

pronation (13) (Fig. 9.5C). In addition, the tibia rotates medially at heel strike, carrying the talus with it and enhancing pronation. Pronation increases as the foot is loaded, unlocking the talus on the calcaneus. Subtalar joint pronation also unlocks the midtarsal joint so that the cuboid and naviculum become more parallel and the forefoot bones become more mobile. During this initial phase of gait, the foot is a loose adapter to accommodate uneven terrain and to absorb shock. Pronation decreases the functional length of the stance leg thus lowering the impact force of loading. Pronation also attenuates other forces, including compression, rotation, anterior shear, and medial shear (5).

A reversal of motion occurs at midstance when the foot is flat. The tibia begins to rotate laterally, moving the talus into abduction and dorsiflexion, as the calcaneus inverts (Fig. 9.5C). The gastrocsoleus, posterior tibialis, extrinsic, and intrinsic toe flexor muscles are all active in this phase, contributing to heel inversion (3). The subtalar joint supinates, locking the midtarsal joint and stabilizing the 1st ray (17). The foot continues to supinate throughout the rest of the stance phase, with the subtalar joint reaching its neutral position at heel off. The bones now serve as rigid levers upon which the extrinsic muscles pull. The synergistic contractions of the peroneus longus and posterior tibialis muscles stabilize the 1st ray. The peroneus brevis and tertius muscles also act to stabilize the 5th ray, exert proximal traction on the cuboid, and effect forward propulsion of the lateral malleolus (18).

As the body weight rolls forward over the forefoot, the heel rises and the toes extend. By increasing tension in the plantar aponeurosis and intrinsic foot muscles, dorsiflexion of the 1st MP joint assists supination and pulls the calcaneus toward the stabilized metatarsal heads (13). The posterior tibialis muscle assists the ligaments and intrinsic muscles in raising the longitudinal arch.

Neurology

Motor Innervation. Branches of the sciatic nerve supply the ankle and foot. The tibial nerve, in direct vertical continuity with the sciatic nerve, extends from the arcade of the soleus muscle to the calcaneal canal (16). In the leg, it supplies the gastrocnemius, plantaris, soleus, tibialis posterior, flexor digitorum longus, and flexor hallucis longus muscles. Between 1–2 cm proximal to the tip of the medial malleolus, the tibial nerve bifurcates into its terminal branches, the medial and lateral plantar nerves (Fig. 9.8C). Near the area of bifurcation, the tibial nerve passes through the tarsal tunnel, under the flexor retinaculum. Various structures and conditions may produce medial tarsal tunnel syndrome, a compression neuropathy within the tunnel (19).

The medial plantar nerve supplies the flexor digitorum brevis, abductor hallucis, flexor hallucis brevis, and 1st lumbrical muscles. This nerve is comparable to the median nerve in the upper extremity. The smaller, lateral plantar nerve supplies the quadratus plantae

(accessorius), flexor digiti minimi, abductor digiti minimi, adductor hallucis, lumbricals II–IV, and interosseous muscles. The digital nerves that branch off of the medial and lateral plantar nerves are susceptible to compression where they pass between the metatarsal heads (Morton's neuralgia).

The common peroneal nerve branches laterally from the sciatic nerve at the apex of the popliteal fossa. It crosses the fibular head superficially, where it is susceptible to injury from blunt trauma or external pressure, i.e., an ill-fitting cast or brace. The common peroneal nerve divides into the superficial and deep peroneal nerves. The superficial peroneal nerve supplies the peroneus longus and peroneus brevis muscles. The deep peroneal nerve innervates the tibialis anterior, extensor hallucis longus, peroneus tertius, extensor digitorum longus, and extensor digitorum brevis muscles.

Sensory Innervation. The saphenous nerve, the terminal branch of the femoral nerve, courses the length of the leg in a posteromedial position. Its branches supply the medial ankle, foot, and hallux. The medial sural nerve arises from the tibial nerve in the popliteal space. It anastomoses with the peroneal communicating nerve, becoming the sural nerve which enters the foot beneath the lateral malleolus. The terminal branches of the sural nerve supply the posterolateral ankle and lateral border of the foot (Fig. 9.8C). The calcaneal nerve branches from the tibial nerve in the distal third of the leg. It supplies the plantar surface of the heel. Sensory branches of the superficial peroneal nerve supply the skin over the anterior ankle and dorsum of the foot.

The medial plantar nerve provides sensory branches for the dorsal and plantar surfaces of the 1st, 2nd, 3rd and medial half of the 4th toes and the medial aspect of the plantar foot surface anterior to the calcaneus (19). The lateral plantar nerve supplies the dorsal and plantar surfaces of the lateral half of the 4th and 5th toes and the lateral aspect of the plantar foot surface anterior to the calcaneous (19).

The deep peroneal and saphenous nerves innervate the ankle joint anteriorly, and the tibial and sural nerves innervate it posteriorly. The deep peroneal nerve also provides sensation to the dorsal aspect of the foot joints, whereas the medial and lateral plantar nerves supply the plantar aspect of these joints. The ankle joint reflex is initiated from the S1-2 nerve root levels.

Angiology

Arterial Supply. Three arteries supply blood to the ankle and foot: the posterior tibial, anterior tibial, and peroneal (Fig. 9.8A and B). The posterior tibial artery supplies the posterior leg. It gives off the peroneal artery, which supplies the lateral leg. Its terminal branches, the medial and lateral plantar arteries, supply the sole of the foot. The anterior tibial artery continues into the foot as the dorsalis pedis artery that provides blood supply to the dorsum of the foot.

Venous Supply. From the dorsal venous arch, the short saphenous vein branches laterally and runs as proximal as the knee before joining the popliteus vein (Fig. 9.8*B*). The medial branch of the arch, the great (long) saphenous vein, runs superficially in a proximal course along the medial aspect of the leg. Cardiovascular surgeons commonly use the great (long) saphenous vein as a replacement graft in coronary artery bypass surgery. There are also pairs of deep veins (venae comitantes) which accompany the major arteries and assist in the return of deep blood flow.

ANKLE AND FOOT EXAMINATION

History

The examiner first obtains identifying data, and then proceeds to question the patient regarding his present episode or illness. Using a body chart to assist specific location of symptoms, the patient describes the location, severity, and nature of his disorder (Fig. 9.9). He also estimates the impairment that it imposes. Pain is the most common and significant complaint of persons with foot disorders (7). The location and character of pain are pathognomonic for certain conditions. Plantar fasciitis presents as medial calcaneal pain upon initial weightbearing. Metatarsalgia produces a dull, burning, diffuse foot pain. An intermetatarsal neuroma is associated with an acute episode of forefoot pain, with pain and paresthesias radiating into the toes (10). Tarsal tunnel syndrome produces burning pain and paresthesias on the plantar aspect of the foot and great toe. Ankle ligamentous injuries result in localized pain over the injured structure.

Symptom behavior also characterizes certain syndromes. Intermittent lower limb pain, which occurs

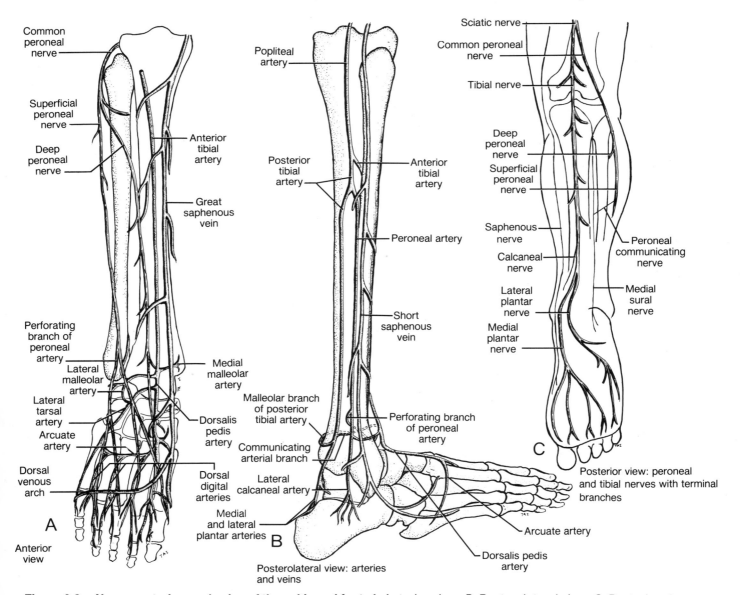

Figure 9.8. Nerves, arteries, and veins of the ankle and foot. *A,* Anterior view. *B,* Posterolateral view, *C,* Posterior view.

A. HISTORY

1. Identifying Data

   Name _____ Age _____ Gender _____ Date _____

   Provisional diagnosis _____ Precautions _____

   Chief complaint _____

   Dominant side R _____ L _____ Prior condition of involved part _____

2. Present Episode or Illness

   a. Description of symptoms

      1) location: / / / / = pain
                    = = = = = paresthesia
                    ° ° ° ° = numbness
                    xxxx = other _____

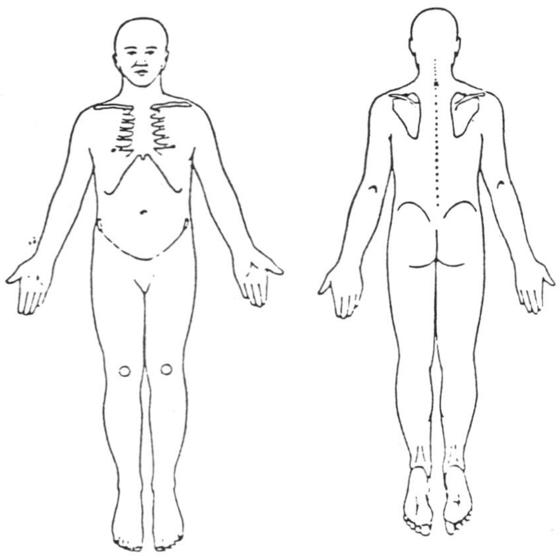

      2) severity:

         _____

         none   worst

      3) impairment:

         _____

         annoying   completely disabling

      4) nature:

         cramping _____ aching _____

         shooting _____ burning _____

         throbbing _____ tingling _____

         stabbing _____ sore _____

         other _____

      5) behavior:

         constant _____ intermittent _____ duration _____

         occurs when _____ elicited by _____

         aggravated by _____ relieved by _____

         24-hour pattern _____

         highly irritable _____ mildly irritable _____ not irritable _____

      6) joint characteristics: catches _____ , locks _____ , swells _____ , gives way _____ , dislocates _____ ,

         other _____

Figure 9.9.   Examination form part 1: History.

only after walking a particular distance, and is quickly relieved by rest, may signal a systemic circulatory disorder in which claudication is a key factor. In contrast, foot discomfort that increases with both standing and walking, and is best relieved by removing the shoe and massaging the foot, may stem from an intermetatarsal neuroma. Most foot problems of mechanical etiology are aggravated primarily by gait; static stance does not reproduce the abnormal stress to a degree to cause pain.

The examiner next probes for information on the condition's background and associated findings (Fig. 9.10). He notes significant dates relating to injury or onset, hospitalization, treatment, etc. He establishes the status of the condition. Ankle and foot injuries are often discrete, so that the patient can accurately describe the injury mechanism. For instance, the history of an inversion ankle sprain usually includes the foot turning under as body weight is imposed upon it, accompanied by immediate pain, difficulty in weightbearing, and sometimes a "snap" or "giving way" sensation (20). Insidious conditions are more difficult to associate with a cause. It is useful to question the patient about a change of footwear or occupation which may produce subtle variations in foot mechanics. Conversely, has the condition resulted in a change of footwear or occupation?

When obtaining a past history, the examiner inquires about systemic disorders that commonly produce foot pain, such as vascular insufficiency and inflammatory arthritis (Fig. 9.10). A patient's life-style also has important ramifications upon foot function. Occupations or activities that demand long periods of weightbearing may cause ligamentous strain and muscle fatigue. Locomotion magnifies mechanical abnormalities, such as an abnormal pronatory motion or pronatory position which is responsible for more chronic low-grade foot and postural symptoms than any other type of foot problem (10). Documentation of current medications, recent radiographs, and the therapist's interpretation and plans for an objective examination complete the history portion of the examination.

Physical Examination

Inspection. The posture of weightbearing joints varies between conditions of loading and unloading. The examiner should, therefore, inspect the lower limb both when it is weightbearing (WB) and when it is nonweightbearing (NWB). Alignment of the pelvis, hip, and knee influences ankle and foot function, so one assesses these proximal "links" as part of an integrated system (Fig. 9.11). Mechanical defects of the lower limb bones or joints manifest directly as abnormal stress or compensatory changes in the ankle and foot. For example, femoral anteversion or retroversion produces compensatory toeing-in and toeing-out respectively. Tibial torsion alters the normal 15–20° of posterolateral obliquity of the ankle axis. The patella is normally aligned between the 2nd and 3rd toes, but

medial tibial torsion moves it into alignment with the lateral toes and lateral torsion with the medial toe(s).

The body normally displays equilibrium during static stance (Fig. 9.12). Only the gastrocnemius muscle contracts to produce a plantarflexion force at the ankle. No muscle support is necessary to maintain structural integrity of the foot. During relaxed standing, the following relationships should exist (10, 21):

1. The distal one-third of the legs and posterior bisection of the calcanei are vertical and parallel to one another.
2. The talocrural and subtalar joints are parallel to the supporting surface.
3. The subtalar joints are in their neutral positions (see palpation).
4. The midtarsal joints are locked in maximal pronation.
5. The forefoot plantar surface parallels the rearfoot plantar surface and supporting surface.
6. All metatarsals bear weight, and their heads lie in the same transverse plane.

The vertical axis of the calcaneus should align with the lower one-third of the leg in the frontal plane when viewed from behind. If the vertical axis of the calcaneus is inclined medially from the long axis of the tibia, the condition is described as hindfoot varus; if inclined laterally, it is hindfoot valgus. In the sagittal plane, the anterior end of the calcaneus is inclined about 20°. Abnormal plantarflexion of the calcaneal axis is equinus; abnormal dorsiflexion is calcaneus (Fig. 9.11).

Normally, the forefoot parallels the hindfoot. If the forefoot long axis diverges medially, the forefoot is adducted; if it diverges laterally, the forefoot is abducted. If the forefoot rotates on its long axis so that the plantar surface faces the midline, the forefoot is in varus (inverted); if the forefoot faces away from the midline, it is in valgus (everted). In the sagittal plane, a line from the medial malleolus to the head of the 1st metatarsal should pass through the top one-third of the navicular tubercle. If the tubercle is above the line, the forefoot is dorsiflexed, and the condition is cavus (high-arched foot); if below, it is plannus (low-arched foot).

The toes should be parallel to the long axis of the foot. Hallux valgus is a common disorder in which the axis of the first toe diverges laterally. If there is restricted motion of the first MP joint, the condition is hallux rigidus. A hammer toe deformity is characterized by PIP joint flexion and DIP joint extension. A claw toe deformity occurs when there is excessive MP joint extension and IP joint flexion.

Since loading and unloading may alter a foot's shape, the patient should be examined in both situations. A practitioner can visually recognize gross congenital abnormalities in children, but will want to extend his examination with palpation to ascertain the presence of fixed versus flexible deformities. Fat deposits in the soles create the appearance of low arches in infants;

b. Background and associated findings

Date of present injury _____ or onset _____ insidious _____

Dates of hospitalization _____ and/or other health care

Treatments; dates; results _____

_____

Status of condition: acute _____ or chronic _____

constant _____ or intermittent _____

better _____ or worse _____

Nature and mechanism of injury or events precipitating present episode _____

_____

Results of injury (if applicable): deformity (describe) _____

corrected _____ disability (type and cause) _____

loss of motion (specify) _____ when occurred _____

loss of strength (specify) _____ when occurred _____

swelling (specify) _____ when occurred _____

bleeding (specify) _____ when occurred _____

3. Relevant Past History and Family History

History of similar condition: dates _____ nature _____

_____

Treatment _____

Other relevant illnesses or disorders _____

General health status _____

Health problems of immediate family _____

4. Life-style

Occupation _____ ADL _____

Regular (3 times/week minimum) physical activities requiring: strength _____ agility _____ endurance _____

flexibility _____ other _____

What patient does to promote wellness _____

Patient's concept of cause of condition _____

Patient's concept of functional and/or cosmetic deficit(s) _____

Anticipated goals _____

5. Other

Current medications _____

Recent radiographs _____

6. Therapist's Interpretation and Plans for Objective Exam _____

_____

Figure 9.10.   Examination form part 2: History, continued.

B. PHYSICAL EXAMINATION

   1. Inspection

      a. Posture

	frontal plane (from back or front)		sagittal plane (from side)	
	WB	NWB	WB	NWB
pelvis				
hip joint/femur				
knee joint/patella				
tibia				
ankle joint/malleoli				

		WB	NWB		WB	NWB		WB	NWB		WB	NWB
hindfoot	varus			valgus			equinus			calcaneus		
forefoot	add.			abd.			cavus			plannus		
forefoot	varus			valgus								
toes	hallux valgus			hallux rigidus			hammer toe			claw toe		

          toe rotational deformity: 1 ___ 2 ___ 3 ___ 4 ___ 5 ___ Other _____

      leg length (R) _____ (L) _____

      b. Shape

      deformity (describe) WB: _____

      NWB: _____

      asymmetry _____

      swelling or masses _____ atrophy _____

      c. Use (gait)

	with shoes	R	L
begin swing	without shoes		
	with shoes		
end swing	without shoes		
	with shoes		
heel strike	without shoes		
	with shoes		
midstance	without shoes		
	with shoes		
push-off	without shoes		

      d. Skin

      color when dependent _____ elevated _____ temperature _____

      lesions _____ scars _____ calluses _____ corns _____

      e. Aids

      assistive device _____ orthosis _____ shoe insert _____

      shoe modification _____

      shoe appearance _____

Figure 9.11. Examination form part 3: Inspection.

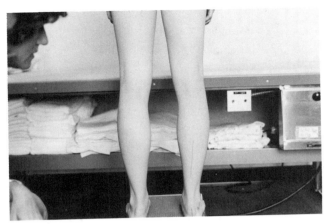

Figure 9.12.   Posterior observation of lower limbs and feet: The examiner measures the angle between lines bisecting the calf and calcaneous to assess rear foot alignment.

therefore, one must mobilize the foot to confirm motion in the major joints (3). A fixed pes plannus (flatfoot), caused by abnormal bony coalition restricts joint motion, and usually must be corrected surgically. In contrast, a flexible pes plannus demonstrates normal or excessive joint mobility. This may occur only during weightbearing, and is aided by foot orthoses, postural, and muscular training.

Swelling usually occurs around the ankles or on the dorsum of the foot where the skin is loosely attached and more synovial tissue exists. The location of the swelling, may be misleading; therefore, the examiner must inspect the foot closely to determine its true source. If swelling is bilateral, cardiovascular or lymphatic problems may exist. Unilateral swelling usually indicates a localized traumatic condition.

Since the primary function of the ankle and foot is locomotion, gait evaluation represents this component of the examination (Fig. 9.11). The patient should walk a designated path, both with and without shoes while the examiner observes in different planes. As the toe leaves the ground and the limb initiates the swing phase of gait, the leg is maximally rotated laterally. Halfway through the swing phase, the leg begins to medially rotate. At heelstrike, the foot's long axis should approach the plane of progression (3). The foot pronates as it is loaded, and the leg medially rotates until the midstance (foot flat) phase of the cycle. A reversal of motion occurs at midstance, as the leg begins to laterally rotate and the foot supinates. As the heel rises, it inverts. Most of the body's weight shifts onto the 1st ray at the push-off phase of the cycle. The shoes should not rotate or slip on the floor.

Changes in skin color, from purplish when dependent to blanching when elevated, may be signs of peripheral vascular disease. Skin lesions may indicate traumatic, infective, or systemic disorders, so the examiner should describe their characteristics very thoroughly. Calluses (diffuse areas of hyperkeratosis) represent the skin's reaction to excessive forces over

a long period of time (22). Corns are areas of callus that have become molded into a nucleus. Plantar warts (hyperkeratotic epithelial tissue surrounding thrombosed capillaries) usually develop on weightbearing areas of the feet. Presumably of traumatic or viral origin, they present a painful, dermatologic condition. Gouty tophi (deposits of uric acid crystals in the tissues around joints) commonly develop at the first MP joints, causing pain as well as deformity (23).

Aids used or worn by a patient to alleviate the effects of an ankle or foot disorder may indicate the severity of the condition. Shoe appearance is also an important parameter in foot examination. Shoes function to prevent irritation from the ground, absorb impact, improve foot control, and increase traction. Modifications and the wear pattern clue the examiner to certain pathologies. Excessive lateral heel and sole wear occurs when the foot is excessively inverted, or when a pes cavus or hallux rigidus exists (7). Medial heel and sole wear results from foot eversion or pes plano-valgus (7). Rotary slippage of the shoe at push-off indicates decreased subtalar joint motion, muscle imbalance, or increased obliquity of the ankle joint axis (3).

Palpation.   The skin and subcutaneous tissue of the foot is normally thick over weightbearing areas. Rheumatoid arthritis, however, often causes deterioration of the fat pads over the metatarsal heads, resulting in excessive pressure of the bones on the skin. Plantar callosities may develop on the skin in areas of force concentration. Such callosities commonly occur on the plantar surface of the 2nd metatarsal head.

Signs of inflammation arise superficially from conditions varying from trauma to gouty arthritis (Fig. 9.13). Bursitis commonly occurs in the retrocalcaneal bursa between the calcaneus and Achilles tendon or in the subcutaneous bursa between the Achilles tendon insertion and the skin (pump bump). Tendinitis in the tibialis posterior tendon or flexor hallucis longus tendon is tender to palpation at the posterormedial aspect of the ankle and medial longitudinal arch. The Achilles tendon is particularly subject to localized trauma and inflammation, and may be painful anywhere along its length, particularly when squeezed.

The examiner performs bony palpation systematically in a proximal to distal direction, progressing from the medial to lateral to plantar surfaces of the leg and foot. Medial landmarks include the tibial shaft, medial malleolus, medial talar tubercle (just posterior to the medial malleolus, where the deltoid ligament inserts), sustentaculum tali (2 cm distal to the medial malleolus), talar dome (just anterior to the medial malleolus, it becomes prominent with eversion), navicular tubercle (distal to talus), and 1st metatarsal head. Lateral landmarks include the fibular head, fibular shaft, lateral melleolus, anterolateral talar dome (just anterior to the lateral malleolus, it becomes prominent with inversion), sinus tarsi area, anterior calcaneus, and base of the 5th metatarsal bone. Plantar landmarks are the posterior calcaneus, medial calcaneal tubercle (plantar surface where the plantar aponeurosis

2. Palpation (note location and nature of abnormality)

   a. Skin and subcutaneous tissue: tenderness _____ temperature _____ swelling _____ decreased mobility _____ trigger points _____ other _____

   b. Muscles and tendons: tenderness _____ temperature _____ spasm _____ loss of continuity _____ decreased mobility _____ other _____

   c. Tendon sheaths and bursae: tenderness _____ temperature _____ swelling _____ crepitus _____ other _____

   d. Bones and joints: tenderness _____ temperature _____ swelling _____ bony prominences _____ other _____

   e. Arteries and nerves: dorsalis pedis artery _____ posterior tibial artery _____ peroneal nerve _____ sural nerve _____ tibial nerve _____

3. Movement assessment

   a. Functional assessment

     bear weight on affected extremity alone _____

     walk on heels _____

     walk on toes _____

     walk on medial borders of feet _____

     walk on lateral borders of feet _____

     squat _____

Key: C = completes task

       D = completes task with difficulty/discomfort

       N = does not complete task

   b/c/d. Physiologic movement

	ACTIVE			PASSIVE			RESISTIVE	
	ROM	Symptoms	Quality	ROM	Symptoms	Endfeel	Strength	Symptoms
Dorsiflexion (knee 0°)								
Plantarflexion (knee 0°)								
Dorsiflexion (knee 90°)								
Plantarflexion (knee 90°)								
Heel Inversion								
Heel Eversion								
Forefoot Abduction								
Adduction								
1st MP Flexion								
Extension								

Figure 9.13. **Examination form part 4:** Palpation and movement assessment.

attaches), sesamoids over the 1st metatarsal head, and metatarsal heads.

Heel spurs commonly occur on the calcaneus, on the dorsal surface at the Achilles tendon attachment, and on the plantar surface at the plantar aponeurosis attachment. They may incite a soft tissue inflammatory reaction. Joint and ligamentous pathology typically produce localized tenderness to palpation. Symptoms usually increase with stress of the involved structures. Palpation may reveal joint subluxation, malalignment, bony prominences, etc.

The examiner palpates the dorsalis pedis arterial pulse on the dorsum of the foot between the extensor hallucis longus and extensor digitorum longus tendons. Peripheral vascular disease often causes diminution in this pulse. One locates the posterior tibial arterial pulse just posterior to the medial malleolus. The peroneal nerve crosses the posterolateral aspect of the fibular head, where it is accessible to palpation. Its cutaneous branch is susceptible to trauma about the 1st and 2nd tarsometatarsal joints; tapping over the dorsum of the metatarsals may elicit Tinel's sign (22). Tinel's sign of the sural nerve may be elicited by tapping over the base of the 5th metatarsal. The tibial nerve may be compressed within the tarsal tunnel; if so, Tinel's sign results from tapping just posterior to the medial malleolus.

Movement Assessment. The examiner performs a cursory assessment of general functional activities, such as walking on heels, toes, etc., to determine the extent of function before examining the specific movements of each joint (Fig. 9.13). The therapist evaluates physiologic movement of the ankle with both the knee extended and the knee flexed, to differentiate effects of the gastrocnemius muscle that crosses both the knee and ankle joints. Heel inversion and eversion represent the frontal plane component of subtalar motion. To measure heel movement accurately, place the patient prone with his knee flexed 135° to align the subtalar joint axis with the horizontal plane. A gravity or regular goniometer over the plantar heel surface provides a measurement of the degrees of inversion and eversion (3). One measures forefoot abduction and adduction by determining the angle between the forefoot and rearfoot, with a fulcrum at the midtarsal joint (23). Since metatarsophalangeal joint extension (especially at the first MP joint) is critical to normal gait, its measurement contributes to the examination. Interphalangeal joint motion, however, has minimal significance in gait, and is customarily not measured.

The examiner tests accessory movement using techniques described in the joint mobilization section of this chapter (Fig. 9.14). He records both the mobility and symptoms produced by testing. Hypermobility is a common finding due to both traumatic and weight-bearing stresses upon the ankles and feet. Injury to the distal fibular syndesmosis produces a passive increase in fibular glide and deep ankle pain. Abnormal pronation with associated stretch of the spring ligament allows the talar head to drop into the space between the sustentaculum tali and naviculum, and creates excessive hypermobility of the foot.

Special tests include inversion and eversion stress to assess lateral and medial ankle stability (Figs. 9.15 and 9.16). The examiner stabilizes the leg and moves the foot in the respective directions. When evaluating an acute ankle injury, these tests most accurately depict ligamentous tear if performed immediately after the injury before the onset of swelling and muscle spasm. An anterior drawer test assesses the anterior talofibular ligament. With the patient supine, the examiner stabilizes his leg and draws his foot anteriorly with a hand cupped around his heel (Fig. 9.17). A Homan test provokes the pain of deep vein thrombophlebitis by passive ankle dorsiflexion (Fig. 9.18). A Thompson test assesses continuity of the Achilles tendon. With the patient prone, the examiner squeezes the calf in an attempt to elicit passive plantarflexion (Fig 9.19).

The subtalar joint neutral position is a reference position from which maximum function can occur, and where the examiner can make reliable foot and ankle measurements. In this position, the foot is neither supinated nor pronated. To obtain the subtalar joint neutral position, the examiner applies dorsiflectory pressure over the 4th and 5th metatarsal heads to align the foot so that the medial and lateral borders of the talar head are equally palpable (Fig. 9.20).

Neurologic Evaluation. Key muscle strength and reflexes indicate the status of nerve root levels L4–S2 (Fig. 9.21). Numerous systemic and localized disorders may affect the sensibility of the ankle and foot. Peripheral neuropathy or neuritis may produce burning or numbness in the distal distribution of the involved nerve. Diseases such as diabetes, syphillis, and syringomyelia typically cause proprioceptive loss with resulting instability and joint deterioration. Chronic joint sprains may stretch ligaments and capsule, and induce pain and reflex muscle spasm. An interdigital neuroma (Morton's neuralgia), a fusiform enlargement of an interdigital nerve, produces pain and sensory changes, most commonly between the 3rd and 4th metatarsals.

Motor neuron pathology produces muscle imbalance by increasing tonicity in muscles that may eventually shorten, or flaccidity in muscles whose antagonists may eventually shorten. Loss of innervation affects coordination as well, and may produce an ataxic or pathologic gait.

Recommendation of Other Tests. Radiologic studies help confirm other examination findings, such as asymmetry in ROM. Since there are numerous foot joints, a patient may have difficulty localizing pain to a particular one. A radiograph may detect early arthritic changes before a patient can localize the symptoms. Stress films assist in documenting ligamentous injury or laxity.

When all the data has been compiled, the examiner can proceed with interpretation, and planning management. Table 9.1 lists a summary of the differential diagnoses and treatment of common ankle and foot disorders.

e. Accessory movement

	Mobility	Symptoms
superior tibiofibular joint glide		
inferior tibiofibular joint glide		
talocrural joint traction		
glide		
subtalar joint traction		
glide		
intertarsal joints naviculum		
cuboid		
1st cuneiform		
2nd cuneiform		
3rd cuneiform		
intermetatarsal joints 1–2		
1–3		
3–4		
4–5		
metatarsophalangeal joints 1		
2		
3		
4		
5		
proximal interphalangeal joints 1		
2		
3		
4		
5		
distal interphalangeal joints 2		
3		
4		
5		

f. Special tests

	+	−	Comments
inversion ankle stress test; talocrural and subtalar joints			
subtalar joint			
eversion ankle stress test			
anterior drawer test			
Homan test			
Thompson test			
subtalar joint neutral position			

Figure 9.14. **Examination form part 5:** Accessory movement and special tests.

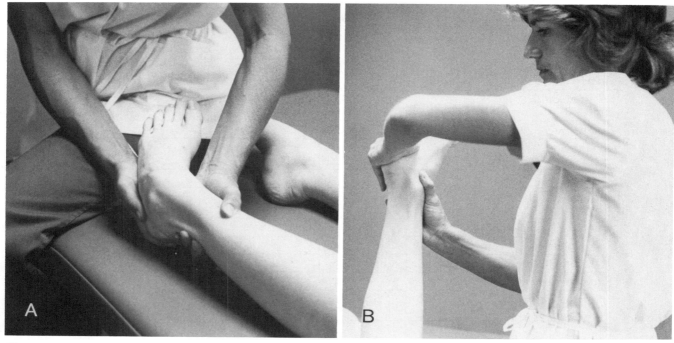

Figure 9.15.   Inversion ankle stress test: *A,* If passive inversion of both the talocrural and subtalar joints reproduces lateral gapping and/or pain, the test is positive for laxity or tear of one or more of the lateral ankle ligaments. *B,* If passive inversion of the calcaneus on the stabilized talus reproduces symptoms, then the lesion lies at the subtalar joint.

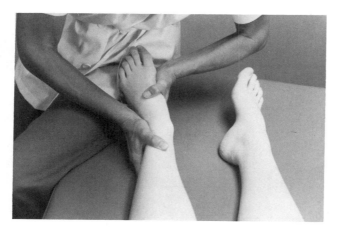

Figure 9.16.   Eversion ankle stress test: if passive eversion of the talocrural and subtalar joints reproduces medial gapping and/or pain, the test is positive for laxity or tear of the deltoid ligament.

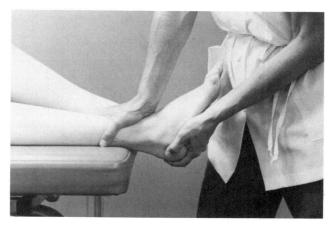

Figure 9.17.   Anterior drawer test: if anterior force on the hindfoot reproduces anterior shear of the talus on the tibia, the test is positive for laxity or tear of the anterior talofibular ligament.

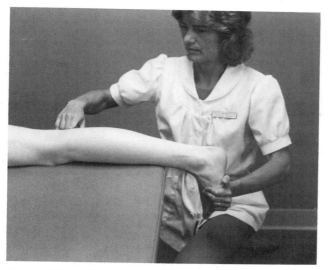

Figure 9.18. **Homan test:** if passive dorsiflexion of the ankle produces deep calf or popliteal pain when the knee is extended, the test is positive, implicating deep vein thrombophlebitis.

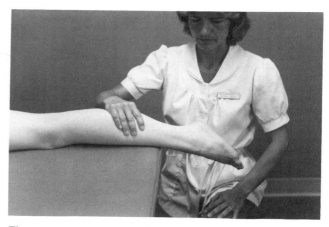

Figure 9.19. **Thompson test:** if squeezing a patient's calf fails to produce ankle plantarflexion, the test is positive, implicating rupture of the Achilles tendon.

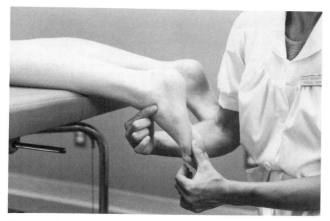

Figure 9.20. **Subtalar joint neutral position:** with a patient prone and foot relaxed, the examiner positions the foot with pressure at the 4th and 5th metatarsal heads until the medial and lateral borders of the talar head are equally palpable.

4. Neurological evaluation

    a. Key muscles (strength grade 0–5)

        L4 = tibialis anterior muscle _____

        L5 = extensor hallucis longus muscle _____

        S1,2 = gastrocsoleus muscle _____

    b. Key reflexes (graded +1 through +3)

        S1,2 = Achilles tendon reflex _____

    c. Sensibility

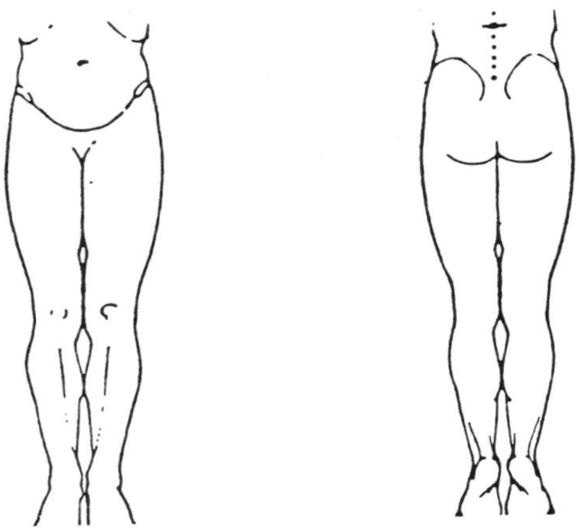

Key: lacking
A = light touch sensation
B = sharp/dull discrimination
C = temperature discrimination
D = proprioception

    d. Motor control: spastic _____ flaccid _____ rigid _____ clonic _____

    e. Coordination (sitting)

        toe tap _____

        heel tap _____

        reciprocal toe tap _____

Key: C = completes task
D = completes task with difficulty/ discomfort
N = does not complete task

5. Recommendation of other tests

    a. Radiography _____

    b. Laboratory _____

    c. Electrodiagnostic _____

    d. Arthroscopy _____

    e. Arthrography _____

    f. Other _____

Figure 9.21. Examination form part 6: Neurologic evaluation and recommendation of other tests.

Table 9.1.
Summary of Differential Diagnosis and Treatment of Common Ankle and Foot Disorders

Disorder	Chief Complaint	Onset	Symptom Characteristics	Static Physical Changes	Dynamic Physical Changes	Special Tests	Treatment[a]
Achilles tendon rupture	Severe distal calf pain	Sudden dorsiflexion stress while gastrocsoleus muscle contracted; or direct blow	Acute lower leg or ankle pain; sense of snapping	Swelling and ecchymosis within 12 hours	Weak plantarflexion; no push-off during gait	Palpable defect; Thompson	Short leg cast with foot plantarflexed, NWB 6 weeks, then WB 4 weeks in cast; or surgical repair and 4 weeks immobilization; both methods require subsequent rehab for gastrocsoleus strengthening and stretching
Ankle sprain (inversion)	Acute ankle pain	Forceful inversion of weightbearing foot	Acute pain and localized tenderness to palpation and stress of involved ligaments	Ankle joint swelling and ecchymosis; spasm	Laxity with inversion or plantarflexion (may be masked by swelling)	Anterior or posterior drawer; inversion stress; radiographs	I-C-E; contrast baths; protective taping; plaster immobilization if complete rupture; rehab for enhanced proprioception, strengthening, and functional activities
Bursitis a. Posterior calcaneal b. Retrocalcaneal	Posterior heel pain and swelling	a. Irritated by shoe b. Repetitive dorsiflexion	a. Local pressure increases pain b. Ankle movement increases pain	a. Tender bump on posterior heel b. Swelling around Achilles tendon insertion			Open-heel shoes or modifications for pressure relief; minimize WB; corticosteroid injections; ice or heat
Flatfoot a. Flexible (supple) b. Rigid	a. "Fallen arches" b. Gait and mechanical problems	a. Insidious, mechanical compensation for foot or limb abnormalities; congenital ligamentous laxity b. Congenital	Foot fatigue; symptoms relate to abnormal stresses and excessive pronation	a. Medial arch flattens & foot pronates with WB, but reforms with NWB or toe rise b. Talus adducted and plantarflexed on everted calcaneus; inflexible, depressed arch	a. Foot & limb changes to compensate abnormal pronation b. Deformity persists both WB, NWB, and during active supination; compensatory changes and gait deviation		a. Symptomatic, i.e., orthoses, intrinsic or supination strengthening, etc. b. Repeated manipulation and casting; surgical correction; arthrodesis; attempt to accomodate with orthoses
Foot strain	Chronic aching of foot	Flatfoot or ill-fitting shoes are predisposing factors	Mechanical foot pain of ligamentous or joint origin, increased by activity	Stretched plantar aponeurosis, excessive WB on middle metatarsals	Pronation, with compensatory changes during stance		Strengthen supination and intrinsic foot muscles; appropriate shoes and orthotics
Hallux rigidus	Pain with big toe extension and gait	Chronic; osteoarthritis	Foot pain stemming from changes to compensate decreased toe extension	Fused or partially fused 1st MP joint	Toe off phase of gait altered by increased supination so that pressure on lateral toes	Excessive wear on lateral shoes	Acute pain relief with immobilization, heat, or decreased WB; mobilization; orthosis with 1st metatarsal plantar pad, valgus support and tarsal pad to stabilize ankle
Hallux valgus	May be asymptomatic; occasional pain around 1st MP joint	Chronic; predisposing factors include metatarsus varus, abnormal foot mechanics, pointed toe shoes	Secondary lesions such as bunion, bursitis, corn, or callus	Lateral deviation of big toe; bunion over 1st MP joint; secondary changes in other toes	Excessive pronation and compensatory changes		Appropriate shoes and orthotics; strengthen abductor hallucis muscle; mobilization; night splint; surgical correction; symptomatic management of secondary symptoms
Interdigital neuritis (Morton's neuroma)	Burning and aching on plantar surface of foot, 3rd, and 4th toes	Unilateral; common in 25 to 50 year-old women, predisposed by chronic pronation	Tenderness between 3rd and 4th metatarsal heads; paresthesias and pain increased by WB	Flattened transverse arch; calluses over 3rd and 4th metatarsals	Antalgic gait; pronation with compensatory changes		Orthotics to restrain pronation and provide digital padding/relief; wide shoes; surgical excision of neuroma
Metatarsalgia	Soreness of middle metatarsals	Abnormal mechanical stress; arthritis	Plantar foot pain and fatigue with WB	Callus over middle metatarsals; hypermobile or pronated foot	Antalgic gait; pronation with compensatory changes		Deal with primary cause, as well as treat symptomatically, i.e., orthotics, mobilization, strengthening
Plantar fascitis	Heel pain with WB	Inflammation of insertion of plantar aponeurosis	Point tenderness over medial calcaneal plantar tuberosity; pain worse upon initial WB after rest			Calcaneal spur (may not be related to pathology)	Cortisone injection; cushion heel and use lift to reduce stress on plantar structures; ultrasound
Tibial neuritis (medial tarsal tunnel syndrome)	Burning pain on plantar surface of foot and toes	Direct trauma or chronic irritation	Continuous burning pain and paresthesias, increased by WB activities; tenderness over tarsal tunnel; sensory loss and weakness of toe intrinsic muscles	May be associated with valgus heel and pronated forefoot; swelling, tumor, or bony deformity that restricts tarsal tunnel		Tinel's sign	Modalities to reduce edema or fibrosis; orthotics; anti-inflammatory medication; surgical release followed by 2 weeks PWB, progressive ankle exercise and functional activities

[a]WB, weightbearing; NWB, nonweightbearing; MP, metatarsophalangeal; PWB, partial weightbearing.

ANKLE AND FOOT MOBILIZATION

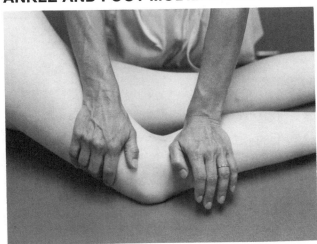

Figure 9.22.   Ventral Fibular Glide, Proximal Tibiofibular Joint.
Patient Position: Side lying with hip and knee flexed 45° and knee resting on table.
Therapist Position: Standing on side opposite of P's leg; S hand supports distal femur; M hand rests on dorsum of fibular head.
Technique: Apply force with thenar eminence of M hand perpendicular to fibula, to glide fibula in ventral direction.
Comment: Use as test or treatment for fibular pain or hypomobility.

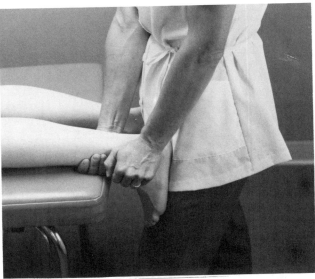

Figure 9.23.   Ventral Fibular Glide, Distal Tibiofibular Joint.
Patient Position: Prone with leg resting on table; foot overhanging end and foot resting against P's thigh.
Therapist Position: Standing at foot of table, facing P's head; S hand holds distal tibia; M hand rests on dorsum of fibular malleolus.
Technique: Apply force with thenar eminence of M hand perpendicular to fibula, to glide fibula in ventral direction.
Comment: Use as test or treatment for fibular pain or hypomobility.

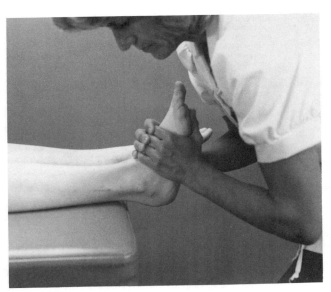

Figure 9.24.   Talocrural Joint Traction.
Patient Position: Supine with leg resting on table and foot overhanging end.
Therapist Position: Standing at foot of table, facing P's head; S hands overlapped over talus and thumbs on plantar surface maintain 0° dorsiflexion.
Technique: Apply force with body weight, parallel to long axis of tibia.
Comment: Use as test or treatment for general ankle pain or hypomobility.

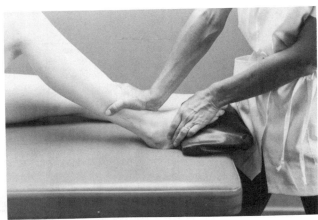

Figure 9.25.   Dorsal Tibial Glide (Ventral Talar Glide).
Patient Position: Supine with hip and knee flexed, heel resting on table with foot supported by sandbag.
Therapist Position: Standing at foot of table facing P's head; S hand holds foot; M hand grasps distal tibia.
Technique: Apply dorsal force to tibia perpendicular to long axis of tibia.
Comment: Especially effective for increasing plantarflexion.

ANKLE AND FOOT MOBILIZATION

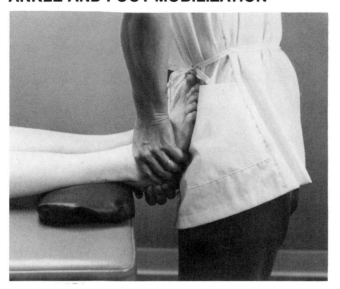

Figure 9.26. Dorsal Talar Glide.

Patient Position: Supine with distal leg supported on sandbag; foot overhanging end of table and resting against T's groin.

Therapist Position: Standing at foot of table facing P's head, S hand holds heel; M hand grasps talus.

Technique: Apply dorsal force to talus perpendicular to long axis of tibia; maintain traction on calcaneus and talus during technique.

Comment: Especially effective for increasing dorsiflexion.

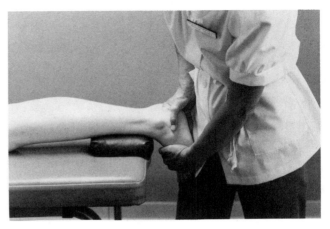

Figure 9.27. Ventral Talar Glide.

Patient Position: Prone with distal leg supported on sandbag; foot overhanging end of table and rests against T's thigh.

Therapist Position: Standing at foot of table facing P's head; S hand holds foot; M hand grasps calcaneus and talus.

Technique: Apply ventral force to calcaneus and talus; maintain traction on calcaneus and talus during technique.

Comment: Especially effective for increasing plantarflexion.

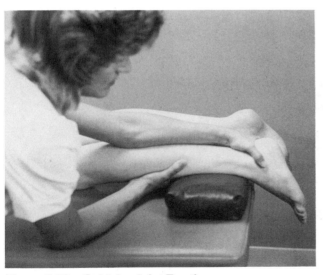

Figure 9.28. Subtalar Joint Traction.

Patient Position: Prone with distal leg supported on sandbag and foot overhanging end of table.

Therapist Position: Standing at P's side, facing feet; S hand secures leg; M hand web space grasps calcaneus, with forearm resting on dorsal aspect of P's leg.

Technique: Apply force 45° to plantar surface of foot.

Comment: Effective as test or treatment for pain or subtalar hypomobility (especially inversion or eversion).

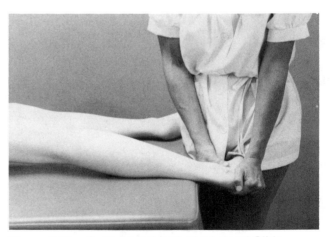

Figure 9.29. Subtalar Joint Medial-Lateral Glide.

Patient Position: Side lying with leg resting on table; foot overhanging end of table, maintained in dorsiflextion by contact against T's groin.

Therapist Position: Standing at foot of table facing P's leg; S hand secures distal leg; M hand grasps calcaneus.

Technique: Apply force to calcaneus perpendicular to long axis of foot.

Comment: Especially effective for increasing inversion and eversion.

ANKLE AND FOOT MOBILIZATION

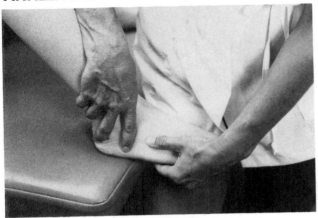

Figure 9.30. Calcaneocuboid Joint Mobilization.
Patient Position: Supine with hip and knee flexed; heel resting on table with fulcrum at calcaneocuboid joint.
Therapist Position: Standing at foot of table facing P's leg; S hand secures distal leg and ankle; M hand grasps cuboid between thumb and index finger.
Technique: Apply dorsal and ventral forces perpendicular to long axis of foot.
Comment: Especially effective for increasing abduction and adduction.

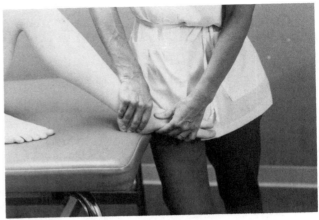

Figure 9.31. Talonavicular Joint Mobilization.
Patient Position: Supine with hip and knee flexed; heel resting on table with fulcrum at talonavicular joint.
Therapist Position: Standing at foot of table facing P's leg; S hand secures distal leg and ankle; M hand grasps naviculum between thumb and index finger.
Technique: Apply dorsal and ventral forces perpendicular to long axis of foot.
Comment: Especially effective for increasing abduction and adduction.

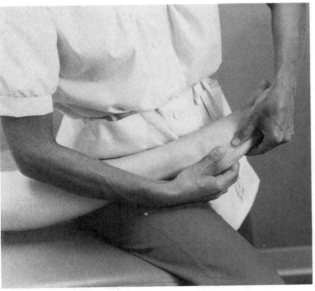

Figure 9.32. Cubometatarsal Joint Mobilization.
Patient Position: Supine with distal leg resting on T's thigh.
Therapist Position: Seated at end of table; S hand holds distal leg and fingers grasp cuboid; M hand grasps 5th metatarsal base.
Technique: Apply dorsal and ventral forces perpendicular to long axis of foot.
Comment: Effective for mobilizing the 5th ray.

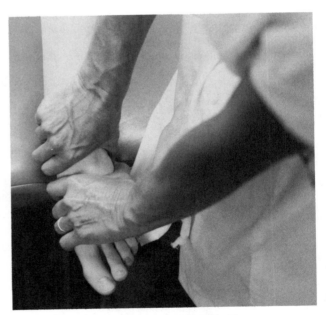

Figure 9.33. Cuneiform Joint Mobilization
Patient Position: Supine with hip and knee flexed; heel resting on table with fulcrum at cuneiform bones.
Therapist Position: Seated at end of table; S secures rearfoot on table; M hand grasps cuneiform bones.
Technique: Apply dorsal and ventral forces perpendicular to long axis of foot.
Comment: This technique can also be used to mobilize metatarsal bones on cuneiform bones by adjusting hand placement.

ANKLE AND FOOT MOBILIZATION

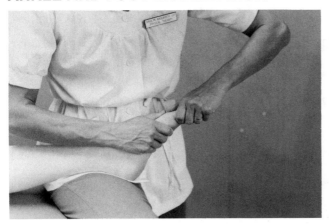

Figure 9.34. Metatarsophalangeal Joint Traction.
Patient Position: Supine with distal leg resting on T's thigh.
Therapist Position: Seated at end of table; S hand fixates metatarsal; M hand grasps proximal phalanx as close to joint as possible; T's arms are parallel to P's foot.
Technique: Apply traction force to phalanx, parallel to long axis of P's foot
Comments: Effective for test or treatment of general hypomobility or pain as indicated; same technique is applied to IP joints by moving T's hand placement distally.

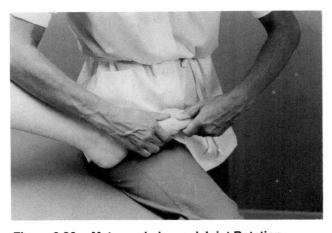

Figure 9.36. Metarsophalangeal Joint Rotation.
Patient Position: Seated with foot resting on T's thigh.
Therapist Position: Seated at end of table; S hand fixates metacarpal; M hand grasps proximal phalanx as close to joint as possible and flexed DIP joint is fixated between middle and ring fingers to insure firm grasp; T's arms are parallel to P's foot.
Technique: Apply rotation force to phalanx through thumb and index finger contacts; maintain traction also during this technique.
Comments: Effective for treatment of pain or any restricted motion; same technique is applied to IP joints by moving T's hand placement distally.

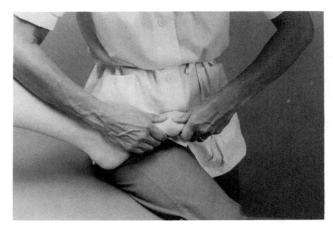

Figure 9.35. Metatarsophalangeal Joint Medial-Lateral Glide.
Patient Position: Seated with foot resting on T's thigh.
Therapist Position: Seated at end of table; S hand fixates metacarpal; M hand grasps medial and lateral aspects of proximal phalanx as close to joint as possible; T's arms are parallel to P's foot.
Technique: Apply medial and lateral forces to phalanx through thumb and index finger contacts, perpendicular to long axis of P's limb; maintain traction also during this technique.
Comments: Effective for treatment of pain or restricted motion, especially abduction and adduction; same technique is applied to IP joints by moving T's hand placement distally. This technique may also be used to produce dorsal and ventral glide by imparting dorsal and plantar forces, which is especially effective for increasing extension and flexion respectively.

References

1. Radakovich M, Malone T: The superior tibiofibular joint: The forgotten joint. *J Orthop Sports Phys Ther* 3:129–132, 1982.
2. Kaumeyer G, Malone T: Ankle injuries: Anatomical and biomechanical considerations necessary for the development of an injury prevention program. *J Orthop Sports Phys Ther* 1:171–177, 1980.
3. Inman VT, Mann RA: Biomechanics of the foot and ankle. In Mann RA (ed), *DuVries' Surgery of the Foot*. St Louis, CV Mosby, 1978, pp 3–21.
4. DiStefano VJ: Anatomy and biomechanics of the ankle and foot. *Athletic Training*, Spring 1981, pp 43–47.
5. Donatelli R: Normal biomechanics of the foot and ankle. *J Orthop Sports Phys Ther* 7:91–95, 1985.
6. Kapandji IA: The Physiology of the Joints, Edinburgh, Churchill Livingstone, 1974, vol 2.
7. Neale D (ed): *Common Foot Disorders: Diagnosis and Management.* Edinburgh, Churchill Livingstone, 1981.
8. Kotwick JA: Biomechanics of the foot and ankle. *Clin Sports Med* 1:19–34, 1982.
9. Ogden JA: The anatomy and function of the proximal tibiofibular joint. *Clin Orthop* 101, 186–191, 1974.
10. Root ML, Orien WP, Weed JH: Normal and abnormal function of the foot. In *Clinical Biomechanics.* Los Angeles, Clinical Biomechanics Corp, 1977, vol 2.
11. Warwick R, Williams PL (eds): *Gray's Anatomy*, 35th British Edition. WB Saunders, 1973.
12. Cailliet R: *Foot and Ankle Pain.* Philadelphia, FA Davis, 1968.
13. McPoil TG, Knecht HG: Biomechanics of the foot in walking: A functional approach. *J Orthop Sports Phys Ther* 7:69–72, 1985.
14. Perry J: Anatomy and biomechanics of the hindfoot. *Clin Orthop* 177:9–15, 1983.

15. Boissonnault W, Donatelli R: The influence of hallux extension on the foot during ambulation. *J Orthop Sports Phys Ther* 5:240–242, 1984.

16. Sarrafian SK: *Anatomy of the Foot and Ankle.* Philadelphia, JB Lippincott, 1983.

17. Hughes L: Biomechanical analysis of the foot and ankle for predisposition to developing stress fractures. *J Orthop Sports Phys Ther* 7:96–101, 1985.

18. Viel ER, Desmarets JJ: Mechanical pull of the peroneal tendons on the fifth ray of the foot. *J Orthop Sports Phys Ther* 7:102–106, 1985.

19. Kushner S: Medial tarsal tunnel syndrome: A review. *J Orthop Sports Phys Ther* 6:39–45, 1984.

20. Mack RP: Ankle injuries in athletics. *Clin Sports Med* 1:71—84, 1982.

21. Root ML, Orien WP, Weed JH, Huges RJ: *Biomechanical Examination of the Foot.* Los Angeles, Clinical Biomechanics Corp, 1971, vol 1.

22. Sammarco GJ: Soft tissue conditions in athletes' feet. *Clin Sports Med* 1:149–155, 1982.

23. Hoppenfeld S: *Physical Examination of the Spine and Extremities.* New York, Appleton-Century-Crofts, 1976.

Index

Page numbers in *italics* denote figures; those followed by "t" denote tables.